"*Wise Childbearing* is a comprehensive birth manual that is empowering and respectful to the reader. *Wise Childbearing* also refers the reader to evidenced-based information and notes the rights and responsibilities of parents to educate themselves in order to make truly informed conscientious decisions during the childbearing year."

—Paulina (Polly) Perez, RN, BSN, FACCE, LCCE, CD
Author of *Special Women, The Nurturing Touch at Birth,* and *Doula Programs*

❁

For years, this book has been used in childbirth classes
and for personal home study with rave reviews.
This is a book that would wisely be read years *before* ever giving birth.

❁

From expectant parents in Association for Wise Childbearing classes concerning the first copy of *Wise Childbearing* that was used in classes, and originally only available by loan:

From a mother: "I enjoyed the manual so much. I had to take a lot of notes before giving it back."

From a father: "Enjoyed it a lot."

From a father: "Lots of great info. Entries were brief enough to keep it interesting.... The info given by the instructor and the manual about how natural the whole process is [was one of the most helpful things I learned in class to help prepare me for our birth]."

From a mother: "Lots of helpful info... [I feel]...informed, empowered to make my own decisions."

From a mother: "I enjoyed doing the reading every week."

From a father: "Would like to be able to keep [the book for my own]."

From a father: "Nice work!"

From a mother: "I would have liked to have [been able to keep the book.... The class] made me feel more in control of my birth."

From a mother: "Well thought out and researched out."

From a mother: "[My favorite thing about the class was that there was] lots of good information on both sides of everything."

From a father: "[This class was] very informative."

From a father: "Knowing that there is a lot more I can do during birth than I thought before [has prepared me the most for our birth]...The class was very good."

From a father: "Good book, teach you what you need to know....Thank you. It be very helpful class."

From a student doula: "Reading [the] manual on stages of labor, birth options, positions to give birth [are some of the things that have prepared me the most]."

Wise Childbearing

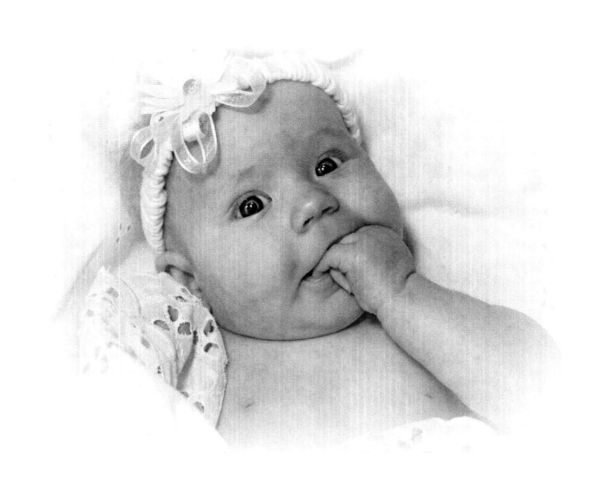

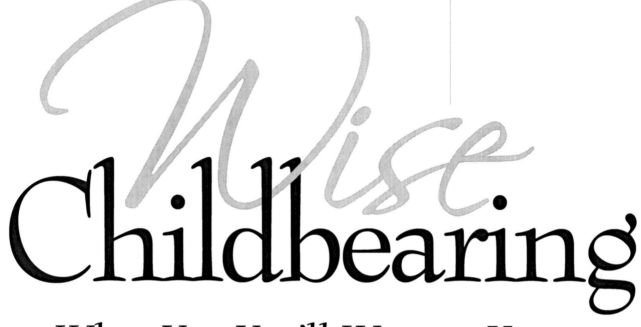

Wise Childbearing

What You You'll Want to Know as You Make Your Birth Choices

Jennetta Billhimer

CCBE, HBCE, CD(DONA), BS

CACHE MOUNTAINS PRESS

The publisher and author of this book assume no liability or responsibility for any difficulties, medical or otherwise, that those taking advice from this book sustain by following the suggestions or treatments described herein. This book should not be substituted for the personal care of a qualified physician or midwife. It is to be used to become familiar with the wide range of options available to birthing families. Readers are ultimately responsible for decisions that are made for themselves and their children, and they have the responsibility to decide on the proper courses of action for their own needs and circumstances. Readers apply anything within this book, or from suggested resources, at their own risk and assume all responsibility for their care during pregnancy, birth, and the postpartum period.

Cache Mountains Press
HC 60 Box 643
Ruby Valley, Nevada 89833

FIRST EDITION

Library of Congress Cataloging-in-Publication Data

Billhimer, Jennetta
Wise childbearing, what you'll want to know as you make your birth choices/Jennetta Billhimer. – 1st ed.
Includes bibliographical references and index.
ISBN 978-0-9823586-0-3
1. Pregnancy, physical and psychological preparation. 2. Holistic childbirth preparation. 3. Fathers and birth companions. 4. Comfort measures for labor. 5. Parent preparation. 6. Postpartum. 7. Baby and child care.
2009912897

Index by Sally Bishop
Cover Photography by Christine Lauder Hall
Text design and composition by John Reinhardt Book Design

Printed in the United States of America

A Note of Thanks...

TO OUR CREATORS. Their love and concern for their daughters is marvelously evident.

To my husband and sweetheart Carl E. Billhimer, for whom I am eternally grateful for his wisdom, insight, patience, and devotion to me and to this cause.

To all those who have come before me, who have lit the pathways for me; to those I now stand among with my own candle, lighting the ways for others as they make their own journeys.

To Mylie and Clint Laing for their dedication and support.

To all of those who have graciously helped with the creation of this book; those who have shared their photographs with me, those who have agreed to be photographed, even during their births. I am grateful for and pleased to acknowledge the Michael and Estee Wilson family; Travis and Raina Jones family; Matt and Kim Clark family; Jared and Karin Hardman family; Emmett and Ashlee Corrigan family; Julia Gill family; Mike and Holly Bradford family; George and Hannah Joekel family; Kirk and Bec Dahle family; Rob Brown and Suzann Kienast-Brown family; and the John and Liz Maurer family, and Christie Weaver as well as those wishing to remain anonymous.

I would also like to recognize the fabulous team of photographers that assisted me with the creation of this book, namely Christine Lauder Hall and Tina Pierson Photography.

I owe special thanks to my designer John Reinhardt, just as much for his patience and enthusiasm as for his clever ideas and ingenious eye for design.

Dear Reader

I am excited to share with you what I have learned from my many years of experience and in-depth studies as a childbirth educator, labor and birth doula, and mentor to women and families. I am fortunate to have learned a great deal over the years from brilliant leaders and reformers in different fields of Childbirth.

I am also a woman who has had a variety of my own birth and life experiences from cesareans to four vaginal births after cesarean, difficult births, miscarriages, waterbirths, pain-free births, easy births, spiritual and ecstatic births and more. As you might be thinking, yes my own experiences are what inspired me to begin my own search. And what a wealth of information I found! I knew I needed to do something to help other families realize their possibilities too. When I first begin having my six children, I didn't know I had choices. I was a busy college student who thought I didn't have a lot of time to be studying about how to have babies. Little did I realize that there wasn't anything I could be studying that would be of more importance.

Over the years through my training in various childbirth capacities, in my work with numerous families, and from continuing experiences, I came to recognize that everyone is unique, with their own needs. Not only that, but each pregnancy and birth is so different from another, even for the same woman. I am honored to share with you what I have learned over the past nineteen years as a parent and as a professional. I am happy to offer you the knowledge to arm yourself with the wisdom and the confidence in yourself that you will need to make decisions that are right for *you*.

The world's birth statistics should be improving. But are they? On the one hand, it is a wonderful time to be born, with numerous favorable options to consider. On the other, the majority of women today do not even know they have choices. Many emerge from this rite of passage less than satisfied with their experience and the care that was provided them. Most of their counterparts are having the same experiences, and so it is taken for granted that this is how giving birth must be.

I have also observed that when women realize they are free to exchange the standard way of doing things for another, they often find their eyes opened to other amazing paths as life continues, ones that they wouldn't have otherwise considered as options. I see mothers and fathers who become stronger and wiser parents and who are surer of themselves. Whether this birth is your first or your last, or somewhere in the middle, this book contains new and exciting reasons and how-tos for hope.

Will you read with a mind and heart that are open to possibility? I have given you 100% here in this book. I ask you to do the same and to be engaged 100% in your study. If you will not only read this book, but will study it wholeheartedly, you will be able to make your choices armed with facts and data that can give you the backbone you need. I encourage you to study in other places too. Don't take my word alone. Read, weigh, and consider all you have learned. Ponder and pray. There are many great resources, some of which are listed inside.

Come, let's begin the journey together—a period in your life you will always remember! My very best to you,

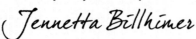

Contents

Read not to contradict and confute;

nor to believe and take for granted;

Nor to find talk and discourse; but to weigh and consider.

Some books are to be tasted, others to be swallowed,

and some few to be chewed and digested:

That is, some books are to be read only in parts,

Others to be read, but not curiously, and some few

To be read wholly, and with diligence and attention.

—Francis Bacon

Foreword

CHILDBEARING is a vitally important part of the life cycle. Women and families need to prepare for childbearing in the best way possible.

This book is an excellent way to prepare as it is scientifically accurate, clearly written and covers all the areas and issues in childbearing. Too many books for pregnant women urge the woman to trust their doctor but this book gets it right by consistently urging the woman to trust her own body and her own wisdom.

And this book emphasizes the joy of childbearing and how the pregnant woman and her family can get what is best for them at the time of the birth of their child.

— Marsden Wagner, M.D., M.S.,
Former Director of Women's and Children's Health,
World Health Organization

1

Welcome to the World of the Association for Wise Childbearing!

SO MANY PARENTS I have met with over the years have wished that they had this information when they first began their families.

I think you will find that this book is much different than many others you could choose to read during your pregnancy.

Numerous books on pregnancy and birth tell readers only what they can expect from their pregnancy, birth, and postpartum experiences within our culture's traditional way of doing things.

Wise Childbearing, in contrast, offers a fresh, new perspective.

Our babies, our families, the United States, and the world deserve better than we are now getting!

It doesn't have to be just one cookie-cutter, out-of the mold way. It can be your way. The decisions can, and should be, yours to make.

Wise Childbearing will show you how it really is possible to expect *more*, and that it doesn't have to be just one, cookie-cutter, out-of-the-mold way. It can be *your* way. The decisions can, and should be, *yours* to make. Right here, all together in our book, you have a concise, yet wide, amount of the information to help you to make good decisions for you and your family.

This book is for women and their families who are getting ready to give birth and welcome a new baby into their lives and hearts.

It is for **parents who are willing to believe that birth can be a *wonderful* experience without sacrificing any safety.**

This book is for **parents who want to make choices based upon evidence and truth rather than fear.** It's for those who are willing to resist the idea that birth has to be a horror story.

It is for **those who are not afraid to put their baby's needs and, yes, their own, above anybody else's** at this most significant time!

This book is for those women, as well, who may feel cheated by what they got from their births in the past. Perhaps these women will never have the chance to give birth again. **It is for the woman who did the best with what she had and who wants more for those women she loves most—her daughters, her sisters, her friends.**

It is for those who have been searching for just the right information to help to prepare those special mothers and fathers in their lives to have the most beautiful and safe birth experiences possible. It's for the caregivers, childbirth educators, professional labor doulas, postpartum doulas, lactation consultants, and others who watch over and care for these families at this time.

Ideally, one has the opportunity to study long before ever conceiving a baby and believes in being educated and prepared ahead of time for this important experience.

Why does this all matter so much? When you think about it, can you possibly really comprehend how much of an influence on the future of the world that we actually have as parents? The way we give birth to our children makes a difference in how we will parent them, in their future lives, and in the world as a whole. This time is not at all insignificant, as illustrated here throughout *Wise Childbearing* in numerous ways. You are urged to ponder on those aspects as you read on.

To varying degrees, the birth of a child has a profound effect on the lives of all of the family members and participants in the birth including, perhaps most immeasurably, the baby—the individual whose birth this is.

Besides touching those immediately involved, the ripples of this time extend out and out and out in ways we, ourselves, may never realize. On and on, as birthing families, our choices influence the nation and even the world in innumerable ways.

Of great importance is our child's conception, her life in the womb, and her birth. These are the beginnings of her earthly experience. **This human being, who will be entering the world for the first time, this** person with already extremely acute senses, deserves as compassionate, tender, and gentle an entry as is possible to give her.

Her first experiences, whatever they may be, her life as a baby and how she grows up, most certainly do affect the kind of individual that she will become. The choices you make *now* play an important role in the kind of life she will have.

Do you respect your baby, even now before she is born? Will you demand that she is treated with respect throughout her growing-up years? How about *now*? Will you be the advocate and supporter she needs *even now*, choosing only those things that have been shown to be the *best* for babies and their mothers?

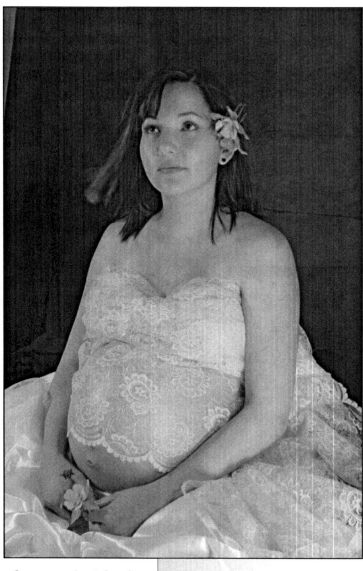

For the Mother

It may seem that the small, private experience of giving birth would hardly make much of a difference in the world. Yet, **this whole period in a woman's life has an important effect on her as a mother and on the kind of woman that she will emerge from all of this as.** This entire time, particularly the moments surrounding the birth of her child, is very significant in the life of a woman. It is one that she remembers forever. It will play an important role in her concept of herself, and even in how powerful and capable she feels in a great many other aspects of her life. **As insignificant as she may sometimes feel, the incalculable difference for good or for ill that one woman makes in the world should not be underestimated— particularly by herself.**

When you are old, and far past your childbearing years, what will your memories of this time be? What kind of stories will you pass on to your granddaughters; the women of the future? Will you be one of those strangers on the bus that, even with good intentions, fills young women's minds with horror stories that make childbirth seem the most horrific experience possible? Or will you be speaking with misty eyes to your posterity one day about the beautiful, sacred events that brought your children to you?

No matter how many times you give birth, *this* birth will become a part of you and it will be something you will remember in detail,

It may seem that the small, private experience of giving birth would hardly make much of a difference in the world...

forever. *How* you do it *will* make a difference. Many women only get one or two chances ever, to do it.

What if your baby's birth really can be one of the most wonderful, beautiful, exhilarating experiences of your life? Are you willing to give what it takes?

For the Father

Not all women have a real man to stand beside them. The world needs more great men, like you, who are willing to learn about all of this and to be an enthusiastic participant in their child's life, beginning with their birth.

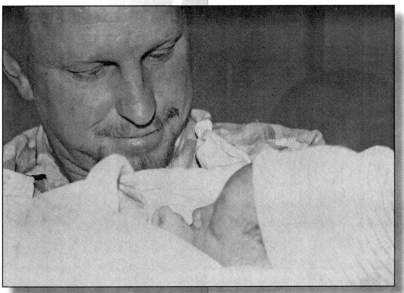

You are also going through one of the most life-changing experiences of *your* life, one that can be enormously consequential as to the kind of father you will be to this particular child, and to the kind of man you are continually becoming. Unfortunately, fathers are often forgotten—even pushed aside in the very moment of their child's birth.

But, your woman and your child need you at this vulnerable time to be gentle, sensitive, and attentive. Even more, they need your protection. If it is important to you to be a protector and guide to this child throughout her growing up years and beyond, it is not at all too early to start. Your child needs you now perhaps more than ever, to be as strong and knowledgeable and well-informed as you can be. What father doesn't naturally have some fears surrounding this important time in their lives? It is entirely normal, but many men have gone through it and survived and found it to be a growing, wonderful experience despite their initial list of reservations.

It is important to understand that particularly during the actual labor and birth, you will not necessarily be able to depend on the mother of your child to be able to take care of situations that arise. It will be important at that time that you have done your homework and are prepared. This book will help you to do that.

Mainly, your child and his mother need you to be there; to *really* be there. You are so important to them. **What you make of this time will matter so very much not only to them, but also to yourself in the future.**

The world needs men who are enthusiastic participants in their children's lives, beginning with their births.

The Very Best for Your Baby

The decision to have a better birth and give your baby the best start cannot be put off. The day is getting closer that you will hold your sweet baby in your arms. When it's all said and done, you won't be able to re-write the events of that day.

Is there really anything that you are doing right now that could be more important than finding out what your best options are and then deciding how to make them happen?

Every parent can do his/her best to give the child of their body the *very best start* in life possible.

Wise Childbearing?

Fortunate many times over is the baby who is born to wise parents. Wisdom is a combination of knowledge and understanding, and the ability to apply both of them effectively. Someone who is wise is able to foresee the likely end-results of potential actions.

An individual who possesses wisdom, seeks effective solutions to challenges by obtaining and using the best sources available. Your responsibility as a parent is to gather, from all of the excellent sources that are available to you, that which serves *your* family.

Be willing to keep an open mind and let curiosity be a guide as you discover new things that just might be worth your time.

Fortunate many times over is the baby who is born to wise parents.

How to Use This Book

You may be reading this book as part of your consumer-oriented childbirth class, taught by a knowledgeable and caring instructor/mentor who is strictly there to serve *you*—someone who is not paid by, or affiliated with, any birth place or caregiver. **Independent instructors are worth every penny you pay and more.** Chances are that she will be one of the most important resources you will find. An independent instructor may even offer doula services, and taking this class from her will be a wonderful opportunity for you to get to know one other.

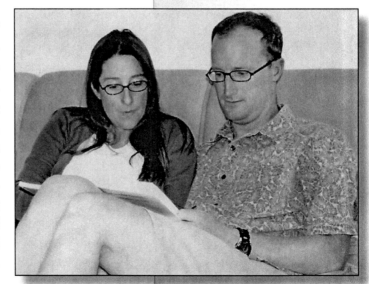

She probably also has a great deal of insight about, and additional resources for, midwives, doctors, birth centers, hospitals, doulas, lactation consultants, and other specialists in your area.

Ideally, you are privileged to be able to be learning alongside others who are also getting ready to birth soon. This type of class is often kept small so you have the opportunity to get to know, and talk and learn with other class members. This kind of setting also gives the chance for activities that will afford you rich discovery experiences not available in larger, ordinary classes.

Even still, if you don't have the opportunity to take a truly great class, you nevertheless have within this book the text of an excellent course. **It is designed to accompany excellent classes.**

And yet, you have a *vast* amount more useful information within these pages than if you had taken a run-of-the-mill, ordinary class that chiefly teaches consumers how to be good patients. If this book is all that you are able to read during your pregnancy, you will have a much, much richer preparation than a great many women and families are presently receiving.

In Appendix B is a listing of traits that characterize classes of quality.

We strongly encourage both parents to read this book, most preferably *together*.

A large part of what *Wise Childbearing* was created to do was to provide easy-to-follow, well-documented, key information for parents who want to make *wise*, **informed** choices for themselves and their baby.

As you are reading and making your decisions, if you own the copy of the book you are reading, **you are highly encouraged to highlight or underline information throughout the book that you personally want to remember. Write notes in the margins. Mark in the "Worksheet for Preparing Your Birth Wish List" in chapter 6 as you go along.** Make this book work for *you*.

You will find bolded quotes throughout. These "stand outs" are to help you to see at a glance information that is particularly essential to understand and remember.

By making *Wise Childbearing* an often-referred-to-resource of your personal library, we are confident that you will find that it has become a truly-valued, if eventually "dog-eared" friend that sees you faithfully through one (perhaps more) of the most important times of your life.

The Association for Wise Childbearing and I are happy to assist you at this time. We wish you a wonderful journey as you read, prepare, give birth to, and continue to parent your baby! *Make* it all it can be!

Is It Possible?

What if your baby's birth really could be one of the most wonderful experiences of your life? What if it could be a beautiful memory you will want to carry with you forever? What if you were to claim the right to birth in your *own* way, because this is *your* body, *your* baby, and *your* birth, and because it is your right to birth the way your body was made to give birth? What if you give birth powerfully—with your *own* power? What if your experience is joyful and full of ecstasy? What if it is one of the most fulfilling experiences of your life? What if your baby's experience really could be gentle and peaceful? What if your baby could be received by your loving touch and embrace and allowed, in those first long moments, to simply be with you and meet you face-to-face? What if your baby could meet with wonder a world of calm and love and comfort—one that is worth trusting? What if your baby could meet it devoid of mind and body-altering drugs and chemicals? What if your baby really could be born gently, treated with the utmost respect by all in attendance, even honored on this significant occasion for all that he has the potential to become? What if it is an experience that is so beautiful, that you want to share it with others so that they too can know the joy and fulfillment you have known? What if others also begin to expect respectful, gentle, evidence-based care? What if the world stops allowing others, particularly those in authority, to take away our rights and privileges? What if you really can reach your potential, and all that you were made to do?

Dare to believe

2

Association for Wise Childbearing, Our Philosophies

BIRTH IS A NORMAL FUNCTION of the body which, like other ordinary processes of the body, seldom necessitates the use of instruments, machines, medications, or drugs. Both women's and babies' bodies were unmistakably designed for childbirth, and to make it through the process without harm.

In spite of the fears that have long woven their way into our culture's way of viewing childbirth, a woman can still give birth with a faith and trust in the design of her body, in her own inner knowledge, and in herself.

A woman is already an expert at having a baby, whether she knows it or not. She does not need to be "delivered" of her baby by someone else under normal circumstances. She is capable of surmounting the challenges of labor and birth.

Of great importance is our child's conception, her life in the womb, and her birth.

Birth is an experience of great significance and consequence for the baby, woman, father and the other members of the family. That which results from the experience endures for a long time. The well-being of the woman, the child, and the father; the very family unit, is of significant consequence to our civilization. We should approach birth with nothing less than reverence.

When women are in control of their births, and when they succeed in their wishes and take on obstacles that confront them, they draw from this momentous life experience emotional strength and a great sense of achievement that is taken with them into innumerable aspects of their future lives.

All of the spiritual, emotional, psychological, and sexual elements of labor and birth are profoundly important. The atmosphere in which a woman gives birth is even more crucial than the proportion of her pelvis or the size of the baby.

Emotional healing is important for those who have had a prior difficult and wounding birth and for those who have suffered previous sexual abuse as these, if left unresolved, can negatively influence future birth experiences.

There are many different ways and places in which to birth. It is a woman's right and responsibility to make the choices necessary to birth in the best possible ways for her baby and herself. These decisions are not for her caregivers to make. They belong to her, and it is up to her to make them wisely.

Not all choices are created equal. There is almost always one choice that is superior to another. Also what may be right for one woman may not be right for another. If a woman doesn't know her options she really doesn't have any.

Interventions would wisely be saved for the exceptional circumstance when nature needs a little help, and not as routine management for every birth and every mother and baby. The process of birth can be, and often is, upset or even halted by physical interventions and disturbances.

The birthing family is not only the consumer, but is the employer of those who will serve them at their births. If they do not like what a particular caregiver or birth place is offering, they would be wise to seriously consider hiring a different caregiver and/or place of birth.

The psychological nature of the process of birth makes this a vulnerable time for the mother. It is also an emotionally vulnerable time for the father. Both may be more willing to accept the decisions of others, particularly those in authority, at this time. It is therefore essential to ensure beforehand, that all of the members of their birth team share the same philosophies and desires for this birth.

When someone plans to attend a woman in labor, they must be sure that they have resolved any "hang-ups" within themselves. A woman in labor can easily pick up on, and be affected by the fear and the psychological issues of members of her team.

Those who attend birth have the opportunity to recognize the sacred nature of the event and act with reverence and respect.

The woman is in charge of deciding who will be at her birth, and she has the right to not invite or to dismiss anyone.

The support of a caring doula can be of immeasurable assistance to the mother, father, and other members of the birth team.

Good nutrition is fundamental to a healthy pregnancy and birth. It can have a profound impact on the health of the baby and the kind of birth the woman and baby will have. Restrictions on healthy food can be seriously harmful to both and the outcome of the birth.

The woman is in charge of deciding who will be at her birth, and she has the right to not invite or to dismiss anyone.

3

Women Were Made to Give Birth!

ONE OF THE FIRST and most important aspects to understand is that women were *made* with the ability to give birth! When women give birth, they are doing something as natural as pumping blood, breathing, and digesting food. **There is a knowledge of how to give birth within each woman, a knowledge that doesn't even require conscious thought.**

Whether it's fictional, true, or a little of both, a TV show or novel that includes childbirth has all the elements to make any good—or bad— book or movie much more exciting. Gripping scenes show screaming women being rushed to the hospital. There they are saved by mask-faced

Within every woman is the knowledge of how to grow a baby and how to give birth.

13

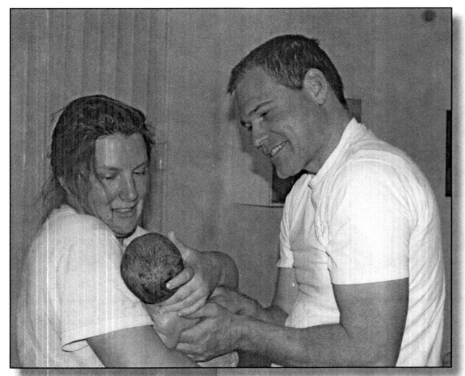

This baby is welcomed by her parents during a gentle and serene homebirth.

heroes. Or maybe the helpless damsel-in-distress is delayed in transit and must be rescued instead by some other savior. Most people in America never witness birth as a natural and healthy part of life as people in other places do. Much of our education about childbirth comes from too many white-knuckled, made-for-screen births before we've even completed grade school. Is it any wonder that we tend to be frightened of birth? **We certainly aren't coming away with the realization that mothers and babies were magnificently designed to come through birth unharmed.**

On the contrary, young girls learn that they cannot trust their bodies, that a birthing woman is a helpless patient, and that she and her baby will certainly die unless carefully monitored.

So we accept this when we approach our own, real-life births. Although things are changing a bit, women in our country are still often made to stay in bed, hooked to machines—as if to suggest that a disaster might occur at any second and that she should let her caregivers make all decisions rather than working together with them in a partnership. After all, "doctor knows best"—right?

Women do not need to be "delivered." Women were made to give birth to babies.

Birth Is a Natural Process

What is missing in this whole picture is that **it is not midwives or doctors that deliver babies. Women give birth to babies!** Women have been giving birth for a long, long time. All over the world mammals give birth without technology—and they do so without a shortage of either people or animals. Birth works! **Birth is as natural and normal a process as is any of our other bodily functions, from digesting food to circulating blood. Women were made to be strong and capable of birth.** This part of their body works too!

You may be surprised to know that even with access to all the latest manmade technology, the U.S. does not rank well in comparison to other developed countries when mortality and morbidity (meaning death and injury) rates, during and shortly after the birth, are considered.

In fact, **the U.S. is consistently ineligible for placing within the top** *twenty* **countries**. There are *many* countries in which it is safer to give birth to babies than here in the United States. (Population Reference Bureau 1996)

Why is this so?

We assert that birth, like other aspects of nature and the natural world is something that does not routinely require instruments, chemicals, drugs, or technological gadgets. In fact, the utilization of invasive procedures on a healthy woman with a healthy baby can actually be very detrimental.

Could the failure that United States obstetrics is experiencing actually (and ironically) have to do with the technology routinely used at U.S. births today?

Marsden Wagner MD, former head of Women and Children's Health for the World Health Organization for fifteen years says emphatically that, "yes, it is" the routine technology used in the U.S. birth culture today that is causing the alarming chaos we are seeing.

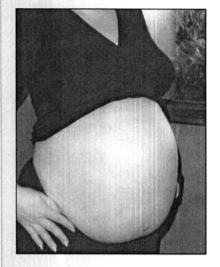

Yet, we are beings of a technological age. We've witnessed the wonders of technology. We depend upon it for a great many tasks in our daily lives.

In a way, however, it is easy to make technology a kind of god. We forget sometimes that man's knowledge and man-made machines are not perfect—that man sometimes makes mistakes. We forget that there are always better machines coming out, better computers, better phones, and better dishwashers. Looking back, we are surprised at how much better things are now than they used to be just a few years ago. Years down the road, we will predictably feel the same when comparing then with now, and so on and so on.

What we forget is that the human body is one of the greatest "machines" ever created. No scientist, not even the most brilliant, has ever been able to duplicate it.

Heavenly Father

Birth is as natural and normal a process as is any of our other bodily functions. This part of the female body works too!

All of nature, including the human body, was organized to follow pre-planned patterns and designs. Trees know how to grow tall and full. Birds know how to make nests. Salmon that are far downstream know how to find their way back home. Newborn horses know how to get to their feet soon after birth. Seeds in the garden know how to grow into plants of their own kind.

Within your body another human being has begun from just two cells. From there your body continues to help build a whole new person. Without any thought required at all by you, bones, muscles, a brain, fingernails, fingers and toes, skin, sight, hearing, an entire circulatory system, respiratory system, and so, so much more are created. Even a new reproductive system is formed—providing the way for this same process to happen time and time again. Then, immediately after you give birth to this new individual, your body begins to create the perfect food for him or her. And other processes are set into motion for this new being to *thrive*.

Has the human mind ever been able to re-create anything this magnificent?

Not only this, but part of woman is her knowledge of how to birth. It's part of her physiology, part of her psyche. Yet, a great many birthing women today are themselves, incredibly enough, treated like machines needing to be monitored, tested, and improved upon by man's technology, by doctors' latest techniques, and by pharmaceutical companies. What we have also forgotten is that **birth has been working for *ages*. It was made the right way the first time!**

What would make us think that when it comes to birthing our babies that something about the process has become defective? The human race has never even approached extinction because the birth process didn't work. What has caused us so much fear and doubt? History can tell us a lot about why we are so fearful and so distrustful, and about the beliefs we hold as a culture. We will discuss how we arrived at such a point a bit later.

In her book *Gentle Birth Choices*, the founder of Waterbirth International, Barbara Harper tells of one doctor's journey as he came to an understanding of these truths: "In his former days as a traditional obstetrician, Dr. Rosenthal viewed the birth process as a medical event to be controlled on a time line. Since then he has learned to stand back and empower the woman to give birth. 'When women control the birth process and actively participate free of traditional interventions, they derive emotional strength and a great sense of achievement,' states Rosenthal. 'At the Family Birthing Center, we feel strongly that women are giving birth. They're not coming here to have their babies delivered. Part of our effort is to restore control of birth back to women. We take the term 'nonintervention' in a very literal sense. It often means that women give birth without me using my hands.'" (Harper 1994)

What an inspiring example of a caregiver who trusts in the process and in women's ability to give birth!

There is remarkable empowerment in giving birth rather than being delivered. But in our day and age many women may feel disconnected from their instincts. "Will I really know, and be able to do, what it is that needs to be done to birth my baby?" they might wonder. They are afraid to trust that they really do know how.

But the answer is yes! A woman's body does know what to do! In labor, without willing it herself, the wisdom of the woman's body will come forward, and the power within her will demand her attention. As long as she isn't interfered with, she can begin to concentrate on the sensations within her body and work with them, allowing her to more easily give birth.

While American women today are striving to be strong, assertive, convincing, open-minded, organized, energetic, meticulous, powerful, and able to work more effectively with those they deal with each day, when it comes to birthing their children many women still

A mother and baby may be less safe in the hospital if the pregnancy is normal.

passively do whatever they are told whether or not they fully understand the logic behind it. Many have their babies taken out for them rather than pushing them out themselves. They give up all power over their bodies, their births, and their babies. They decide on drugs before they ever know what it feels like to experience labor—drugs that besides decreasing any discomfort, reduce the power and effectiveness of the body. At the same time, the *joy* and *pleasure* that are inherent accompaniments of truly experiencing childbirth in its fullness are also greatly diminished. Who is telling them that unhindered childbirth, under decent circumstances, can actually be *enjoyable*?

History and the present appalling birth statistics in our country have shown us that we cannot afford to just climb onto the conveyor belt any longer. We and our babies deserve better.

Women's bodies are designed to give birth and to do it well! Isn't it time we took back the power?

Yes, But Can My Body Give Birth?

Chances are good that you have already heard comments such as, "Your body frame is just so small. You're really going to have a hard time having a baby." The same old myths and fears have been floating around for much too long. Even some caregivers believe them. Our past plays a significant role in this belief, as you will soon read. Ironically, though it is a prevalent fear in our society, the width of the pelvic opening cannot be determined by the outer dimensions of the pelvis and even an ultrasound is not a good means of determining inner pelvic dimensions.

Some of the best friends a pregnant woman has are the hormones which her body naturally releases during this time. Just as hormones are causing a remarkable transformation in her breasts as well as the rest of her body during her pregnancy, those hormones are also causing a woman's pelvis to soften, become loose, and to give. The now softened cartilage and elongated tendons and ligaments that hold the bones of the pelvis together have become loose and pliable. This is one reason she may sometimes feel so uncoordinated when walking during pregnancy! Later, as the baby descends during birth, the pelvis widens and spreads into the right positions. During the birth, it can stretch to amazing proportions.

Of interest are the numbers of women who have cesareans, due to errant judgment and interference, who later go on to vaginally give birth to a larger baby the next time. Big babies often just fit better because they can more easily move into and stay in a great position for an easier and more efficient birth. We love to use the example of a woman we know who had her almost thirteen pound baby in about forty-five

Joy and pleasure are inherent accompaniments of childbirth. Unhindered childbirth can actually be "enjoyable."

minutes. This woman is not particularly large, either. She is, though, a woman who believes in her body's ability to birth her babies. There are many such examples.

The vagina also naturally expands into huge dimensions. If unhurried, the woman's body gradually opens naturally to accommodate the baby. It is not uncommon when babies are allowed to gently descend, rather than being strenuously pushed out, that mothers only realize the baby has descended through the vagina when they feel the baby's head at the opening. The "watermelon fitting through an olive-sized hole" analogy doesn't hold any water! Women's bodies were designed to accommodate their babies. They were created to open and s-t-r-e-t-c-h, then to return to near normal afterwards (this of course is dependent on the woman being in reasonably good health and upon her nutrition). Our bodies were remarkably created.

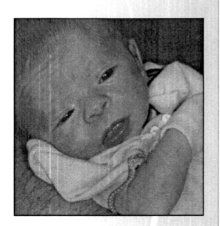

Babies Were Made to Be Born!

Likewise, babies were designed to be born! For this very purpose, their skull bones are not yet fused together and have space between them so they can overlap, reducing the circumference of the head during birth. Afterward, they soon return to normal. Babies were made to be born without forceps, vacuum, or surgery.

Of course when the baby is in an optimal position in the womb, labor is naturally more comfortable and efficient. Knowledge of this and how to encourage it is important and is discussed later in the book.

Using upright positions is one of the best ways for a woman to open and allow her baby to be born. Having a woman flat on her back may be easier for her caregiver, but this position also collapses the pelvis, making it less able to perform its job the way it was designed to. This also is not what is most comfortable for the mother! (See Positions...in **chapter 13**.)

Incredibly, a woman's body will give birth whether or not she is even aware of it! There are reports of women giving birth undetected when they were in a comatose state. It did not require any thought-process at all! In fact getting our minds out of the way, once we have educated ourselves and made good decisions for our care, so that we can just *let our bodies do the work*, is one of the best things we can do!

Did you know big babies often just fit better because they can more easily move into and stay in a great position for an easier and more efficient birth?

Facing Our Fears

Birth is a normal function of the body, just as digesting food is. Seldom is there a problem when we eat something. Bad food or stress can give us an upset stomach, but usually digestion works as it was created to. So does birth.

Yet, in our culture we are *terrified* of birth. Think about it. Why, for example, don't we insist that everyone who operates machinery or snowmobiles in the mountains or who eats dinner be within ten minutes of a hospital? There really is risk in almost everything we do. To avoid the chance of choking, should we all stop eating and get feeding tubes put into our noses?

It seems that women are at a higher risk of dying on the way to the hospital (20 in 100,000 women of childbearing age die in car accidents) than they are when simply giving birth (6 in 100,000). Do we install IVs in the cars of all women of childbearing age "just in case"?

If we were as paranoid about all aspects of life as we are about simply having a baby, we would likely make up nonsense rules in other areas besides childbirth.

Why is our culture so obsessed, so fanatical, in this particular area? One reason, surely, is that so much is at stake. Good care should certainly be readily available to both mother and baby in the case that something might go wrong. Yet sadly, the extent that we have gone to out of *fear*, is very unfortunate because the question must then be asked as to whether our culture's attempts to protect mothers and babies have been productive. Routine use of technology at birth has *not* improved outcomes. Babies born in the U.S., surrounded by technology, have been shown statistically to be born in *less* safe conditions than babies in a great *many* other industrialized countries. (Health 2003)

The fact is that we take risks all the time, and giving birth is no different. Birth is really as safe as life gets—just like anything else.

Once again, understanding the history of childbirth in our culture gives some answers and insight into what this insanity is really all about.

Parents can decide to make choices based upon evidence and truth rather than fear.

4

Our Evolving Birth Culture

IN THE PAST there have been many childbirth practices that once were thought to be helpful to the birthing process and that since have been abandoned. Understanding the history of childbirth and how practices have changed can help us to see where we actually are now and to decide if what is presently offered is really what we want for ourselves and our children.

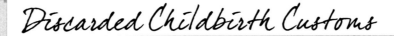

Discarded Childbirth Customs

One practice that had some of most devastating effects on our birthing culture was Twilight Sleep. An older relative or friend may be able to tell you about her own experience with a Twilight Sleep labor. Women were given morphine for pain, amnesiac scopolamine, which caused a woman to forget the trauma, and chloroform or ether. Rather than experiencing the absence of pain, however, women often simply didn't remember the experience. Women were described to behave like deranged animals in this state. They were tied to their beds, on their backs. They could do nothing for themselves and appeared to be out of their minds. Hallucinations, such as believing one was actually tied up and was being tortured, were not uncommon for a woman laboring under the influence of Twilight Sleep.

What's more, when the woman awoke, she was often told she had a baby but then was not allowed to even see the baby for an extended period of time. Sometimes it was because a woman needed time to recover. Other times it was due to bruises and other injuries to the baby caused by forceps delivery and other procedures to get the baby out. These things were common since the mother could do nothing, such as walking and using different positions, to help to birth her baby. These injuries to the baby often necessitated observation in the nursery. *It took forty years before Twilight Sleep was abandoned because it was finally judged to be unsafe.*

It is also, thankfully, no longer standard practice to hold a baby by the feet and spank her. Approaches have become a bit gentler over all (though gentleness varies greatly from caregiver to caregiver).

Another illustration of a practice that has since been judged to be unsafe and unnecessary is that of shaving the perineum. This was once thought to lessen infection, when in actuality it promoted infection.

How about the giving of an enema? A few caregivers may continue to require the unnecessary, uncomfortable practice of cleansing a woman's bowels prior to birth, even to this date.

Responsive Revisions

Things are continually changing on the childbirth scene. **Informed parents have been responsible for many of these changes. Good caregivers listen to their clients.** They continue to learn even after they have finished formal schooling. They read studies and take continuing education classes. They practice evidence-based care. They welcome information on how experiences can be improved; made safer, more comfortable, and better for their clients.

One example of doctors and hospitals listening to the needs of their clients is that in many hospitals, women can labor in a homier-looking room with its own shower. While most hospitals still very much consider the comfort and convenience of the doctor and the hospital first, there are hospitals that are becoming more accommodating. In some hospitals now, Jacuzzis are even included in the floor plans. In a number of hospitals they are included in each room, because the staff is seeing how helpful they are—and because they are listening to birthing families.

The birthing environment our daughters and sons will know will undoubtedly be different than it has been for us.

So then, ask yourself the following questions: If you could live in *any* time or place, where and how would you choose to give birth? Why? How can you create that kind of birthing atmosphere *today*, with the resources available to you? What, if anything, is holding you back? What can you do to overcome those barriers? **What can you do to make a better birthing culture for your children when they give birth to your grandchildren?**

*If you could live in **any** time or place, where and how would you choose to give birth?*

Childbirth Practices throughout History

Let's take a look as far back as 2,000 B.C. Back then women were revered as givers of life. Many of the statues unearthed from this time were very womanly. And at the time of birth people would gather around the mother in the temple for this celebration of life. **Birthing was apparently a *sacred* and *beautiful* religious rite, and not the agonizing ordeal it was later to become.** Apparently this joyous perception of birth prevailed for a very long time. Curiously, Hippocrates, Aristotle, and Soranus gave no indications in their writings that childbirth was considered by the people of their time to be a painful experience except during complications. Even then, women were brought into a relaxed state with herbs so that they could be treated. Women appear to have been well-cared for by birthing attendants, and also to have had the support of labor assistants. The dominating mindset surrounding childbirth seemed to be *joy*.

Many years later, however, childbirth began to be considered the result of carnal sin. In fact, midwives and doctors were forbidden from attending women in labor. Translation of the Bible from the original word "etzev" (meaning to labor, toil, or work), introduced instead words like pain, sorrow, anguish, or pangs in its place.

So at this point in history, while laboring women were forced to labor without skillful care and labor support, if there were complications they were forced to be attended by field hands. If those attending them deemed it necessary, they could cut a mother open to save a live baby, or to baptize a dead one—whether or not the mother was alive and without the use of any pain-killing herbs.

Women were taught that this was their punishment for the sin of Eve. It is not surprising that women now very much perceived birth with fear. The "Fear-Tension-Pain Syndrome" (see Hypnobirthing in **chapter 13**.) became deeply established.

Finally, midwives were again given the right to attend women. However physicians were not because only women were allowed to take care of the "disgusting" business of childbirth. Because of the prevailing belief of the times that childbirth was intended to be a punishment, laboring women were also denied the use of chloroform when it was first introduced.

When physicians were finally allowed to attend women, the environment in hospitals was horrifying. Obstetricians were often not well-trained. Large numbers of women actually did, you might say, pass through "the valley of the shadow of death." That diseases could be spread from one person to another was not yet well-known. Many mothers who simply went in to have a baby, died of infections spread from diseased patients who shared the hospital and from doctors naively going straight from autopsies of infected cadavers to birthing rooms without washing their hands. Maternal death rates due to infection were high. When what was happening was discovered, it was not reported immediately, or broadly, to other hospitals. After all, what a horrific thing to admit to—so many women had died needlessly because of this mistake. Florence Nightingale, who had begun training midwives, saw what was happening and noted the much lower rates of maternal death at homebirths in comparison with those in the hospital. She worked to improve the situation for birthing women after studying what was happening.

Now that death and pain in childbirth were both believed to accompany childbirth hand in hand, anesthesia became accepted for use in childbirth. With acceptance came more usage. **Drugged births, where the baby had to be pulled out with instruments, became the way that physicians believed was the *only* way.**

Methods from those days have been handed down through obstetric medical school training to the present day.

Sadly, this type of thinking *still* prevails in a great many physician practices. This way of attending a woman who is giving birth still remains all that most doctors and nurses have ever had experience with.

Remember the old saying that we must learn from history or we will be doomed to repeat it? **With the direction things are moving presently in our U.S. birthing culture, we would do well to take a good look.** The following is a brief overview of the history of birth in the last one hundred years or so.

Early 1900s—Checking into a hospital to give birth becomes the thing for the middle-class woman to do. After all, being surrounded there by doctors and the best machines available must certainly be the safest place to have a baby!

1914—Twilight Sleep is developed. Just after the introduction of this invention, the U.S. infant death rate *grows* to six in 1,000, *the highest in the industrial world*. A woman must labor alone, without other knowledgeable women that had once cared for and supported her. The woman is put to sleep, and when she awakes, she has a baby. This is often all that she remembers, although a number of women recall experiencing a horrific and torturously painful dream-state while under the influence of the anesthesia.

1931—Statistics show that those countries in which midwives attend the majority of births are those that actually have the lowest infant mortality rates. How could this be, with the finest technology available in the 1930s right at doctors' fingertips? The first nurse midwifery education program is started in the United States.

1940—The use of total anesthesia during childbirth becomes the "modern" way to give birth. "Scientifically" managed, scheduled bottle-feedings begin to be promoted by pediatricians.

1952—Lamaze and Vellay present their version of psycho-prophylactic obstetrical practices that were being used at the time in Russia. This method uses distraction as a form of coping during labor, including practicing structured breathing. The doula is omitted when the practice is introduced into the United States. Thus the method proves less than wholly successful at this time of introduction.

1960—Cesarean birth rates in the U.S. reach about 7 percent.

1965—Concerns about the effects of medication begin to be considered. Large numbers of women begin to take classes and successfully give birth without drugs. Bradley introduces the concept of fathers as labor "coaches."

1974—Almost all women in the U.S. are giving birth in the hospital with only about 29,413 births attended by midwives.

1977—A major study by Lewis Mehl, MD indicates that home births are actually *safer* than hospital births when good nutrition and prenatal care are present.

1978—The cesarean rate approaches 18 percent.

1980—The rate of hospital births declines slightly following a statement by the American Public Health Association asserting that "births to healthy mothers can occur safely outside the setting of an acute-care hospital." Endorsements to expand midwifery are given by The Institute of Medicine of the National Academy of Science, The Office of Technology Assessment of the U.S. Congress, and the National Commission to Prevent Infant Mortality.

The timeline was adapted with permission from cited sources by Mongan and O'Mara.

In the chapters that follow, we will illustrate today's general customs and practices. You will have the opportunity to consider the results you want for *your baby, yourself,* and *your family.*

1982—More routine interventions come into common usage, but the rates of maternal mortality (death of mothers) in the United States do not improve.

1986—*Silent Knife* by Nancy Wainer Cohen, about cesarean prevention, is published. She receives over 100,000 letters in response. Birthing centers are introduced.

1988—132,670 births in the U.S. are attended by midwives.

1989—The HypnoBirthing® program is developed by Marie Mongan, offering women much more gentle and comfortable birthings while still being conscious and active participants in their births.

1989—Studies show that low-risk women birthing at freestanding birth centers actually have lower rates of cesarean birth, less neonatal mortality, and *no* maternal mortality.

1990—One in every four U.S. women (25 percent) gives birth by cesarean section.

1991—Approximately 5 percent of births occurring in the hospital are attended by midwives. In the Netherlands, more than 33 percent of births are homebirths attended by midwives. Infant mortality there is much lower than that of the United States.

1992—Doulas of North America (DONA) is established after a number of new physician-led studies reveal greatly enhanced outcomes at births where a doula is present. Outcomes include a 50 percent reduction in cesarean rates and a 60 percent decrease in requests for epidural when doulas attend births.

1995—The rate of cesarean births in the United States declines a little—20.8 percent and the vaginal-birth-after-cesarean rate surges to 35.5 percent.

1997—The majority of insurance carriers initiate coverage for midwife-attended hospital/birth center births.

1998—The number of midwife-attended births is now increasing rapidly. The percentage of midwife-attended hospital births is growing even more quickly, having increased by 1,000 percent since 1975. One study shows greatly reduced infant-mortality numbers for births with certified nurse midwives as the attendants.

2009—Cesarean rates rise to over 30 percent as women are led to believe that cesarean sections are a more refined, sophisticated, easier, and safer way of giving birth.

The World Health Organization has stated that in the future it hopes to see no more than 10 to 15 percent of all births being cesareans, induction for birth occurring no greater than 10 percent of the time, and upright positions being used for labor and birth. They hope, as well, that there will be a discouragement in the routine use of electronic fetal monitors, analgesics, anesthetics, and artificial rupture of membranes, and an emphasis on breastfeeding immediately after birth.

Unfortunately, a great many medical caregivers do not want to change to conform to these goals of WHO. Nor are they accountable to anyone, and no one regulates them. In fact, believe it or not, there is *no one* in place to whom care must be reported or to whom accountability, verification, or justification must be given!

The United States has the potential to be the best, safest place to give birth. But it is a *far cry* from that at present.

The future depends on the consumer. Will more and more consumers begin to stand up and insist on more than what is status-quo? **Will *enough* families demand that the United States begin to study why it is so much safer to be born in so many other countries than it is here?**

On a more personal note, what about for you? Will your birth experience be reflective of present birth statistics? We believe that if individual women and families will stand back and take a good long look at the past, at other cultures, and at potential futures, they will be able to decide what kind of birth they want for their babies—regardless of the time in which they live. Using wisdom, they can create something more joyful and gentle for their baby and for themselves than most people are currently getting.

It is possible to create something more gentle and joyful than is presently being offered...

5

Where Do I Want to Give Birth?

Where you give birth is one of the most important choices you will need to consider. That initial decision will also be fundamental in determining what kind of subsequent choices you will be making from here on out.

Think for a moment about what *your* ideal birth would be like. All over the world at this very moment, women are laboring in many different places and circumstances. Perhaps it's in a grass hut in the mountains, on a houseboat, in a tide pool, in a field, by the fire, under fluorescent lights, in a bedroom by candlelight, or in a grove of trees. Women birth in different places according to the traditions and the culture in which they live—just as birds and animals instinctively build their nests with whatever is available to them.

Typically, we in our culture think of three places for giving birth: the hospital, at home, and a birthing center. Let's look more closely at each of these three options.

The Hospital

The hospital is an option available to just about everyone in the United States.

Hospital rooms have been made to look much homier in past few years. There are beautiful bedspreads, a TV, pictures, and wall paper.

There are Jacuzzis (perhaps just one for the entire Labor and Delivery wing) available in a number of hospitals. These range in size from quite small to quite large. Often there is a shower in the bathrooms, though showers and bathrooms are sometimes shared by more than one room. Some hospitals will allow you to bring in your own birthing tub. Some caregivers and hospitals are more accommodating to this than others. In some less-informed hospitals, it is against policy to birth in the water. You may still be able to *labor* in the water, however.

Hospitals are not for those who expect a "home-like" atmosphere. They must be run efficiently to be cost-effective.

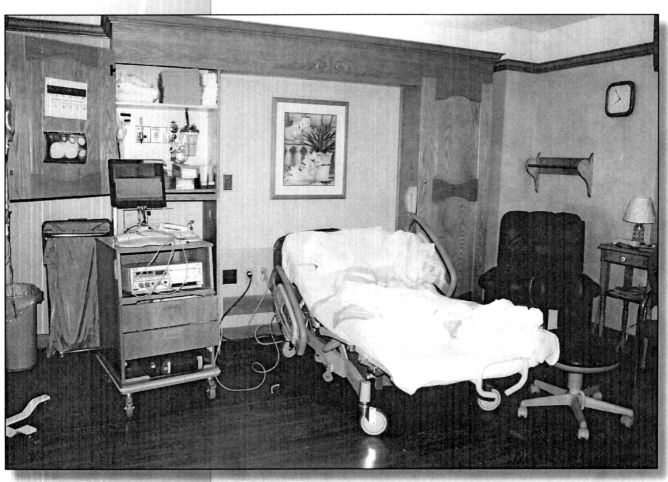

Amount of privacy is most often less than desirable in the hospital. A number of people, including the nursery staff, the doctors, a number of nurses, medical students, even the janitor, may all attend your birth. You may also feel less free to be noisy or to move around out in the halls because of other people on the Labor and Delivery floor.

When giving birth in the hospital, the best technological help is nearby, and precautionary measures are in place, just in case something does not go right. A helicopter may be available to take your baby, if necessary, to a larger hospital equipped with more advanced, lifesaving technology.

Simply being in the hospital with the IV in place, the monitor on, and nurses nearby makes some people *feel* safer.

Some families who do feel safer birthing in the hospital, labor at home as long as possible and then check out as early after the birth as they can. For some, this is because they find it difficult to get much rest in an unfamiliar, brightly lit, and noisy facility, with nurses making frequent assessments of them and their baby for their records.

What is crucial to consider, is whether you and your baby are indeed safer.

If you have problems that truly put you in a high-risk category, this might be the case. (See "High Risk?" in **chapter 9**.)

Hospitals are generally safer for women and babies undergoing a pregnancy that is indeed a high-risk pregnancy. Statistics report, however, that mother and baby may be *less safe* in the hospital if the pregnancy is normal.

Homebirth, birth center birth, and hospital birth have all, by and large, been shown in multiple studies to be about equal as far as mortality (death) rates go. Hospitals do have higher rates of morbidity (injury) than do the other two, though.

Nurses are usually as helpful and friendly as possible, though typically they are much too busy to offer a lot of support (for this, couples are very much encouraged to bring a doula).

It must be understood by those wishing for an unmedicated birth, that in many hospitals members of the staff are most familiar with the scenario of women having epidurals. Therefore, they may not be as considerate of the needs that naturally birthing women have for outside quiet and the lowest amount of interruption possible. Some may talk to, or require things of, a woman while she is working through a contraction. There may be a number of other distractions as well, such as having to stay in bed (often not a comfortable thing to do in labor) for monitoring of the baby. (See "Electronic Fetal Heart Monitor" in chapter 7.)

Likewise, usually of lesser consideration to the hospital staff than other components of the birth are the spiritual and psychological aspects of the experience. In some larger hospitals especially, so many births occur daily that after a while the staff naturally becomes, shall we say, a bit callused? It is not uncommon for less-professional doctors and

Hospitals are generally safer for women and babies undergoing a pregnancy that is indeed a high-risk pregnancy. Statistics report, however, that mother and baby may be less safe in the hospital if the pregnancy is normal.

nurses to visit and joke together during the birth, perhaps about the latest hospital gossip or about what is happening in the news. It must also be said, regretfully, that there are those doctors that are not very respectful to the rest of the birth team, particularly the nurses. Would these types of uncontrollable atmospheres make a difference to you? To some families this sort of thing wouldn't bother them. Others consider their birth to be a sacred moment and wish for all of the attendants to be attentive to this. Is it possible that a few well-chosen words in your birth wishes would create more of the atmosphere you desire?

Hospitals are *not* for those who expect a "home-like" atmosphere. Hospitals aren't home. They must be run efficiently to be cost-effective. That is simply the way it is in most hospitals.

Choosing the services of a hospital requires abiding, to a large degree, by the hospital's policies. There are rules about such things as what you can and cannot do with your baby, even about *when*, *where*, and how you are allowed to have your baby with you after he is born. If opposed to any of the rules because they seem to serve the hospital more than the family, consumers would do well to let the hospital know of their dissatisfaction for the benefit of others in the future. Yet they must realize that this is what their choice of birth place is currently offering at this time and policies will probably not change a great deal during their own pregnancy.

So do be sure to consider if you choose to birth in a hospital, whether your beliefs about birth parallel the kind of care women and babies receive in the one you are considering. Do you feel like you will be supported there in your wishes, or will you be fighting every step of the way for what you want for your family and your baby? Will you feel safe there? Is this a hospital in which you will be treated as more than just another woman on "the conveyer belt of birth"? Will you have the privacy you need?

We suggest taking a tour of the labor and delivery ward of the hospital you are considering. While there, think about the questions above.

You can also ask your childbirth educator, if you have one, for more information about the specific hospital you are considering.

The largest percentage of women have given birth in the hospital for the last century. And so we cover hospital birth carefully throughout this book. The hospital may best option for some, particularly for those who are genuinely high risk.

Choosing the services of a hospital requires abiding, to a large degree, by the hospital's policies...

Where will I feel the most support?

At Home

We will spend a little more time on homebirth here than hospital birth due to it being a lesser known option in the United States culturally.

Most people raised within our culture are surprised to hear that homebirth really is as safe a choice as birth center birth and hospital birth for the majority of birthing families today. With all of the horror stories that have been included in entertainment shows today, one would hardly think that this could actually be true—a regular, commonplace, everyday birth is definitely not as exciting as the kind scriptwriters and novelists can invent. But it *is* true. **Studies have shown again and again that there are *very few* women for whom homebirth may not be a good option. After all, the world was well-populated long before modern obstetrics!**

Researchers studying data from U.S. birth certificates have found a 20 percent increase in American births at home from 2004 to 2008. (Wyckoff 2011)

Women today, just as all of their grandmothers before them down through the ages, still have the power to birth their babies. They do not need a lot of manmade instruments to be able to do it, and it is

Most modern day women that have experienced a planned homebirth will report great satisfaction with their experience, often describing the beauty and sanctity of this special event as well as how it was more relaxed and less stressful than it otherwise could have been in a hospital atmosphere.

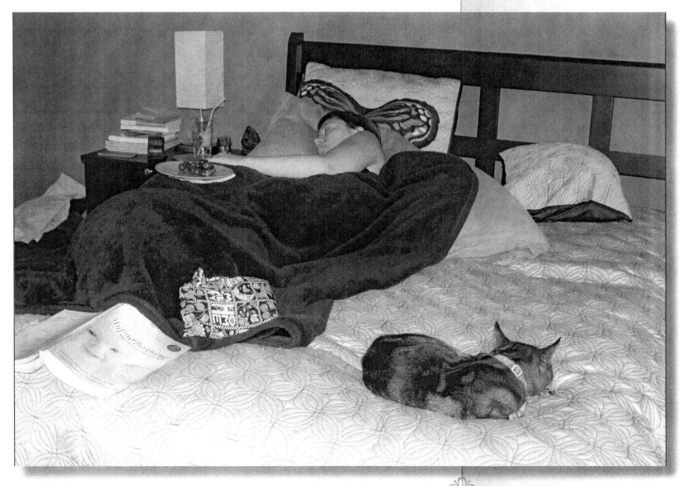

typically unnecessary, despite what we have grown up being told, to be in a hospital to have a baby. Women's and babies' bodies were *designed* to come through birth unharmed. If we have the courage to just leave them alone and *trust the process*, they will have a much better opportunity to do just that.

In more and more places in the United States, families can have the best of both worlds—homebirths with exceptionally-trained midwives or doctors, as well as within minutes appropriate hospital technology in case of a special circumstance.

It might also be hard for those who have been raised in our culture to believe, but **transfers from a homebirth to the hospital take place only a small percentage of the time.** One popular midwife says that she transfers women to the hospital on average only about four times a year. When her mothers do have to go to the hospital, it rarely involves an emergency. Transfers are often for non-emergency reasons such as a long, exhausting labor or failure-to-progress. Typically the couple drives to the hospital with their midwife, in their own vehicle, without having to run any red lights. It is unusual for an ambulance or paramedics to be necessary. During that time, a swift transport can be made to the hospital from a nearby planned homebirth. When a true emergency occurs in the hospital, it takes a certain amount of time for the hospital to set up and perhaps even call the doctor to the hospital. Have you ever sat for long periods in the emergency room of your local hospital? How are "emergencies" handled there? Is it anything like the frantic, panicked rush you see on the TV show "ER"? Hardly! Most of the time, if there are any, problems in labor develop slowly. Watchful midwives can see them coming from miles away.

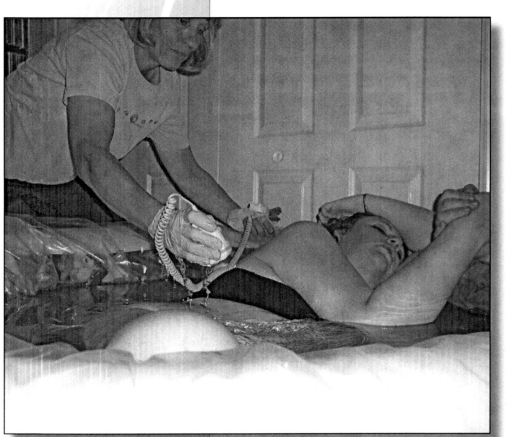

Almost all homebirths are attended by midwives. There are a variety of avenues through which midwives are educated. Some are trained by apprenticeship with experienced, well-seasoned midwives. There are also a growing number of midwifery colleges and programs available which train midwives in normal, natural birth as well as complications.

Why wouldn't most medical caregivers recommend homebirth? As good-hearted and as honest as many obstetricians are, in general most have no experience with normal homebirth whatsoever. Laws vary from state to state, but the majority of doctors and CNMs (certified nurse midwives) in the United States are restricted from attending homebirths—they could lose their licenses for doing so, in fact. Most have also never been educated or taken the opportunity to become well-informed on the issue.

Homebirth is still illogically alegal and even illegal in some states. People who understand the issues from all directions are needed to make sure that quality homebirth care is available to all women in the United States that would choose it.

In the hospital setting, most often the doctor or certified nurse midwife is called in only at the end, to come for the actual birth, although a certified nurse midwife will sometimes be able to stay for more of your labor. Nurses, who give the primary care in the hospital labor-and-delivery, can have several women that they are in charge of and they have other responsibilities as well, so they aren't able to be with the woman a lot of the time. This is one reason women are put on a monitor in the hospital. It makes it easier for the nurse to watch the monitor at her desk as she takes care of other responsibilities such as paperwork.

By watching and caring exclusively for one woman at a time, homebirth midwives typically attend a birth from active labor until well after the birth when the family is all "tucked in together."

In the hospital, a family usually does not have the opportunity to meet with the people that will care for them during their labor. This can be a bit stressful for both parents and staff as they all test the waters and set out to sail together on this most significant journey.

Most nurses probably entered the profession because they wanted to help mothers and babies. There are many wonderful, open-minded nurses, but if a couple is assigned a nurse or nurses whose philosophies do not match theirs–and if requesting a different nurse doesn't help— they will need to be able to deal with the unpredictability of what they get. Some nurses are unreceptive and even aggressive toward new or different concepts.

At home, much of the paperwork has already been done, and optimally the midwife has known and seen the couple throughout the pregnancy, is aware of any special needs, and is there exclusively for *them*. The "hands on" assistance that midwives can give at a homebirth is invaluable. Midwives can also give more one-on-one attention at prenatal visits. When it comes time to give birth, a family can feel very comfortable with this woman they have developed a relationship with. Because homebirth midwives are there throughout the pregnancy, making themselves personally available in person and by phone, midwives

By watching and caring exclusively for one woman at a time, homebirth midwives typically attend a birth from active labor until well after the birth when the family is all "tucked in together."

have many more hours of experience dealing one-on-one with women, and caring for their needs, than do most physicians. Usually in a doctors' office it is the office nurses who spend the most time with women during their visits and who answer questions and concerns by phone. Time restraints imposed upon doctors make it impossible for them to spend but a few minutes at a visit with their long list of clientele. This unfortunately makes it close to impossible to learn a great deal about each individual woman, let alone remember all of the important details that pertain to each one in his/her care.

Too, during their births most women would much rather be watched continuously by a knowledgeable, caring attendant than be hooked to a machine and have someone check the readout every once in awhile. Some wonder why we do not change the way that birth is handled in the United States by increasing individualized midwifery care to women. This would thereby allow doctors to focus on people that are in the high-risk category. Logically, this would decrease each doctor's work load, allowing her to do what she was trained to do—be a doctor.

Most modern day women that have experienced a planned home-birth will report great satisfaction with their experience, often describing the beauty and sanctity of this special event as well as how it was more relaxed and less stressful than it otherwise could have been in a hospital atmosphere.

One of the chief reasons that so many families are beginning to choose to birth outside of the hospital is because of all of the irrational policies, rules, and routine interventions that serve the facility and staff first and foremost—before the safety and comfort of the birthing family. **Birth first moved from home to the hospital out of convenience for the caregiver, not out of safety for the mother and baby as we have assumed.**

More families are standing back and taking a good look at what has become the ritual way of birthing in our country. Study after study has shown that the inventions and implementations of all of the machines and protocols have made birthing in our country anything but safer. Years now after hospital births have been instituted, U.S. maternity care results are incredibly grim in comparison with many other places in the world. People are starting to stand up and refuse what this system is offering.

It is interesting to note that in the 1920s birth began moving to the hospital, though, in the mid-1940s the majority of births still occurred at home. When birth was moving to the hospital, infant mortality rates were decreasing. While it appeared that hospitalization was the reason for this, the improved nutrition and health of parents and the availability of antibiotics actually played more of a role in the decrease of mortality rates than being in the hospital for birth did. Maternal death rates *increased* however, and there was a high rate of "childbed" fever in mothers who birthed in the hospital stemming, as discussed previously, from terrible and unsanitary conditions that were professed to be "sterile."

In the 70s a lot of people began to opt for birth at home again. Homebirth rates began to steadily rise. In 1978, however, a report was issued concluding that out-of-hospital births caused a 2–5 times greater risk on a baby's life. The report was misleading, however, because outcomes of planned, attended homebirths involving full-term, low-risk mothers were put together with such births as those that occurred on the way to the hospital, high risk mothers, those who hadn't received prenatal care, or whose babies were preterm. *Amazingly, even miscarriages and stillborn babies were included!* (American College of Obstetricians and Gynecologists, homebirth 1978)

Later though, in a study conducted by Dr. Mehl of 1,046 women who planned hospital births and 1,046 women who planned homebirths, all of them low risk, *hospital birthing women were shown to be more likely than those who gave birth at home to have high blood pressure in labor, nine times more likely to have a severe perineal tear, three times more likely to have postpartum hemorrhage, and three times more likely to have had a cesarean section. Infants were six times more likely to have fetal distress during labor, four times more likely to have needed assistance to start breathing, and four times more likely to have developed an infection. There were no birth injuries at home. Thirty suffered birth injuries in the hospital.* (Mehl)

More recently, and which should be noted with great significance by U.S. caregivers, on June 18, 2005, the largest study on homebirth ever done was published in the British Medical Journal.

The study found that "**Planned home births for low risk women in the United States are associated with similar safety and less medical intervention as low risk hospital births**... In the largest study of its kind internationally to date, researchers analyzed more than 5,000 home births involving certified professional midwives across the United States and Canada in 2000. Outcomes and medical interventions were compared with those of low risk hospital births."

The study also reported:

"Rates of medical intervention such as epidural, forceps and caesarean section, were lower for planned home births than for low risk hospital births. Planned home births also had a low mortality rate during labour and delivery, similar to that in most studies of low risk hospital births in North America. A high degree of safety and maternal satisfaction was reported, and more than 87 percent of mothers and babies did not require transfer to hospital." (*emphasis added* Johnson and Daviss, BMJ, *2005*)

"The countries with the lowest [death and injury] rates are those countries where midwifery is an integral part of obstetric care and where home birth is commonly practiced.... The Netherlands has had a consistently high ranking among all countries since the 1970s.

"*A high degree of safety and maternal satisfaction was reported*"
~British Medical Journal

In 1987 [fetal/infant deaths] in the Netherlands was 9.8 deaths per 1,000 live births, whereas in the United States, it was 10.8 deaths. This may not seem like a significant difference until the numbers are sorted out a bit more. For midwife-attended births this [death] rate is only 2.1 deaths per 1,000 live births. In the Netherlands midwives attend more than 70 percent of all births; 40 percent of all births are home births. While there are additional factors, such as socialized medicine and prenatal care, to consider when comparing both outcomes between the Netherlands and the United States, **there is a strong case for home births attended by midwives.**" (*emphasis added* Harper 1994)

Yet another very important plus for homebirth is a **much lower risk of infection** at home versus the hospital. It's appalling to know that hospitals are not obligated to release information about infections patients had developed during their stay—and most don't tell. *Infections caught in hospitals are the fourth leading cause of death in the United States.* In July of 2002 The Chicago Tribune reported that 103,000 deaths in 2000 were linked to infections caught in the hospital, though the National Centers for Disease Control and Prevention calculated that number to be closer to 90,000. Many of the deaths originated in unsanitary accommodations, by contaminated instruments, and by germ-covered hands. Since 1995, over 75 percent of all hospitals have been found to have had serious breaches of cleanliness and sanitation rules. Some surmise that hospital cutbacks, carelessness, and serious infringements of the standards that are in place in most hospitals for infection-control were all explanations for this. (Berens 2002)

At home, you and your baby will encounter your own bacteria, that same bacteria shared by your family, which you and your baby are already familiar with. This is not true at a facility that treats a variety of sick and diseased patients every day.

But what about pain medication—what if a woman decides she wants some during labor? Mothers that have chosen to remain at home to birth their babies have stated that in the comfort of their own environments with skilled and loving support, the freedom to move as they pleased and follow what their bodies were telling them was needed, greatly lessened anxiety and thus discomfort as well. Labor was able to move along more efficiently, and there was no hasty, uncomfortable trip to another location to meet strangers who would have been assigned to their care. Those chosen to nurture her often help to make things much more comfortable for her with suggestions for positioning for both her and the baby. They prepare water for her to soak in, make her a cup of tea, massage her body if she wishes, and give emotional encouragement. In fact, many women at home never even consider pain medication. Not often, but once in awhile, midwives transfer a mother because she has decided she would like some medication. In

At home, you and your baby will encounter the bacteria which you and your baby are already familiar with. This is not true at a facility that treats a variety of sick and diseased patients every day.

labor women usually just move into the mode of simply having their babies. Without distractions, birth often happens much more easily.

Are you a candidate for homebirth? Homebirth isn't for everyone. Homebirth is for women who are healthy, eating a sound prenatal diet, and are non-smokers. Do you wish to forego drugs? Do you live where midwives are available, and do you live within thirty minutes of a hospital? Women who have chronic problems like diabetes, high blood pressure, or prenatal problems such as preterm labor, those who would rather not face the raised eyebrows, those who fear and mistrust the birth process, or those who just feel psychologically safer in the hospital may be better candidates for a hospital birth.

Those who have views that may differ from those of the staff at the hospital and are not "high risk," those who would rather not be fighting battles over rules and regulations (which is not fun for either the family or the staff), would do well to give homebirth further thought. At home, the family itself is in charge of their own birth. Battling for what you want at such a time is not at all conducive to easier birthing. A woman needs to feel safe to trust her body and be allowed to do the work of birth.

In the hospital environment it can be difficult to believe that birth is normal, to be confident that your body really can give birth. Monitors, IVs, restrictions on what you can eat and drink, how active you can be, and nurses and doctors hurrying around and in and out of the room, can leave you with the impression that things are not going to go along very easily. In some hospitals, women may walk during labor, use showers and Jacuzzis, listen to music and wear their own clothes. *Some doctors/hospitals will allow for no IV or electronic fetal monitor.* When a woman is able to truly control her environment herself, however, it is easier for her to relax, be comfortable, and to feel safe and confident. These are all reasons some women choose to give birth outside of the hospital, at home or in a birth center.

On the other hand, sometimes a woman plans to have a homebirth, and is unable to give birth there, but soon after crossing the hospital threshold, the baby is born. It is reasonable that women who hold unresolved fears that the hospital is safer will have difficulty giving birth at home. Some couples just feel more comfortable in a high-tech hospital environment. From where do these beliefs stem? Are they based on fact? Facing the fears and the facts are important things to do before giving birth.

Others shy away from homebirth because they live close to neighbors and they know they would feel inhibited to make much birthing noise at all with their paper-thin walls. But then, of course, they will have "neighbors" in the hospital too. Most often neighbors have no idea anything is even going on until after the baby is born.

What about "the mess"? Natural birth is quite neat. More than two cups of blood is considered a hemorrhage (and hemorrhages are

> *Without distractions, birth often happens much more easily.*

unusual). Babies are born with clean amniotic water. A bit of meconium (The baby may have its first bowel movement in the bag of water before it is born—more about meconium later.) is not unusual but also not difficult to clean up. If tissue isn't cut, as often it isn't at a homebirth because midwives have good rates of successfully protecting the perineum, birth is usually wet but not very messy. Most midwives clean up any birth-related "mess" and get laundry started.

For women desiring a **VBAC** (vaginal birth after cesarean), home may be the only place available to her as hospitals and birth centers turn women away not for her own safety or her baby's, but *for that of their own.* (See Cesarean…) A look at the larger picture shows that home is now the safest place for the majority of low-risk women having a VBAC.

Why are many midwives and doctors who work in the hospital adamant that the hospital is the only safe place to birth? **The American College of Obstetricians and Gynecologists** (ACOG) admits that their recommendation is based on their own opinions and on concurrence between doctors rather than on scientific fact. Hospitals and physicians depend on women coming to their hospital to birth. How many billboard signs advertising a variety of hospital obstetrical care units dot the sides of the freeways you travel? Obstetrics is big business in today's hospitals. Labor and Delivery units bring in a great deal of revenue for them.

Giving birth in the hospital may cost somewhere around $4,000 to 6,000. For complicated births, they can cost much more. Homebirth may cost somewhere around $1,000 to $3,500, depending on the midwife and where you live. This includes prenatal care, birth, and postpartum visits. Insurance companies have been including coverage for more and more homebirths submitted by midwives. **Overall, homebirths are usually much less complicated and costly. This benefits the family as well as insurance companies.**

~

Having a competent, experienced midwife with the proper equipment and being within reasonable proximity to a hospital is important. Finding a direct-entry midwife may be more difficult than finding an obstetrician or CNM. If numbers are not listed in the phone directory, you might try contacting out-of-hospital childbirth educators or doulas in your area. Doing a search on the Internet might prove useful.

Interviewing homebirth midwives and homebirth doctors (though rare to find) together as a couple is important. Make a list of questions of your own that you would want to know about your midwife.

See Questions for Your Homebirth Midwife/Doctor in **Appendix D**, and Resources in **Appendix E** for websites on homebirth.

The Birthing Center

There are different types of birth centers. There are large ones and small home-like ones. Centers vary in services provided. Small birthing centers can give some of the intimacy of home away from home. Sometimes birth centers include a garden tub and private bathroom for each room. Some might be equipped with large beds that accommodate mom, dad, and baby.

One of the major factors to consider is who runs the birth center— Direct-entry midwives? Nurse-midwives? Doctors and nurses?

Some centers are privately operated. Others, though, within, attached to, or belonging to the hospital, still function under restrictive institutional protocols. These may be called "birth centers" but really are just another labor and delivery unit.

Similarly, when considering private birth centers, those looking for a non-medicalized, non-hospital-like birth do need to be careful about choosing a center that *looks* homey, but that actually has a lot of paraphernalia hidden behind the beautiful cabinetry—equipment that is just begging to be taken out and used. This kind of birth center is also simply another kind of mini-hospital.

Advantages of birthing in a birth center generally (depending on the type) include the following:

- Birth centers are purposely associated only with maternity care.
- They are an alternative for parents who prefer not to give birth in a hospital.
- Clients can more likely get to know the entire staff before the birth.
- Requests for pain medication by the mother are reduced.
- Chances of cesarean section are also greatly reduced.
- Birth centers cost less to use than hospitals, yet provide more personalized care.
- Interventions as well as policies that limit choices are reduced.
- The mother invites only those she wants.
- The mother may eat and drink during labor, and the likelihood of using a birth position of her own choice is increased.
- Researchers report that death rates of babies born in birth centers are as low as those found in studies of comparably low-risk childbearing women birthing in hospitals. There was, however, greater personal satisfaction reported by mothers giving birth in a birth center than in the hospital.

There are a variety of reasons families choose birth centers as their birth place.

Some disadvantages are as follows:

- Though birth centers generally have more flexible policies, a mother is still not on her own turf and in charge as she is when she is at home.
- There is oftentimes rigid screening that eliminates healthy low-risk mothers because they have given birth by cesarean section in the past, are over thirty-five, or plan to birth in the birth center but whose membranes release without starting labor for a period of time—all regardless of other more significant factors.
- Too, a great many birth centers still use intervention-oriented care, though thousands of women are leaving hospitals because they want to avoid just that.

There are examples of other birth place choices in the U.S., such as Bellanatal in Orem, Utah. Bellanatal is not a birth center, as the care that is given therein is separate from the facility in which the care is received—it is simply a place where women can go to give birth. The woman and the caregiver are responsible for her care; the facility is not. There are no in-house policies or interventions that must be routinely carried out such as those that are set in place to protect regular birth centers and hospitals. All of that is left up to the woman and her caregiver. It is cozy and homey with a stocked kitchen, fireplace, TV, and toys for waiting siblings and other family and friends.

Families might choose a birth center or a place like Bellanatal because they do not have a midwife in their area and they are willing to travel to where one is available. Or perhaps a woman does not want to give birth in her own home for whatever reason—perhaps because she lives in an apartment (though many babies are born at home in apartments) and is afraid that neighbors might be disturbed by "labor noises." Some families are just not ready for a homebirth, but do not want to give birth in the hospital. There are a variety of reasons families choose birth centers as their birth place. Being choosy when selecting one is key.

See Resources in **Appendix E** for more information about birth centers. You can also go online to check out a variety of birth centers here in the United States.

Being choosy when selecting a birth center is key.

6

Birth Wishes

T HE DAYS of the factory conveyor belt birth are becoming a thing of the past for a larger percentage of families. Because they have educated themselves, more parents know that they really can *expect more* from their birthings than what is known today as standard care. Since the standard, mainstream classes, books, and other such resources have essentially offered little in preparing past families for better birthings, today's families are judiciously searching elsewhere. They want off of the old conveyor belt. They want a more personalized birth experience that fits their own particular desires and needs, one that will provide their baby with a *much* gentler, *kinder* welcome than babies are receiving in a typical birth today. And what's more—they don't feel at all like that's asking too much!

So how *do* you avoid the typical, routine birth that is not evidence-based and proves over and over not to be in the best interests of the baby, mother, and family? How can you create a safer, gentler, more personalized experience?

First, you must decide whether you willing to take the steps needed to find out what you do want. It does take some work—and it's *worth it*. Your baby is worth it, and you're worth it.

One of the ways to accomplish what you want is to study, while creating a list of those things you desire. This can be the start of preparing birth wishes that fit *your own* needs.

Why Make Birth Wishes?

You have probably heard the term "birth plan." We like to refer to birth plans as "birth wishes" because birth, just like a lot of other things in life, is unpredictable. We may be called on to alter, or entirely change, our plans.

Then why even make birth wishes?

First, making birth wishes helps a woman to define in her mind which of all the choices she prefers, and what she needs to have in place to get the kind of birth she wants. Writing down your choices and having them in front of you helps you to figure things out and remember what you have chosen and why you did so in the first place.

Second, you can use your birth wishes to activate communication with your caregiver. This can help her/him to know your desires. It will help you to know if this is the caregiver who will best help you to obtain your desires. And having a written copy helps a chosen caregiver to remember, at a glance, what is important to a particular woman/family.

Third, for those who birth in a hospital, it lets the nursing staff know what you want. If your doctor has initialed your wishes at the bottom of the page, the nurses will know that they have been approved by your caregiver.

Do you respect your baby, even now before she is born? Will you be the advocate and supporter that she needs now, choosing only those things that have been shown to be the best for babies and their mothers?

Fourth, it can help your doula to know exactly what you want. She can help you to know whether your wishes are reasonable, and then be your ally and advocate as she works together with your birth team.

Getting the Kind of Birth You Want

Can you actually get the kind of birth you want? That depends. Women's desires should be considered a great deal more than they presently are. At the same time, some well-meaning individuals and publications tell a woman that she ought be able to expect *anything* she wants, wherever she births. But can she really? Truthfully, hospitals in particular are not set up for languid, nurturing, spiritual births. It's a busy place. Sometimes there are even women waiting in line for a labor and delivery room. Yes, lots of families have had beautiful experiences in the hospital with wonderful caregivers. But unfortunately, many have gone into the hospital with a birth plan only to leave disappointed in particular aspects of their care, simply because what they wanted was not what was being offered as "standard care."

Look at it this way: **It only makes sense that if it's not on the "menu" at a particular place of business, your chances of receiving that item there are indeed slim.** If you were to go into a Chinese restaurant and order a big, hot plate of tacos, beans, rice, coleslaw, chips, and salsa along with a virgin strawberry daiquiri, you are probably going to be disappointed. That's just not what they offer there. They'd probably laugh, and if you kept insisting, they might become rather upset. You *might* be able to get them to agree to leave the sauce off your order of stir-fry. But then again if it's a busy night, they might either forget or simply tell you that it just isn't possible.

The cook at a Mexican restaurant may want to be helpful if you asked to make your own salad, but you would probably soon be told that—well, that sort of thing simply isn't done there. He/she probably wouldn't allow you to do so until perhaps a lot of other people begin to voice their desires for a buffet salad counter. Then the restaurant might eventually decide to add one to please customers.

Likewise, if you would like to use upright positions because you have learned that they are more comfortable and help to better facilitate easier birthing, you need to find out if your caregiver, for example, has any experience with women who have given birth in a kneeling position. If not, if she is very accommodating and you have a good relationship with her (and if it isn't an extremely busy day) she might be willing to let you give it a try. If you don't want your caregiver to tug at

If you don't want what others are getting, it makes sense to look around for something different.

the cord to speed up the delivery of the placenta (which can cause hemorrhage), pick someone who doesn't perform this routine procedure!

Don't kid yourself. At the risk of sounding unsympathetic, don't set your heart on anything too out of the ordinary. Frankly, if you care about safety and the kind of birth you will have, **if you don't want what others are getting, do something different!**

Figure out what you really want. Some things that can help you to figure that out are writing, talking it out, or making art. *Birthing from Within* (see Resources in **Appendix E**) is an excellent book about using art as a fun, effective way to figure things out. Or perhaps simply find a place to be relaxed and quiet so that you can really listen and tune in to your thoughts. These activities have proven enormously helpful for many expectant mothers and fathers who are in the process of making thoughtful decisions about where and with what they want to build their own "birth nest." It can be very effective as you study, to list in a rough draft, a drawing, or perhaps a conversation what you want and need. Then choose the kind of caregiver, birth place, the team, etc. that will help you to achieve those wishes.

You are wholeheartedly encouraged to go to your Creator/Higher Source/Voice Within as you make your decisions. When you believe you know what you want, if your heart is open to it, you can gain an assurance that you are headed in the right direction. Listen to the feelings and impressions that come to you. If you don't feel negatively or experience a state of confused thought where you can hardly think of the subject at all, you have most likely made choices that are good for you. It should *feel* right.

> NOTE: As you continue to read through the rest this book, refer back to the two lists that follow labeled Personal Notes and Worksheet. You can take notes on these lists about what you want for your baby's birth and why. Ideally, you have your own copy of this book so that you can highlight and write notes throughout that can be referred to later. Although all material in the book is copyrighted, we give our permission for you to copy these two particular forms for your own personal use. Write in what you have learned and mark the checklist as you go along. Doing so should make preparing your birth much easier.

In **Appendix C** you will find examples of what birth wishes might look like.

Though presented side-by-side in this book, not all options for childbirth are created equal. There is almost always a choice that is better than the others.

Making Educated Choices

Throughout each step of your pregnancy, it is so important to ask yourself if each particular decision will help you to achieve your objectives. Your pregnancy and your birth don't have to be just one, cookie-cutter way! Don't discount your feelings about a subject. It's okay to follow your own design, to trust that voice within, to do what is best for *you*. *You* decide.

Though presented side-by-side in this book, not all options for childbirth are created equal! There is almost always a choice that is better than the others.

There are various wonderful resources for finding answers to your questions. Seek them out. You can find good resources in some types of classes, the Internet perhaps, and other good books. Check out the recommended resources we have listed here and on our website.

It is even possible that the choices that are best for you may not be for someone else. Everyone is different with their own set of passions, fears, likes and dislikes, baggage, and particular needs. Do we all live in the same houses because it is easier for the builders, drive the same cars, listen to the same radio station as we drive home from work, and eat the same food when we get there?

What do you know about the different choices? What are the options? **If you don't know what your options are, after all, do you really have any?**

Some choices are more controversial than others. How much does that matter to you if you suspect it may be the best choice for you? Be thoughtful, be creative....Have fun! Most of all, follow that voice within to do what you *know* is right.

Follow that voice within to know what is right for you and your baby.

Personal Notes

First, make a list of details that would be present in your *ideal* birth environment. Think about what you can do to ensure you have this kind of environment (or as close as possible) at your birth. Then, as you study, jot notes about each of the following topics in the spaces that follow.

BIRTH PLACE

Home (pros and cons):

_____

_____

_____

Hospital (pros and cons):

_____

_____

_____

Birth center (pros and cons):

_____

_____

_____

My choice:

_____

_____

_____

NUTRITION DURING LABOR

Notes:

_____

_____

_____

My choice:

_____

_____

_____

ONSET OF LABOR (allow body to go into labor naturally, artificial induction, natural induction…)

Notes:

_____

_____

_____

My choices:

_____

_____

_____

ARTIFICIAL RELEASE OF MEMBRANES (AROM)

Pros and cons:

_____

_____

_____

My choice:

_____

_____

_____

ELECTRONIC FETAL MONITORING (EFM)

Pros and cons:

_____

_____

_____

Alternatives:

_____

_____

_____

My choice:

_____

_____

_____

IV

Pros and cons:

_____

_____

_____

Alternatives:

_____

_____

_____

My choice:

_____

_____

_____

CERVICAL CHECKS BEFORE AND DURING LABOR

Pros and cons:

_____

_____

_____

Alternatives:

_____

_____

_____

My choice:

_____

_____

_____

COMFORT MEASURE CHOICES I MIGHT WANT TO USE IN LABOR (water therapy, a doula, HypnoBirthing, music, etc.)

Notes:

_____

_____

_____

_____

_____

_____

_____

WHO WILL BE PRESENT AT MY BIRTH? What about baby's siblings (if so, who will be there for each of them so dad can be fully there for the birthing mother)?

_____

_____

_____

PHOTOGRAPHY? Who will be in charge of it?

_____

TIME LIMITS SET ON LENGTH OF LABOR

Pros and cons:

_____

_____

_____

Alternatives:

_____

_____

_____

My choice:

_____

_____

_____

POSITIONS I MIGHT WANT TO USE

In Labor:

_____

_____

_____

For the actual birth:

_____

_____

_____

Notes:

_____

_____

_____

EPISIOTOMY

Notes:

_____

_____

_____

My choice:

_____

_____

If I choose not to have this procedure, what can I do to avoid it and to protect the perineum?

_____

_____

_____

_____

PAIN MEDICATION (list pros and cons of each type)

_____

_____

_____

What you want caregivers/birth team to know about your preferences about medication:

_____

_____

_____

BIRTH OF PLACENTA

Notes:

_____

_____

_____

My choice:

_____

_____

_____

CORD CUT RIGHT AWAY?

Notes:

_____

_____

_____

My choice:

_____

_____

_____

METHOD OF MAINTAINING UTERINE MUSCLE TONE AFTER THE BIRTH

Notes:

_____

_____

_____

_____

My choice:

_____

_____

_____

WELCOMING BABY

Suctioning? Immediate contact with parents? Freedom to breastfeed right away? Exams and procedures done right away? Wait to do any of them? Rooming in?
Notes:

_____

_____

_____

My choices:

_____

_____

_____

FEEDING OF BABY

Notes:

_____

_____

_____

My choice:

_____

_____

_____

Who to contact for assistance I might need (Contact before the birth can be very helpful.):

_____

_____

_____

NURSERY PROCEDURES (your notes about pros and cons of each)

Do I wish for my baby to receive any of the following nursery procedures?:

_____

_____

_____

Erythromycin eye ointment:

_____

_____

_____

PKU:

_____

_____

_____

Vitamin K:

_____

_____

_____

Immunizations (Are there any being given by your caregiver/birth place at the time of birth?):

_____

_____

_____

Circumcision:

Pros:

_____

_____

_____

Cons:

_____

_____

_____

My choice:

_____

_____

_____

Other:

_____

_____

_____

GROUP B STREP IN MOTHER (common procedures and options)

_____

_____

_____

BREECH POSITION (pros and cons of common procedures, options for birth)

_____

_____

_____

ENCOURAGING A SLOWED LABOR

Natural options:

_____
_____
_____

Pros and cons:

_____
_____
_____

Medical options:

_____
_____
_____

Pros and cons:

_____
_____
_____

My choice:

_____
_____
_____

PRE-ECLAMPSIA AND TOXEMIA

When is induction truly needed?

_____
_____
_____

What are the best ways to avoid pre-eclampsia?

_____
_____
_____

JAUNDICE (prevention, medical treatments, natural treatment of)

_____

_____

_____

CESAREAN

Pros:

_____

_____

_____

Cons:

_____

_____

_____

My choice:

_____

_____

_____

If chosen or necessary, what options are available during a Cesarean?:

_____

_____

_____

DEATH OF BABY (hold initially, see and hold baby as often and as long as desired, no contact, obtain mementos such as photographs, lock of hair, foot prints, naming, ring for baby for you to wear later, to dress baby, contact with women who help families at this time, autopsy, services of memorial, mother's recovery separate from postpartum unit, early discharge, spiritual and grief counseling, contact with parent support group):

_____

_____

_____

_____

ULTRASOUND

Pros and cons:

_____

_____

_____

My choice:

_____

_____

_____

OTHER ROUTINE PREGNANCY TESTS

Test _____ (pros and cons):

_____

_____

_____

Test _____ (pros and cons):

_____

_____

_____

Test _____ (pros and cons):

_____

_____

_____

Test _____ (pros and cons):

_____

_____

_____

Remember, some of the above procedures might be practiced regularly by your caregiver or birth place, but is each one right for you and your baby?

QUESTION TO CONSIDER

Is there anything that might be standing in the way of making the choices you know are right for you?

_____

_____

_____

Notes:

_____

_____

_____

Worksheet for Preparing Your Birth Wish List

Wise parents will research the pros and cons of each before making their choices.

Use the preceding and following pages to record your choices as you study. The items listed will help you keep track of what you are learning and what you desire for your birth.

Examples of prepared birth wishes are in Appendix C at the end of the book.

In parentheses below, you will find references for information about these choices within this book.

ATMOSPHERE (For all below see: Exploring the Rituals in **chapter 18** and The Body/Mind... in **chapter 15**.)

_____ Dim lighting

_____ Quiet, no background chatter

_____ Family and friends of choice allowed in birthing room

_____ No extraneous staff, privacy

_____ Freedom to use sounding (See Birthing Your Baby... in **chapter 7**.)

_____ Privacy

_____ Music

_____ Freedom of movement (See Electronic Fetal... in **chapter 7**.)

_____ Aromatherapy—essential oils, etc.

CLOTHING (For all below see: The Body/Mind... in **chapter 15**.)

_____ Hospital gown

_____ Own clothes

NUTRITION DURING LABOR (For all below see: Intravenous Drip and Nutritional Needs... in **chapter 7**.)

_____ Easily digestible foods and juice

_____ Ice chips and popsicles only

_____ IV only

COMFORT MEASURES (For all below see: Comfort Measures... in **chapter 13**.)

_____ Help from partner and/or doula (See Dad's Role... in **chapter 14**.)

_____ Relaxation (See Personalized Comfort... and Hypnobirthing... in **chapter 13**.)

_____ Breathing techniques (See Personalized Comfort... and Hypnobirthing... in **chapter 13**.)

_____ Use of hypnobirthing (See Hypnobirthing... in **chapter 13**.)

_____ Bath or shower (See Using Water... in **chapter 13**.)

_____ Jacuzzi (See Using Water... in **chapter 13**.)

_____ This is what number I would rate myself at on the medication preference sheet. (See Pain Medication... in **chapter 7**.)

_____ Bring own things from home

_____ Birth ball

_____ Hot and cold packs

_____ Massage

_____ Freedom to walk and change positions often (See Finding The Power... in **chapter 10.**)

_____ Type of medications preferred (See To Have or Not... and Medications... in **chapter 7.**)

_____ Please don't mention pain medication unless I ask.

ONSET OF LABOR (For all below, except where noted, refer to **chapter 8.**)

_____ Spontaneous even if past estimated due date, as long as baby continues to do well; use of Fetal Movement Counts (See Keeping...)

_____ Natural induction (See Inducing Labor Naturally...)

_____ Artificial rupture of membranes (See Rupturing...)

_____ Stripping of membranes (See Stripping the Membranes...)

_____ Pitocin (See Inducing Labor with Drugs...)

_____ Cytotec, Cervidel, etc. on cervix with stay in hospital over night, Pitocin (See Inducing Labor with Drugs...)

_____ Induction only with tests for fetal maturity and well being

_____ Induced only for medical reasons

_____ Induced for convenience

_____ Enema, shave of the perineum- Can you believe some caregivers still employ these? Find out about your particular hospital to see if these apply to you. (See Discarded... in **chapter 4.**)

LABOR (For all below see: Personalized Comfort... in **chapter 13.**)

_____ In bed throughout

_____ Slow dancing with partner

_____ Standing and leaning forward into labor support

_____ Shoulder against wall during contraction

_____ Sitting upright or leaning forward with support

_____ Kneeling, leaning forward with support

_____ Walking

_____ Stair climbing

_____ Birth ball

_____ Rocking chair

_____ Belly dancing (See Belly Dancing... in **chapter 13.**)

_____ Baby's siblings allowed in room (See Siblings... in **chapter 14.**)

_____ Reminder to concentrate inward and not what is going on around (See The Body/Mind... in **chapter 15.**)

BACK LABOR (For all below see: Back Labor... in **chapter 13**.)

_____ Double hip squeeze, counter pressure, Kingston Maneuver

_____ Climb stairs; walk

_____ Shower, Jacuzzi, tub (See Using Water...)

_____ Hot, cold packs

_____ Straddle chair backwards

_____ Birth ball (rotate hips to get in position and help baby move down, kneel over and have companions use double hip squeeze, counter pressure, and the Kingston Maneuver

_____ Remind everyone to hang in there and have patience!

_____ Visualize baby moving into correct position, talk to baby (See The Body/Mind... in **chapter 15**.)

_____ Avoid having bag of water released (See Rupturing... in **chapter 8**.)

_____ Belly lift

_____ Knee-chest one hour

_____ Someone sits back-to-back with mother

_____ Sterile water injection

RUPTURE OF MEMBRANES (For all below see: Rupturing... in **chapter 8**.)

_____ Spontaneous

_____ To try to start labor

_____ During early labor

_____ Just before birth

MONITORING (For all below see: Electronic Fetal and Ultrasound... in **chapter 7**.)

_____ Continuous

_____ 10–20 minutes of electronic fetal monitoring upon arrival and then 10–20 minutes every subsequent hour

_____ Doppler use only

_____ Fetoscope only

_____ Internal electronic fetal monitoring (inserted into baby's scalp)

IV (For all below, see IV in **chapter 7**.)

_____ None- will take fluids by mouth

_____ Heparin lock

_____ IV from beginning

_____ IV only for surgery and with the use of pain medication

CERVICAL CHECKS (For all below see: Group-B Strep... **chapter 7** and Rupturing... in **chapter 8**, At Home... in **chapter 5** and The Impact... in **chapter 15**.)

____ No exams

____ Frequent exams

____ Only at time of urge to push to be sure of complete dilation

ENCOURAGING A SLOWED OR STOPPED LABOR (For all below see: Encouraging a Slowed Labor... in **chapter 7**.)

____ Pitocin augmentation (See Inducing Labor with Drugs... in **chapter 8**.)

____ Talk about fears (See Body/Mind... in **chapter 15**.)

____ Talk to baby and visualize what is needed (See Body/Mind... in **chapter 15**.)

____ Check out, go home for the night to get some rest or for a walk around the mall. Allow labor to start again naturally on its own (*Note:* Parents have done this. It's better than further interventions and perhaps an unplanned cesarean! Have faith that nature will take its course!)

____ Nothing unless mother or baby is in danger for some reason

____ Patience- sleep, drink, eat, walk, wait for nature to take its course the way it was meant to

____ Natural methods- nipple stimulation, making love, walking, change positions, use gravity (See Inducing Labor Naturally... in **chapter 8**.)

____ Massage by birth companions

____ AROM (See Rupturing... in **chapter 8**.)

____ Rest!

TO EMPTY BLADDER

____ Walk to toilet

____ Catheter—used with epidural for emptying bladder

POSITIONS FOR LABOR (For all below see: **chapter 13**.)

____ Flat on back, feet in stirrups

____ Semi-sitting on bed, feet in stirrups

____ Hands and knees

____ Side-lying

____ Squatting

____ Supported squat "dangle"

____ Squatting bar

____ Using birthing stool

____ Standing, being held from behind by partner

____ Standing, facing partner, holding onto his/her shoulders

ACTUAL BIRTH (For all below see: Birthing Your... in **chapter 7**.)

___ Breathing the baby down gradually

___ Coached pushing

PREMATURE URGE TO PUSH (For all below see: **chapter 7**.)

___ Begin breathing baby down

___ Panting to control the urge to push

BIRTH (For all below see: Rituals... in **chapter 18** and Birthing the Placenta... in **chapter 7**.)

___ Partner to announce sex of baby and cut cord

___ Partner to receive the baby

___ Take baby from own body

___ Delayed cutting of the cord until finished pulsating

___ Mirror to see birth

___ Waterbirth (See Using Water... in **chapter 13**.)

___ Cesarean (See Cesarean... in **chapter 7**.)

EPISIOTOMY (See Episiotomies... in **chapter 7**.)

___ Yes

___ None

___ Perineal massage

___ Only for use with forceps or vacuum

WELCOMING INFANT (For all below see: Rituals... in **chapter 18**.)

___ Suctioning with bulb syringe immediately

___ Baby coughs and expels own mucus

___ Immediate contact

___ Given immediately to mother, covered with blanket

___ No infant hat, will regulate baby's body heat on mother's chest

___ Freedom to breastfeed right away (See Breastfeeding... in **chapter 18**.)

___ Bonding time for family

___ Cord finishes pulsing before cutting

___ Siblings welcome (See Siblings... in **chapter 14**.)

DELIVERY OF PLACENTA (For all below see: Inducing Labor with Drugs… in **chapter 8** and Birthing the Placenta… in **chapter 7**.)

_____ Spontaneous, no traction

_____ Traction on cord okay

_____ Induced with Pitocin

_____ If slow to deliver, use of walking and squatting, breastfeeding

MAINTAINING UTERINE MUSCLE TONE AFTER THE BIRTH (For all below see: Inducing Labor with Drugs… in **chapter 8**.)

_____ Fundal massage by mother as necessary

_____ Fundal massage by nurse or doctor

_____ Pitocin by IV or injection

_____ Pitocin only if obviously necessary

VIDEO OR PICTURES, IF ALLOWED

_____ _____ in charge of video

_____ _____ will take pictures throughout labor—the doula?

_____ Doula to take pictures only after birth

OTHER

_____ No time limits (See Your Own Timing… in **chapter 7** and **chapter 8**.)

_____ Labor to take its individual course without aid of artificial augmentation (See Your Own Timing… in **chapter 7**.)

_____ Thank you for not disturbing during uterine surges, talk to husband and doula only and they will confer with mother (See The Body/Mind… in **chapter 15**.)

_____ Doula to keep track of times and write birth story

NURSERY PROCEDURES (For all below see: Rituals and Nursery Procedures… in **chapter 18**.)

_____ Rooming-in for mother and baby

_____ Modified rooming in

_____ Nursery care

_____ Leave hospital soon after birth

_____ Exams to be delayed

_____ Exams immediately

_____ Baby examined at bed

_____ Weighing etc. to be delayed

_____ Bath right away

_____ Bath delayed for 24 hours

_____ No circumcision

_____ Anesthesia for circumcision

_____ Vitamin K

_____ Eye ointment

_____ PKU testing

_____ Immunizations

_____ If baby shows signs of jaundice which is not severe, breastmilk and sunlight only

_____ Pictures right away

_____ Pictures wait

_____ Others _____

FEEDING (For all below see: Breastfeeding... in **chapter 18.**)

_____ Breastfeeding on demand

_____ Breastfeeding on schedule

_____ Breastfeeding only, no pacifier, no glucose water, water, formula, etc. to be given to baby

_____ Formula or other_____

CESAREAN (For all below see: Cesarean Birth... in **chapter 7.**)

_____ Scheduled

_____ Low horizontal incision

_____ If labor slows or stops, if mother and baby are well, we wish to use natural means to augment labor rather than having a cesarean

_____ Support person(s) present

_____ Partial shave

_____ Complete shave

_____ Epidural anesthesia

_____ General anesthesia

_____ Screen lowered so mom can see baby being taken from abdomen

_____ Screen up

_____ At least one hand free to touch baby

_____ Oxygen mask removed so mother can talk to baby

_____ Family bonding period after surgery

_____ Support person/father with baby in nursery

_____ Support person/father with mom

_____ Pillows under mother's head

_____ Pictures

DEATH OF BABY

_____ See baby

_____ Hold initially

_____ See and hold baby as often and as long as desired

_____ No contact

_____ Obtain mementos (photographs, lock of hair, foot prints, naming, ring for baby for you to wear, dress baby)

_____ Autopsy

_____ Services of memorial

_____ Mother's recovery separate from postpartum unit

_____ Early discharge from hospital

_____ Spiritual and grief counseling

_____ Contact with parent support group

ULTRASOUND DURING PREGNANCY AND BIRTH (For all below see: Ultrasound… in **chapter 7**.)

_____ No ultrasound

_____ Use of fetoscope only, no Doppler use

_____ Ultrasound only if there is a pressing medical reason where benefits outweigh risks

_____ Once to see if all seems to be fine and to find out sex

_____ As often as possible

OTHER EARLY PREGNANCY TESTS (Don't be afraid to look up information in other places than the sometimes sugar-coated handouts that are available from some caregivers. It is important to know all of the facts.)

_____ Every test available

_____ No testing

_____ Other

Tips for Creating Your Birth Wish List

1. We suggest making a separate list of birth wishes for each of the members of your team (midwife/doctor, doula(s), labor and delivery staff, and nursery staff) with information that pertains to them. For example, there are some things that would most appropriately only be listed on the wishes for yourself and your doula. For example, the labor and delivery staff probably won't need to know every kind of comfort measure you may think you would like to use during labor. It is good, on the other hand, for your doula, as your support and advocate, to know both what comfort measures and what interventions you do and do not want for yourself and your baby. It would be appropriate for those birthing in the hospital to give the nurses the same copy they have discussed with their doctor, particularly if he has put his initials on it—indicating to the nurses that he approves of the contents.

2. Keep the list as **neat, short, and simple as possible**. If anything is relatively unimportant to you, leave it off. A page or less of easy-to-read print is ideal. Select only options from the list that apply to you. Do not write that you wish to avoid an enema, for example, if, as in most hospitals, your hospital never does this anymore. If your caregiver is a homebirth midwife, most of the hospital interventions mentioned on the list are not relevant. You may wish to write a separate list of wishes in case of transfer to the hospital (although depending on the reason for transfer some of your wishes would not be approved if more aggressive treatment of some kind were necessary).

3. **Be assertive but polite and pleasant** in your requests. A long list of demands can really turn a staff off. A few positive words of appreciation can be just what you need to elicit extra support and care.

4. Remember that it is important to **stay flexible**; birth is as unpredictable as anything else in life, and therefore cannot be planned. These wishes are not set in stone. That is why they are called a Birth *Wish* List!

5. It can be a good idea to **have your doula look over your wishes** when you have finished them to see if they are actually realistic in her experience of working with your caregiver and/or birth place.

6. The hospital you birth at may allow you to submit your Birth Wish List when you fill out your pre-admission papers. This way it **can be in your file**. Carrying **extra copies** in your birth bag is still a good idea!

Do not be afraid to put your baby's needs and, yes, your own, above anybody else's at this most significant time!

7. Use your birth wishes to facilitate conversation between you and your caregiver. If when you approach your caregiver with your wishes and he seems agreeable about something, but then perhaps teases you about it or laughs and says that—well, he can "try," it is probably a good indication that this is not normally what your caregiver usually offers, and that there is a very good chance that you will not receive what you want. It is important that your caregiver shares your views and philosophies. What is he carrying in his black bag, so to speak? How does he really feel, deep down, about birth? What are his beliefs and philosophies? Don't kid yourself! If your birth wishes do not match the kind of care he gives, do not expect them to be fulfilled, no matter what promises are made! It is essential that you talk specifically about each relevant item in your birth wishes with your caregiver. **Reach deep within for the courage to change to a different caregiver if you know this one is not the right one—** no matter how "nice" they are or how much you do not want to "create a stir."

8. When presenting wishes to your caregiver, let her know, "this is why we chose you, because you are willing to listen and help us with what we need." **Be positive, confident, and well-researched.** Don't say, "I chose this because my childbirth educator (or this book) said to." Show your caregiver that it is important to you to make well-researched decisions. Let them know that you wish to be informed about decisions to be made, that you care.

9. Important note: **If your wishes have become long**, due to the fact that most of it is not what normally happens in the birth place you have chosen, then **perhaps your wishes are actually not very realistic.** There may have to be some give and take in your chosen birth place, some compromising. It just may be that all of your wishes can only be fulfilled in a different place altogether. As discussed before, a certain place of birth is probably not going to completely change overnight simply because you have a sheet of birth wishes in hand. If you still desire to give birth in your originally chosen place, then perhaps leaving some—or most—of your wishes behind may be necessary.

10. **Some women have situations that require them to be in the hospital when they would rather birth at home or in a birth center.** A mother bird carefully builds her nest in a protected crevice of a brick apartment building, high above the bustle of a busy street, being sure to line it with feathers and soft bits of napkin. Just like this mother, who might prefer a gently swaying apple tree in the country, a woman can build her own nest from bits and pieces of things she finds available to her.

A woman can give her situation some thought and decide how to make the best of a less-desired locality. Perhaps she will bring her own pillow; a doula to be an advocate for herself and her husband and to offer physical comfort and support in the forms of aromatherapy, massage, soft music, emotional support, and more; a small memento she can wear around her neck or hold in her hand as she gives birth; or a quilt for her baby to be wrapped in.

Reach deep within for the courage to change to a different caregiver if you know this one is not the right one.

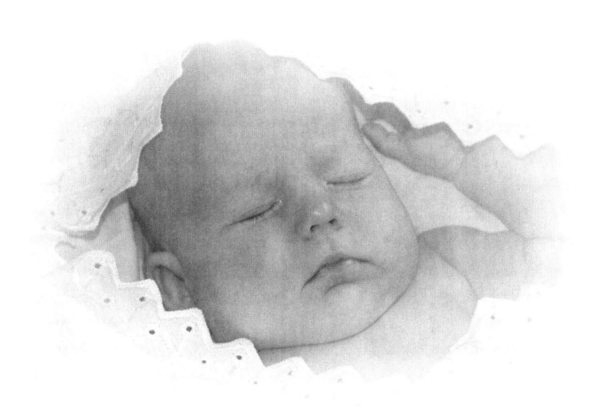

7

Birthing Your Baby in Your Own Way

MUCH OF THIS CHAPTER pertains only to those who will be giving birth in the hospital or perhaps a birth center. But they are things important for *everyone* to know. We'll begin with time restrictions and move through other routine procedures that are a common part of our culture's way of birthing today.

Your Own Timing vs. the Friedman Curve

Finding out she is only three centimeters dilated, 30 percent effaced, and still in early labor can be disappointing for a woman and her birth team. But under most circumstances this is not a good time to be checking-in to the hospital! Taking a walk around your neighborhood or the mall might do wonders to get things moving. Get some lunch. If it's night, go home and get some rest!

For those birthing in the hospital, you may have heard that it is generally a very good idea to wait until well into active labor before heading to the hospital. One very important reason for this is that once you get to the hospital, your labor is immediately placed within a rather strict time-frame. You are "on the clock" so to speak, once you are admitted. This "clock" is called the Friedman Curve. The Friedman Curve is the model used by many hospitals to time labors. If certain milestones have not been reached in certain designated amounts of time, routine interventions such as Pitocin augmentation or AROM (Artificial Rupture of Membranes—releasing the bag of water that surrounds the baby) begin to be implemented in hopes of moving things along. If these do not produce desired results, a cesarean will very likely be the next suggestion.

Some caregivers, however, strongly feel that it is erroneous to put every woman onto the same absurd curve and then judge her labor as "very fast" or "too slow—needing synthetic augmentation" or perhaps even referring to it as having gone by the "textbook"—though a "textbook" labor is itself a fallacy. The book *William's Obstetrics* concedes that the limits that have been set by the Friedman Curve are "admittedly arbitrary."

The illogicality of the whole idea of a "curve" lies in the fact that **every woman and every labor is different!** Even the lengths of different labors for the same woman can be vastly different. Some labors progress within forty-five minutes all told. Others take days. Everyone, and every labor, is different. A lightening quick birth is not necessarily better than a laid-back, leisurely one. A more gradual labor, in fact, can help you ease into the surges so that you have time to figure out what comfort measures work best for you.

Many times in labor there are periods of no apparent progress being made in dilation, but this does not mean that other, unseen, things are not happening. If a mother is conserving and re-building her energy with food and rest, if contractions are manageable and the baby is

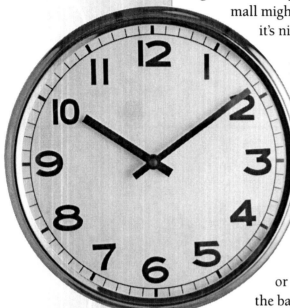

You are "on the clock" so to speak, once you are admitted.

doing well you need not worry. A labor that lasts several days is just another variation of *normal*! Most hospitals, though, would never allow a woman to labor for that long. They are much too busy and need (for their sake) to keep things on the Labor and Delivery floor moving along.

Contractions may or may not cause the mother's cervix to dilate at a *steady* rate. Something that is often not taken into consideration is that the cervix must thin out as well as dilate. **So even if your cervix is not dilating, it is very likely thinning out. Especially the cervixes of many first-time mothers tend to thin before opening.**

The Friedman Curve does allow for a two to four hour pushing stage, but a woman may receive instrumental delivery (vacuum or forceps) or a cesarean after a much shorter amount of time. Truthfully, because of the time schedules doctors are under, there are those who feel they simply do not have time for a three to four hour birthing stage. Although a three to four hour birthing stage is just as "normal" as a three to four minute one, there are those physicians that will assert that instrumental delivery (along with a nice-sized episiotomy to accommodate the instruments) or a cesarean, are necessary.

Interestingly, more cesareans are performed on particular days of the week and month.

How many women actually have labors that fit into the Curve? Why does it even matter? If your labor reaches a point where it does slow down or even stops for a bit, that's okay!

Babies come in their own due time! We do not need to start getting out the Pitocin or forceps or talking about a cesarean if labor or pushing is taking longer than the Curve says it ought to take! If your caregiver is starting to talk this way, you have probably chosen the wrong person to help you birth your baby. What's the hurry? There is simply **no scientific evidence that shows that a rigidly time-controlled labor serves anyone other than the caregiver and his dinner hour.**

It may be wearisome to be a midwife/doctor at times. There may be those days he feels rushed to get back to the office on time or that he needs to get home for his mother-in-law's birthday party. But midwifery or obstetrics is the job she/he chose—with all of the attached pros *and* cons. And it is not your responsibility to put the *safety* and *well-being* of your baby and yourself on the line to make her/his life easier. We'll have our babies when we and they are good and ready, thank you very much! Excellent caregivers understand this completely and would not think of asking you to be induced without good, honest reasons. If they are not willing to give themselves to this kind of service, they could be of better service to society in a different capacity. **Birth was not meant to be set within a rigid time frame. This is a part of the job description for birth caregivers. It takes a patient individual to be good at this work.** Choose your caregiver and place of birth wisely.

Babies come in their own due time! Birth was not meant to be set within a rigid time frame. Waiting is a part of the job description for birth caregivers. It takes a patient individual to be good at this work.

Women around the world birth regularly and safely in places where there are no set time limits.

Think about it. Women around the world birth regularly and safely in places where there are no time limits set. Our great, great grandmothers and their mothers before them labored without being put on a clock, and you can look in the mirror for proof that birth worked for them too.

After planting two different tulip or daffodil bulbs at the same time, we often notice that they both don't emerge from the ground, grow, or open at the exact same time on the very same day. Do we then dig up the bulb that isn't sprouting yet or open a bud that isn't unfolding just when we think it should be? This would most likely result in tearing and scarring of the flower—or worse. Locked within the flower is the knowledge of when and how to come forth. It will not necessarily be when we, with our limited understanding, think it should. It will happen when the time is right.

Animals' birthings are not governed by a clock. But still their bodies work and their babies are born in their own due time. When chickens are sitting on eggs, we don't stand by with a stop-watch. If one egg is taking longer to hatch, do we break the shell and help the chick out? This could be a very detrimental thing to do. Likewise, we have also learned that hurrying a woman's labor can be a dangerous thing for both mother and baby.

Are our bodies so different than these and other examples in nature? Why must we allow someone to poke and prod at our shells?

Simply because your body is following its *own* clock, is not an indication that it has become necessary to go to the hospital for IV hydration either (water or Gatorade by mouth is just fine). Your body knows what it's doing. Trust it, and know that your baby really will be born *soon enough*. If you are really getting some outside pressure, you can try some of the natural induction methods, mentioned in **chapter 8**. Yet nothing will work very well, Pitocin and other more severe means either, if the baby is not ready yet. Your wise body and baby are protecting themselves for the right time.

As long as the bag of waters is still intact and vaginal exams have been kept to a minimum, you are most likely just fine. In fact, your body may be getting a lot of the work done beforehand, if gradually. It is entirely normal to dilate and efface in the weeks or days before the birth. It is also entirely normal not to, and to dilate and efface only the day your baby is born.

Even if your bag of waters has released, there is probably not an immediate chance of infection if objects—*including exam gloves*—are kept out of the vagina. If your body's temperature and your blood pressure remain normal, and your baby is doing fine, know that women have gone for *days* with their water released. Labor typically soon ensues. Sometimes a woman simply develops a "high leak" from which some of the amniotic fluid escapes, and which naturally re-seals itself. Rest assured, too, that a woman's body keeps making more amniotic fluid. Mothers with Strep B need to take extra precautions.

Wishing to avoid being admitted too soon, you may wonder how you will know when it really will be time to go in. *The best indication is when the mother really has to stop and concentrate during contractions.* As a rule of thumb *only*, call your midwife or doctor when you are having around twelve to fifteen contractions in an hour. Or call when contractions are less than five minutes apart, last at least one minute, and make you concentrate. Start heading to the hospital, then, if you are birthing in one. **Most importantly, listen to the laboring woman! Her feelings are often *very* accurate for deciding what to do.** If she is persistent that it is time, don't put her off. Go right in—and don't leave the birth center or hospital if she feels uneasy about doing so.

Encouraging a Slowed Labor to Progress

Here are a few things that can help move labor along:

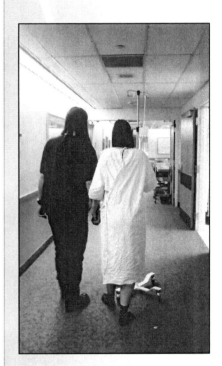

- Walk
- Do belly-lifting and positioning may help to speed labor considerably. Optimal positioning of the baby down on the cervix helps to dilate the cervix evenly. (See Back Labor… in **chapter 13**.)
- Change positions frequently.
- Drink more fluids.
- Take warm showers or baths (*after* five cm, as getting in before seems to slow labor, where getting in after five cm can help relax the mother and move labor along)
- Get some sleep, if at all possible, between contractions as this can help to rest the body and prepare it to continue on with increased energy to complete its work. Often the contractions will slow during sleep, to again regain momentum when the mother is properly rested.
- Consider, too, the psychological factors. What is going through the mother's mind? Is she afraid perhaps, of becoming a mother or having another child, afraid that labor will hurt her baby, or is she possibly finding herself dwelling on a negative past experience? Is she emotionally at odds with anyone? Encourage her to talk and resolve these thoughts.
- Rate the contractions. If she is not allowing labor to become strong, try saying, "On a scale of one to ten, how would you rate the power of that contraction? Make it a (the number next highest to the one she named) this time." Keep increasing the

number until labor is progressing more steadily, or as long as it works.

- Avoid calculating. A woman may think that if she's been in labor for eight hours and is dilated to two centimeters, that because it's taken four hours per centimeter so far, that she has another thirty-two hours to go. Take heart, the latter stages of labor often go much faster than the first. The rule observed by some, that labor should progress a centimeter per hour, is absurd. Every labor is different!

- Once again, avoid going to the hospital too early. Labor can slow when you change to a new and sometimes less comfortable location, and once you are there you are "on the clock."

- *Trust your body.* Do you really need Pitocin or other augmentation? Your body knows what to do! Believe that it *will* accomplish the task at hand in its own time.

To Have or Not to Have Pain Medication

Why wouldn't a woman want medication? You have likely heard all of the reasons why you should—the pros. Therefore presented here are reasons to avoid medications. What is the best choice for you and your baby? Again, it is up to you. The choice is yours!

Choosing an Unmedicated Birth

Does it seem like everybody is telling you, "Don't try to be some kind of hero. Just get the epidural, Honey!"?

Despite the horror stories people love to tell, a number of women throughout the United States are choosing not to have pain medication at their births.

"Why bother to experience birth? Why not plan to feel as little as possible of the labor?" asks Judith Lothian in her article in Lamaze Magazine. "We hear a great deal about the pain of childbirth but very little about the joy and the pleasure of feeling the contractions, bearing down as your baby pushes into the world and feeling in harmony with the rhythms of your body as it does the incredible work of birth. Women who are able to labor and give birth relaxed, confident and with loving support experience an inner harmony that brings with it strength and endurance....Experiencing labor and birth, rather than obliterating the experience, allows you to feel the interweaving of the joy and pain, to work very hard and then delight in your incredible accomplishment. In discovering the power of giving birth you are forever changed." (Lothian 1998)

Some women who have had an unmedicated birth say, "Friends tell me I'm crazy. I guess it's just one of those things you can't explain to someone unless they've experienced it themselves. They just don't get it. It was such a deep, moving, beautiful experience. The strength was amazing and it *was* hard. But I'm so glad I didn't miss out on any of the sensations or any of the power of my birth. It was so incredible!"

One very popular actor who had a baby without pain medications said that she chose this route not only because it was healthier for the baby, but because of what a truly primitive experience giving birth is— that we don't get many of those experiences in life.

What will the awesome and powerful sensations of your body feel like as you experience what it is like to give birth to a new life?

With medication, women relinquish that opportunity to experience the innate wisdom of the body and its ability to birth without physical assistance from anyone else. They surrender their own connection to their power and life-creative force. As they lose much of the physical control of their bodies, with it they also lose the ability to move the baby along in its journey from the womb. Even contractions often slow with the administration of pain medication.

Considering Medication Safety

There are caregivers that assure their clients that medications are totally safe in this day and age! Why then must forms be signed? Why can the medication only be administered in the hospital? Once you have received the medication, why are you hovered over with questions about how you are feeling? Why must you be monitored and receive an IV from there on out?

The truth is that **no medications given during labor have yet been deemed safe**. Listed on the forms you sign are a lengthy number of side effects, *most* of which don't often happen, but which *can* occur—and *have* occurred—to women and babies that were given this medication.

And while you or your baby may only have a small chance of being the one, in that one in 500 or that one in 1,000, who has a particular risk happen to you, **there is a *very* good chance that if you have a medicated birth you will need vacuum extraction or forceps assistance for your birth (probably complete with episiotomy), or a cesarean (with the further inherent risks and side effects of each of these) or other more common problems such as a sleepy, disoriented baby when born.**

Ask yourself whether the trade-offs are actually worth it. Is it possible that some children might be able to sidestep special education classes or

The truth is that no medications given during labor have yet been deemed safe.

prevalent unexplained problems that are rapidly growing in our modern day children by protecting them from drugs during their births?

Is an Unmedicated Birth Possible for You?

You might wonder, if for example you are afraid of merely going to the dentist, whether you could give birth without medication.

Rest assured that the sensations of childbirth are not the same as having a wisdom tooth removed. The sensations of labor and birth are something that can be *worked with* and which do not need to cause suffering.

The popular belief is that having no drugs is equal to having pain and having drugs is equal to not having any pain. Neither is true. Dig a little deeper.

Sensations we feel every day are essential to staying healthy. We know to eat when we feel a certain sensation in our stomach. Hunger is a signal to nourish our bodies. Awareness of it helps to prevent starvation. We know to put sunglasses on when our eyes tell us that it is too bright—thus preventing injury to our eyes. We know to put on a warm sweater when our skin receptors tell us that it is chilly. This helps to keep our bodies from getting too cold. Some might call hunger pangs "painful" but if a new medication came out to eliminate them would it be wise to take it to eliminate the discomfort? The sensations of our body are our daily guides for taking care for it.

Sensations from our bodies tell us what we need to do in labor as well, such as what position to be in to best help rotate a baby into place. Not being able to feel what your body is telling you to do can cause problems.

Before signing up for an epidural it might only be fair to yourself to give your body a chance to experience labor before devaluing your abilities.

Many hypnobirthing families have found that when using the deep relaxation taught in their childbirth classes, that a woman can experience the sensations, but at the same time comprehend them the way she chooses—in a way she can mentally select before labor begins; erasing what she has previously been "programmed" by society to believe labor feels like.

These hypnobirthing families learn that if the body is working in the way it was meant to, *without the birthing muscles being tense from stress*, that a woman does not normally experience pain. In fact, every muscle in the body functions by contracting and releasing. None of the other muscles hurt while functioning as they were meant to. If a muscle is malnourished or dehydrated or injured you may experience discomfort. But do your legs hurt just from walking, your heart when pumping, your eyes when moving? Why would the uterus hurt? It usually doesn't as the cervix opens during menstruation or as it contracts during orgasm.

What will the awesome and powerful sensations of your body feel like as you experience what it is like to give birth to a new life?

The uterus stretches from the size of a pear to be large enough to hold the baby. The uterus was made to do this task, just as it was made to open when the time is right, just as the pelvis and birth passage were made to open to amazing proportions.

Must it be painful? Must a woman suffer? Many, many women throughout time have given birth *easily and comfortably*.

Not the story you've heard all these years? Read on about some things your body has to offer you. True, in modern society it may be more difficult to give birth comfortably for a variety of reasons, all unrelated to the wondrous way your body was made. Therefore we offer things that other women have found very helpful below and in **chapter 13**.

One thing about labor's design is the periods of rest between each surge, moments that allow for resting and re-grouping. Just as it helps to remember in life that you only have to deal with one day at a time, it's helpful to know that you only need to take one contraction and deal with that *one* contraction at a time. Also women are given, when labor is allowed to progress as it will, wonderful **endorphins** (natural pain relievers, your body's natural pain medication). However **catecholamines**, which are stress hormones, counteract endorphins. So the more your needs are taken care of, the more comfortable you are. Reducing things in the birthing environment that will cause fear, and receiving encouragement and reassurance from your support team, can be very helpful for reducing or eliminating discomfort in labor. **Choices you make before labor starts will have a lot to do with how comfortable your birth will be.**

Some people in our society may wonder if it is "civilized" to give birth naturally. When picturing a woman in labor, some people think of the classic sitcom scene where an angry mother-to-be is screaming at everyone, especially her husband. Some women, fearing that they may turn into this, may desire an epidural just to avoid it—and with good reason! But before devaluing your ability to give birth without medication altogether, read some *real* birth stories about *real* people who have given birth naturally. The Internet is one place where people gather. You may be surprised how many people have loved their natural birth experiences and are eager to share them with the world! How do their *true* stories compare with the fictional, made-for-TV births we have grown up with?

When a woman's needs are truly being met by her birth team, she generally doesn't become angry toward any of them. Certainly labor companions are wise not to take anything a woman says in labor personally, but on the other hand, professional doulas seldom experience anything like the sitcom scenes. When her assistants listen and are attentive, a laboring woman usually remains positive and even cheerful in her relations with all those that are there to help.

Many, many women throughout time have given birth easily and comfortably.

In general, if a woman can make her place of birthing a more private, intimate place where she won't be afraid to let go and do what she needs to do, she is preparing for a quicker, easier, lovely birth.

Medications Given During Labor

Medications that may be given during labor can be divided into three groups according to labor's progression: early labor, active labor, and actual birth. Of course, if a cesarean is necessary, drugs will be given then.

Drugs Given in Early Labor

Sleeping Pills are generally the only medications given in early labor. These have no effect on pain, are given to encourage rest, and sometimes to discern whether this is true labor or not. (See Birthing Your Baby…in **chapter 7**.)

Mothers may experience drowsiness, difficulty dealing with contractions, nausea, and with large doses hypotension (low blood pressure), lowered pulse rate, and disorientation. Possible effects on the baby are respiratory depression, impaired responsiveness and sucking ability, as well as decreased muscle tone.

Drugs Given in Active Labor

Drugs most commonly given during active labor include analgesics, narcotics, tranquilizers, spinals, epidurals, and paracervicals.

> **Analgesics and Narcotics.** These are usually given through IV or intramuscularly. Some are given directly under the skin. There are no benefits to the baby. They may cause decreased respiration in the baby. If given after you have the urge to push, the baby may be born at the time the narcotic peaks and the baby may require resuscitation or Narcan to reverse the effects. Also, after birth, the baby can no longer use the placenta to get rid of drugs. The baby's blood-brain barrier, which prevents outside substances from entering the brain, is more permeable, and the liver and kidneys are less able to excrete the drugs. Drugs have been detected in the baby's blood at even eight weeks after the birth. Breastfeeding difficulties and disorganized behavior can occur.
>
> Benefits to the mother include a reduction in pain perception. The medication doesn't eliminate discomfort, although it may give a chance to escape for a little while. A well-timed dose can help to regain the ability to work with labor. The intravenous route

If a woman doesn't look like a Goddess during birth then someone isn't treating her right.
—Ina May Gaskin

is the quickest but doesn't last as long. Intramuscularly administered, the medication doesn't work as fast, but it works longer. If a mother does have it intravenously, she may want to request a heparin lock so she can still be mobile.

Risks to the mother include hypotension; dry mouth; respiratory depression if given through IV; drowsiness; and a fuzzy, uncomfortable, disoriented feeling. It may compromise walking ability. Some mothers feel the amount of pain relief was not worth losing the rhythm of labor she was working with. It may slow labor and cause vomiting, dizziness, and the feeling of being spaced-out. It can reduce clear thinking. Medical personnel have reported interference with the bonding of the mother and infant as a result of *both* being spaced-out. Second doses of Nubain, which has the fewest side-effects, but include feeling spaced-out and sick, aren't very effective.

Tranquilizers. Given intramuscularly or through IV to reduce tension and anxiety, relax muscles, relieve nausea, and enhance effects of narcotics, they can cause sluggishness, trouble concentrating, dry mouth, and hypotension in mother. In the baby they can induce declined responsiveness, sleepiness, and apathy toward learning to feed her baby.

Spinal. A spinal is anesthesia from the breasts down. Onset is rapid, but there is also a risk of rapid onset of hypotension. Mother is awake. There are risks of spinal headache and dense motor block. Small doses work well. There is a limited duration and more medication cannot be added.

Epidural. A needle is inserted at waist level into a space in the spine, and a tube is placed next to the spinal cord. **Analgesia** (which refers to a reduction in pain without loss of movement) or **anesthesia** (which refers to a block of sensation *and* movement) are administered. It takes perhaps thirty minutes to administer and about twenty to thirty minutes for relief. It is usually a highly effective method, although sometimes incomplete. Caregivers often want mothers in their care to wait until they have reached 5 cm before receiving an epidural because particularly early on, an epidural can cause labor to slow or stall. Other procedures such as augmentation by Pitocin, and even cesarean, are often used if this happens. When administered before 5 cm, an epidural makes the slowing or stopping of labor a much more common occurrence.

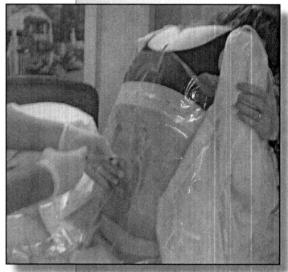

Be aware that your caregiver may also want the epidural to wear off for the actual birth as this allows the mother to use her own power to birth the baby rather than having to depend on potentially harmful vacuum or forceps extraction.

• *Procedure*: You must remain very still while in labor with your back rounded for quite a while. There is a sting as the needle is injected. The anesthesiologist inserts a test dose to determine that you aren't allergic and to be sure the needle is in the right place. Then a catheter is threaded through the needle into the space and the needle is removed. You will start to feel numb. You probably will be turned from one side to the other for the next few hours to be sure the pain relief is even, and you must remain relatively horizontal at first to adjust, due to danger of falling blood pressure. An IV is used so that high doses of intravenous fluid can be administered. Other safety measures need to be taken, such as blood pressure monitoring. The mother and baby are monitored continuously to make sure they are handling the medication okay. The baby's heart rate pattern may begin to decelerate.

• *Risks for the Baby and Mother:* **Families are often told that there are no longer any risks with medications used today. However, there are small chances for a large number of things to occur including maternal breathing difficulty and a long-lasting spinal headache.** Epidurals require skilled personnel to administer it. Large doses are needed. There is a slight risk of systemic poisoning from large doses. There is also the risk of inadequate pain relief, because levels can't always be easily controlled. Managing to numb only the exact, desired area can be difficult. There are cases where the upper

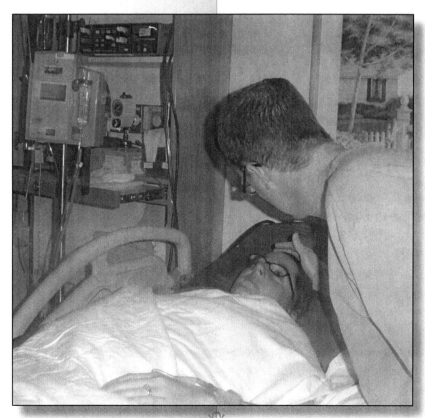

half, rather then the lower half, of the body were numbed, necessitating life support of the mother. Vacuum extraction or forceps use often cause deep vaginal tears which frequently yield subsequent future urinary and fecal incontinence as well as painful intercourse. A urinary catheter may need to be inserted in the mother's urethra, introducing higher risks of infection. Unremitting backache is considerably greater among mothers who receive epidurals. Other technical errors such as inserting the needle in the wrong place can occur.

Shivering, nausea and vomiting, itching, and trouble with urinating are common. Some women experience difficulty breathing. Epidural fevers in mothers are common. Fevers are a typical reason for yet more interventions.

It is difficult to determine for certain, why the mother has a fever. So the case must be watched in case Strep B or some other serious infection is the culprit. Then if the baby has a fever after the birth, it will be required to have blood drawn at least once, and as often as every few hours. They may have to have fluid removed from the spine. This is extremely painful and expensive, interfering with breastfeeding and causing anxiety and further pain.

Epidurals restrict movement and active participation and may prolong the actual birthing stage. Descent and rotation of the baby can be impaired since the mother can't assume helpful positions and is forced to lie on her back causing pelvic diameter to also be decreased. So-called "walking epidurals" really only give some sensation and seldom the ability to walk. There must be a total dependence on nurses, physicians, and support people for basic physical needs during labor. The woman's legs are left useless. Bedpans and catheters become necessary.

Perhaps it is intended kindness that prompts some caregivers today to tell their clients that epidurals are safe and that there is nothing to worry about.

Though it might be easier to just not have to think about the above risks, they must nevertheless be considered for your baby's safety and your own, and in order to make a truly informed decision.

You will most likely be required to sign a form that protects the hospital if complications do occur, because they *do* occur, some things more often than others—thus the form to sign that protects the hospital.

Epidurals do get to the baby. There is a very noticeable difference between a naturally-born and an epidural-born baby. A baby that has been given epidural medication may be very tired, pale, shaky, and irritable. Epidural babies are often noticeably sleepy after birth. One study showed that in the first *month*, a baby may seem more disorganized, irritable and withdrawn, looking away, and suckling less. Mothers may be more likely to perceive their babies as disorganized which can affect mother-infant bonding. Problems with breastfeeding are also a likely natural result of epidural anesthesia. And there may need to be a separation between parents and baby while the baby (or mother) is in intensive care due to complications. Weeks after the birth, residue from the medication has been found in babies.

Benefits of an Epidural: Some benefits of having an epidural are that relief with an epidural is adjustable from slight to full relief in some labors, and that it allows for some movement, although "walking epidurals" are a myth. Onset of hypotension is slow, mother is awake, and more medication

There is a very noticeable difference between a naturally-born and an epidural-born baby.

can be added easily. In the event of a cesarean, the mother can be awake. And once in awhile an epidural even enhances labor progress if the mother is exhausted (although it may also have the opposite effect). More medication can be added easily. Mother can be conscious and aware during labor and birth. She may also still be numb for episiotomy (the cutting of the perineum to enlarge the outer birth passage opening) repair if needed. Though, epidural births often *necessitate* episiotomies to accommodate for vacuum or forceps which are often required to help birth the baby due to the effects of the epidural.

- **Paracervical.** A needle is inserted into the cervix by way of the vagina. It blocks uterine sensation. It can slow down contractions necessitating Pitocin with its risks. (see Risks of Inducing in **chapter 8.**) It also can cause slowed heart rate in the baby.

Drugs Given During Actual Birthing Stage

Drugs that may be given during actual birth include locals, pudendal blocks, spinals, and saddles.

- **Local.** This drug is given just prior to birth, or before episiotomy for repairs. There are not many known side-effects except temporary loss of sensations with inability to know when and how to control the descent of baby to avoid perineal injury. Since the needle is near the baby's descending head, there is a slight risk of injury in this regard.
- **Pudendal Block.** Given immediately before birth, or after birth for perineal repair, administered through the vagina into pudendal nerves as an anesthesia for the vagina and perineum. This eliminates the "stretching" sensation, and is employed for use of forceps. There is a possible partial loss of the sensation of the baby descending. This is not recommended when the baby is in distress.
- **Spinal.** (see above)
- **Saddle.** A saddle provides relief for those parts with which one would sit on a saddle. It is given in a side-lying position or sitting bent over with the back bowed. The purpose is to give complete anesthesia for contractions, birth, and repair of episiotomy. Mom is awake and alert. This medication can be used for forceps and cesarean deliveries. Possible side effects include hypotension, spinal headache, and need of a catheter. Labor may stop and sensation of how to work with one's body may be lost, resulting in need for forceps. For the baby, hypotension in the mother can cause a drop in fetal heart rate and can also cause hypotonia, as well as subtle behavioral changes.

Cesarean

Cesareans are typically done upon administration of an epidural, spinal, or general anesthesia.

- **Epidural.** (see above)
- **Spinal.** (see above)
- **General Anesthesia.** Onset is quick and mother is in a sleep state. General anesthesia can be used if the mother has low platelets or hypovolemia. There is a risk of aspiration, excessive bleeding, and neonatal RSD (reflex sympathetic dystrophy). Mother's airway must be managed with a tube down her throat. There is chance of awareness in the mother of what is happening without her ability to communicate this, and a need for analgesia after surgery.

Tips for Obtaining an Unmedicated Birth

Don't do it alone. Too many women who would like to "go natural" decide to choose medication when in labor. Most often these are the women that have no true labor support from someone that really knows what to do and how to help beyond offering medication. Most nursing programs do not train their nurses in any support techniques or comfort measures for labor other than pharmaceutical ones. It isn't that labor and delivery nurses aren't caring. The reality is that they are often too busy with all of the requirements of their duties to be of much help, despite the fact that many of them probably became labor and delivery nurses so that they could nurture the laboring mother. Offering medication is the best trick they may know of and that is one main reason many are so insistent about it. Too, having all five women that are in her charge tucked comfortably into bed makes it a whole lot easier to get the mounds of required tasks and paperwork done before the shift ends.

You may have heard of women who have wanted to avoid medication, and have indicated this on their birth wishes only to have people continue to offer drugs throughout labor. How does one avoid this?

In some hospitals there is very little encouragement for natural birth. Without support and help when the mother really needs it, without belief in her ability from those around her, it can be very difficult for a woman to birth her baby without medication.

Repeated offers of medication can really wear a woman down. We don't drive alongside a runner in a marathon "just in case," or hover with a helicopter over someone who is climbing a mountain. We do not offer a delectable slice of mousse chocolate cake to someone who is watching their weight. To the dieter, a fit figure is more important than a slice of chocolate cake. How helpful would it be to keep offering the cake and reminding them how much they really *should* want

We don't drive alongside a runner in a marathon so that if he gets tired of it he can get a ride. A woman should be able to have the chance to give it her all if she wishes, without anyone mocking her for it.

it? A woman should be able to have the chance to give it her all if she wishes, without anyone mocking her for it. And mock her many do. Why is that?

It may help, if you have chosen to labor without drugs, to let everyone know that you would rather that they did not mention medication to you. If it is a staff member that is having a difficult time with your choice, you can graciously request a different one that better matches what you need. The nurse that was originally assigned to you may be a lot happier too. You will want people around you that will support you, people that don't have their own agendas for your birth, who want to assist you with the decisions *you* make.

Some people watching a laboring mother may misconstrue what they are seeing only as pain instead of a powerful experience. Dad, with best of intentions, may even encourage the ride to the finish line. But for a woman who wants to avoid drugs, this is when she needs help and encouragement the most.

Instead of suggesting an epidural at the first moan, it would be more supportive and helpful for the woman to be shown comfort techniques such as those covered in **chapter 13**.

Sometimes Mom will mention in labor that maybe she should try medication. **Toward the end of labor, a woman may wonder if she is equal to this. She will look to knowledgeable others around her to know if she possibly can do it. Her support team needs to understand that often this statement is a request for help, a signal that it is time for a fresh, new trick—something different to help her finish the race.**

Certainly if the woman adamantly states that she wants medication after all, those around her should help her to achieve her wishes. But many times it is the assurance that she really is almost there that she really needs. Just knowing that can give her the strength to finish that last quarter of a mile.

Some doulas bring a Pain Medication Preference form (not unlike the one below) to a prenatal interview so that the woman can communicate best just how much she desires to avoid or obtain medication. This aids the support team in knowing just how they can best serve her.

Last but not least, **avoid induction if at all possible**. There are certainly those circumstances when induction is necessary. But induction generally does not make for an easier labor! (See To Be or Not to Be... **chapter 8**.)

Pain Medication Preference Scale

Where are you on this scale below? Let this scale be a tool to assist you in sorting through your thoughts and feelings about medication and to help your birth team understand and discuss your wishes. Do understand that both ends of the scale (+10 and -10) are probably not very practical.

+10   Desire to feel nothing, desire for anesthesia before labor begins!

 + 9   Fear of pain, lack in confidence that I will be able to cope; want medication as soon as possible.

 + 7   Desire for anesthesia as soon in labor as caregiver will allow it.

 + 5   Desire for epidural before transition (period just before birth), willing to cope until then perhaps with narcotic medication.

 + 3   Desire to use pain medication, but would like as little as possible.

   0   No opinion or preference

 - 3   Prefers that pain medications be avoided, but only if labor is short or easy.

 - 5   Strong desire to avoid medication, mainly for baby's benefit; I am preparing and learning comfort measures, but will accept medication for difficult labor.

 - 7   Very strong desire for natural childbirth, for benefit of the baby as well as for a sense of gratification; will be disappointed if I use medications.

 - 9   Want medication denied by staff, even if I ask for it.

-10   Don't want medication, even for cesarean birth!

Adapted from Pain Medications Preference Scale with permission from Penny Simkin.

Intravenous Drip

Intravenous drip (IV) is a routine procedure to administer fluid through a needle into the vein. In many hospitals it is routinely placed in labor so that in the event that it is difficult to find a vein (if a woman were to go into shock for example, which is *extremely rare*) an IV would already be in place to give medications and to provide fluid.

IVs are also used during labor by many hospitals for hydration of the mother.

When a labor is being artificially induced or "augmented" by the use of Pitocin, an IV is employed to administer it.

IV poles typically stand on wheels and a woman may push it with her to the hospital halls in labor. This is certainly doable if necessary, though a bit awkward and cumbersome to a woman who would like to be active and have the freedom to move around in ways she instinctively knows will help to birth her baby.

What are the hazards of an IV? **Besides the fact that some women have adverse reactions to the fluid, excessive dextrose may harm the newborn. It is also far too easy for staff members to add other chemicals and drugs that you would question but which are sometimes simply dispensed through the IV without questioning the desires of the woman. Simply, an IV is often the first intervention in a line of subsequent interventions that may be needed as a result.**

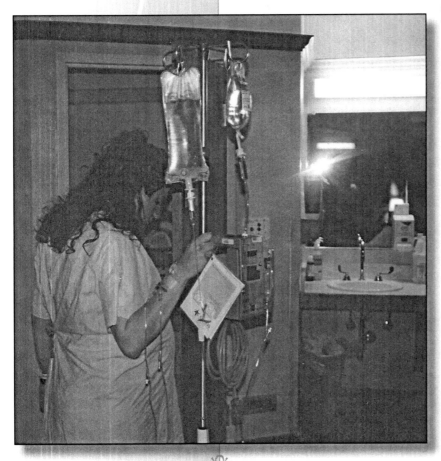

Of course, psychologically, a woman often feels like a sick patient when fastened to an IV, rather than a healthy woman who is simply doing something her body was made to do.

Sick people who cannot get nourishment any other way can receive a formula through an IV. Healthy birthing women *do not need one.*

Requiring IVs for every laboring woman is ridiculous. **Even if it did become necessary to have an IV, there would be warning signs, and there would be plenty of time to find a vein. There are ways to promptly place a line in the rare event that a vein was difficult to find and access.**

Too, if the labor is lengthy, the mother can develop a fluid overload. It can take quite a while afterwards for a mother to excrete all of the fluid that has been pumped into her body during a long labor, and she will probably experience a great deal of swelling in her face and extremities following the birth. Pain and inflammation of the IV site can also occur.

If glucose is used, the baby could develop hyperglycemia.

Here's a thought: Perhaps we ought never eat or drink and just hook up to an IV every time we need nourishment. Perhaps we should also put in an IV every time we get into our car. Why not? Statistically, it is more likely for a woman to die in an accident enroute to the hospital than when actually giving birth. Perhaps it would be wisest for the woman to wear the IV in the car on the way to give birth, just in case, and take it out when she gets there!

Wouldn't you say we are a bit worried that birth must be a very dangerous thing to do?

Why shouldn't a healthy woman be able to eat and drink according to the dictates of her body? Ironically, IV fluid not only does not provide adequate nourishment, it may even cause a negative nitrogen balance, which is a condition of starvation.

Some caregivers may suggest that you wear a heparin lock in your arm. A heparin lock is a small device secured to the arm with a needle already inserted into the vein, ready to be hooked to an IV if necessary. This also would be considered by some caregivers as an unnecessary procedure but may serve as a trade-off for not having to have an IV. When wearing a heparin lock, there are still the psychological implications to you and everyone else of "a-disaster-waiting-to-happen."

Having an IV does allow for the administration of drugs if you think you might use them.

It is mandatory that an IV be used in conjunction with the administration of an epidural due to potential complications, and during surgery as well.

Perhaps we should also put in an IV every time we get into our cars!

Nutritional Needs During Labor

Eating in labor is forbidden by some hospitals. They maintain that if a patient were to regurgitate during emergency surgery under general anesthesia she might inhale the vomit and risk pneumonia. Most cesareans, however, are now done with a spinal or epidural, not general anesthesia, and the odds of this happening to someone are as great as being hit by lightning twice in one year—that is seven in ten *million* births! (Kakuda) Ironically, if a mother were to actually inhale the straight acids of her otherwise empty stomach, these stomach acids would actually be more damaging to the lungs than if she had just eaten some easily digestible food!

It is extremely important that a woman eats as her appetite allows. Taking care of your energy is crucial to the success of your birth.

Other hospitals serve a full and delicious meal to the laboring mother. And a good many caregivers are appalled with the insane practice of forcing a woman to fast during labor. Becoming dehydrated and going without food can actually cause labor to stall. Cesareans are too often a result of this modern practice which leads to fatigue and loss of energy, strength, stamina, and endurance—all of which are so essential for an efficient, more comfortable, do-able labor!

Women in labor are indeed running a kind of marathon.

Do bikers, mountain climbers, and runners need to stick a needle in to stay hydrated?

Nourishment can be taken by mouth! It is extremely important that a woman does eat as her appetite allows, especially in early labor as she does not know how long her labor will last and appetite is most often naturally suppressed in the latter stages of labor.

Popsicles (which produce quick sugar-highs and then plummeting energy) and ice chips are all that is available in many hospitals. Some hospital-birthing women bring their own food.

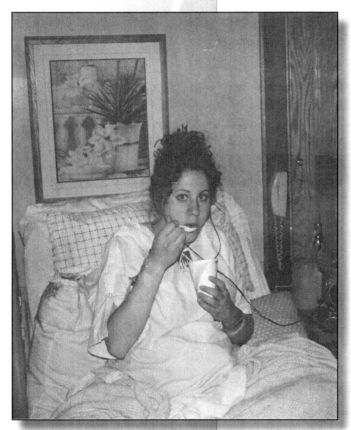

Easily digestible foods that are high in protein are best, such as a high protein soup, perhaps with some toast, a soft-boiled egg, or yogurt. To fend off dehydration, it is important to take a drink every fifteen minutes or so of water, herbal tea (red raspberry is a good option), or clear soup every fifteen minutes or so. Juice popsicles can be refreshing if you are birthing at home or have other access to a freezer. Be aware that the acidity of orange juice tends to make laboring women vomit and is best to avoid.

Even when they originally wanted to avoid one, women birthing in some hospitals may still face the insistence of caregivers to start them on an IV if they are showing signs of dehydration or exhaustion due to low blood sugar. However, thirst, hunger, and exhaustion are *not* prevented by having an IV. All three can easily frustrate a woman's endurance levels and slow or halt the progression of good labor patterns. Taking care of your energy is *crucial* to the success of your birth!

Electronic Fetal Heart Monitor

Most birthing women in hospitals today will be placed on an electronic fetal heart monitor (EFM) for a good part of their labors. Elasticized belts are positioned around the mother's belly to hold a monitor over her abdomen to track the baby's heart rate. The ability to monitor the baby throughout labor *sounds* like technology made in heaven. What piece of mind it *should* give. In reality, we should have risen to the top of the list among industrialized countries because of pieces of technological equipment just like this. We have not. On the contrary, there are twenty-seven other countries that have less infant loss than the United States. That number is worse than it was ten years ago. (March of Dimes 2002)

Unfortunately, expected results of this piece of technology have not taken place over the years it has been implemented.

The monitor is neither very accurate nor easy to read, and a mistaken diagnosis is *not* a rarity.

Originally designed to prevent neurological impairment, the EFM has not decreased the incidence of cerebral palsy. In fact, over the past forty years, the rate of cerebral palsy has not changed from about two per 1,000 live births.

There have been a great many more cesareans performed however, due to incorrect readings of the EFM which seemed to indicate distress, for babies who are found to be pink and breathing without difficulty.

Published works in the American Journal of Obstetrics and Gynecology showed *years ago*, that the EFM raises the cesarean section rate *160 percent*, with no advantages for the baby. (Haverkamp and Langendoerfer, et al. and Kelso, Parson, and Lawrence, et al. 1979) Quite the contrary, as risks of cesarean surgery are high for both mothers and babies.

The electronic fetal monitor is one of the most blaring cases in point that show that old habits die hard, effective or not.

There have also been an increased number of *unnecessary* forceps deliveries.

In a great many hospitals, EFMs from each room can be watched out at the nurses' station. This way the nurse can take care of her other responsibilities at the same time. A nurse may be assigned to several women at once, and this way she can watch them all at once and get her paperwork done. Nurses are often overworked and are usually very busy with required duties. This is one of the most significant reasons that monitors are used. Nurses most often do not have time to sit with or assist a woman in labor.

To further compound these dilemmas, it has become part of the protocol in many hospitals to use the monitor much longer than the following recommendation by ACOG. Consequently, time in the bed for the mother is considerably lengthened.

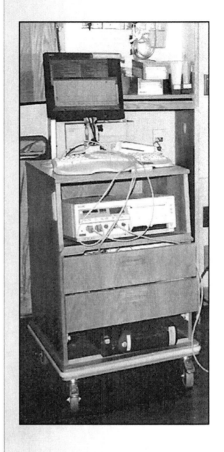

Unfortunately, the expected results of using the external fetal monitor have not taken place over the years this piece of equipment has been implemented.

Although it may be common practice in some hospitals to evaluate at least every *thirty minutes* in active labor and *every fifteen minutes during actual birthing*, ACOG (American College of Obstetricians and Gynecologists) says that only *fifteen minutes during labor*, and *five minutes during actual birthing* is all that is necessary for *anyone, even when risk factors are present*. They define risk factors for a baby as intrauterine growth retardation or illness.

The most important reasons for monitoring, though illogical for the reasons listed, is for protection from all-too-common litigation; to be able to show that "everything that should have been done was done— and here's the proof."

Some of the most convincing evidence against the Electric Fetal Monitor was given by Edward H. Hon, the very *inventor* of the fetal monitor, when he spoke at a 1987 conference on "Crisis In Obstetrics: The Management of Obstetrics." He stated firmly, "Not all patients should be electronically monitored...most women in labor may be much better off at home than in the hospital with the electronic fetal monitor."

Logically it might seem the wisest thing to do; birthing in the hospital where constant monitoring is done. Hon himself emphatically stressed, though, that it was *not*.

Nor has the electronic fetal monitor *ever* been proven safe as far as the ultrasonic waves it emits during use.

One of the most important reasons that routine monitoring is discouraged by many caregivers is that it forces the woman to remain in bed—typically a very uncomfortable position for labor, creating an increased need for pain medication.

The IFM (internal fetal monitor) is used for the same purpose as the EFM, except that it is used internally. The IFM is a device that is inserted through the mother's vagina and may be screwed into the baby's scalp—ouch! There is increased risk of infection from the use of the internal fetal monitor for both mother and baby.

One hospital's protocol states that those refusing the EFM are to be informed of the risk factors associated with the decision not to allow fetal monitoring [scare them]. The physician is to be notified that they have refused fetal monitoring [again read: Intimidate them. After all what woman wants an angry caregiver?], and that the woman should be asked if she will allow a *reassuring* baseline tracing [further scare tactics based upon more fallacious assertions].

The EFM can also distract from the woman herself. It is amazing how family, friends, and others including the baby's father who have come to support the woman seem to be attracted by the EFM monitor and who, instead of giving their attention to the mother, sit themselves in front of the monitor, absorbed in every rise and dip of the lines on the screen.

Caregivers may come in, spend awhile making documentations on the EFM, and after a quick glance at the woman make a brisk exit.

Some women, wishing to avoid the EFM during labor but not wanting to risk irritating anyone by refusing this common procedure will agree to a fifteen minute "strip" (the read-out on paper) when admitted to the hospital. During the strip a baby must show a certain amount of wakeful activity. If the baby is sleeping, a loud buzzer may be put near on the mother's abdomen to frighten the baby into wakeful motion. This is again primarily for proof in the case of litigation. A good number of families have learned, to their frustration, that once the monitor is on the woman it is sometimes not taken off after the initial fifteen (usually much longer than fifteen) minutes. Experience has taught many families to refuse the monitor altogether.

Many caregivers agree that it is just as safe, if not a great deal more safe, to have *continual, watchful care by an actual person* and the occasional use of a Doppler (used at prenatal exams with KY Jelly to find the babies heart beat), or perhaps even preferably the fetoscope (with the added plus that it doesn't use ultrasound). **Both the Doppler and fetoscope are very effective ways to assess the baby's well being.**

An occasional check with a Doppler (or better yet the fetoscope) can alert the caregiver to a problem or can give the assurance that the baby is still doing just fine.

The **Doppler** (also known as the Doptone) *also uses ultrasonic waves.* The baby is exposed to a lower dose however, than when monitored by the electronic fetal monitor for extended lengths of time.

The European Committee for Medical Ultrasound has stated, "The embryonic period is known to be particularly sensitive to any external influences. Until further scientific information is available, investigations should be carried out with careful control of output levels and exposure times. With increasing mineralization of the fetal bone as the fetus develops the possibility of heating fetal bone increases. The user should prudently limit exposure of critical structures such as the fetal skull or spine during Doppler studies...." (Rados 2004)

The **fetoscope** is a simple tool, related to the stethoscope that allows the caregiver to hear the baby's heart. It uses no ultrasound and is just as effective as a Doppler. Some staff members are less experienced in

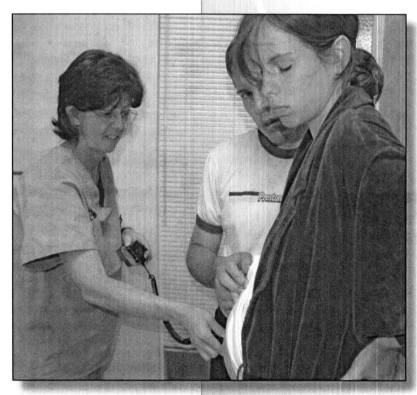

This nurse checks fetal heart tones with a Doppler, allowing the mother to remain in her chosen position of comfort.

using a fetoscope than others. It may also be necessary to give them time to find the facility's fetoscope.

Especially if you are planning to labor or birth in water, or if you wish to be mobile during labor, these hand-held devices can help to ensure a much more comfortable labor.

Why are some caregivers so insistent about something that was once thought an important piece of protocol but that has since been proven ineffective and even harmful? **When something has been a standard procedure for a long time (especially something that makes people *feel* more secure), it often takes something momentous for it to ever change.**

Keep in mind, though, that hospitals are businesses. The more the consumer insists on the best, the better the business will become in an effort to keep the patrons of their facility.

Note that in order to have pain medication, electronic fetal monitoring and an IV are both required.

Ultrasound

The American College of Obstetricians and Gynecologists has stated that it does not support the routine use of ultrasound and recommends only indicated scans be done. It has stated, "No well-controlled study has yet proved that routine scanning of all prenatal patients will improve the outcome of pregnancy."

The American Medical Association, the World Health Organization, and the Department of Health and Human Services have all three discouraged the routine use of ultrasound as it is being utilized today in conjunction with pregnancy.

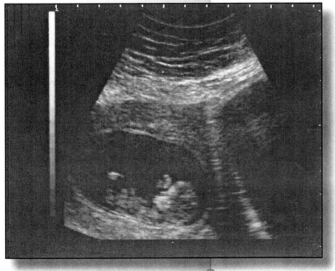
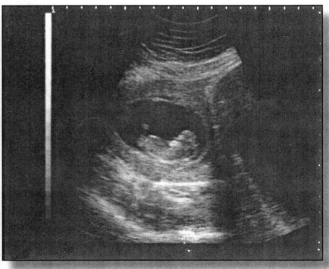

Even the FDA stated in May 2004, "While ultrasound has been around for many years, expectant women and their families need to know that the long-term effects of repeated ultrasound exposures on the fetus are not fully known. In light of all that remains unknown, having a prenatal ultrasound for non-medical reasons is not a good idea...."

Ten professional health organizations and the National Electrical Manufacturers Association were informed by the FDA of its apprehensions concerning using ultrasound on unborn babies. The FDA also said that anyone leasing or selling ultrasound equipment for making keepsake fetal videos could be in violation of the law and that ultrasounds for any reasons other than medical ones should be avoided.

And yet, ultrasound plays a large role in prenatal care in the United States today. Despite all of these assertions, a great many doctors employ ultrasound technology routinely, without presenting it as a choice with precautions.

The convenience of obtaining an ultrasound, whether at her doctor's or midwife's office or at a booth in the mall, makes it an easy process. Some women may have ultrasound scans weekly during their pregnancies.

Yet pregnancy is a normal process performed by our bodies. **By itself, pregnancy does not constitute a medical reason to be exposed to ultrasound. Ultrasound is expensive and is seldom essential to a healthy pregnancy and birth,** *perhaps even to the contrary.*

Not long ago, x-rays were used regularly during pregnancy! A person was even able to check to see if a shoe at the shoe store fit properly by putting their foot into an x-ray machine. Now we know of the dangers of x-ray. But what of those presented by ultrasound? It is frightening to realize that no formal studies have ever been done to prove the safety of ultrasound on an unborn child. Studies *have* shown reduced fetal weight in infants and adverse affects on rats, mice, and monkeys including reduced fetal weight.

There have been reports of miscarriages following early pregnancy ultrasound, but what is the effect on the older unborn baby? We don't really know. In a Canadian study, reported in the *Medical Association Journal,* of 72 children with tardy speech development, those children who were exposed to ultrasound in utero were found to be twice as likely to have speech difficulties as those who were not exposed. The majority of the children in the study group were only exposed to ultrasound *one* time. What will the future show to be the effects of ultrasound on an unborn baby? Will it have an effect on intelligence, personality, fertility, growth, sight, hearing, allergies, or susceptibility to infection? We don't know. Do we risk it? Possible risks must be weighed next to benefits.

The American College of Obstetricians and Gynecologists, the American Medical Association, the World Health Organization, the Department of Health and Human Services, and the Federal Drug Administration have all discouraged the routine use of ultrasound as it is being utilized today in conjunction with pregnancy.

Is the excitement of knowing the sex of the baby, or seeing him/her move worth the risk of exposing him to ultrasound?

When might the benefits of ultrasound outweigh the risks? Ultrasound can be helpful in determining the location of the placenta and in discovering any problems with it, finding out if there has been a miscarriage, or if there is a tubal (ectopic) pregnancy. Ultrasound is also used with Amniocentesis to find the right place to put the needle (A side note—Amniocentesis also has its risks including the very high possibility of causing the miscarriage of a healthy baby while testing for abnormalities).

When might the risks outweigh benefits? Commonly, ultrasound is used to estimate a due date. Prior to eighteen weeks gestation, an ultrasound is more accurate for showing baby's age, but can never predict an exact date. In fact, it can still be *weeks* off track of when the baby would normally arrive on her own. Ultrasound is also not a good tool to use for prediction of weight in the latter stages of the baby's development. It can be off by two pounds either way! Too many women in the United States are induced because of ultrasound results, only to discover that their babies are premature and need care in the NICU (Neonatal Intensive Care Unit)!

Many major physical abnormalities such as Down's Syndrome, cerebral palsy, and heart or kidney problems will very likely not even show up in an ultrasound. A 1989 study by the American College of Obstetricians and Gynecologists found that 51 percent of ultrasounds failed to reveal an existing serious problem.

As far as confirming multiples, the same can be detected by listening with a fetoscope. As an example of the error that ultrasound scans can still have, once in a while even a diagnosis of twins is missed with a resulting significant surprise to the family!

Detecting a baby in a breech position can be done quite simply by an experienced midwife or doctor using their hands on the mother's abdomen to feel the position of the baby in the uterus. This is called palpation.

Sometimes an ultrasound can detect that the placenta is lying over the opening of the uterus. This can cause severe bleeding during labor and can necessitate a cesarean. This is not common, however, and even then nineteen out of twenty cases of diagnosed "placenta previa" correct themselves as pregnancy progresses, before the time of birth.

A study by Uppsala University in Sweden concluded that midwives' measurements were more accurate than ultrasound measurements in determining intrauterine growth retardation (IUGR), a condition in which the baby is not growing in the womb normally. Studies in the U.S. and Europe report the same findings. Perhaps fifty percent of ultrasound screenings for IUGR give false positive results, reports Marsden Wagner who served as the Perinatal Epidemiologist and former head of the Responsible Office for Maternal and Child Health for the European Office of the World Health Organization.

What about the excitement of knowing the sex of the baby, or seeing him/her move? Is this worth the risk of exposing babies to ultrasound? Patience can truly be a gift.

Just as you've heard of babies that have been proclaimed a member of the opposite sex only to surprise his/her parents upon arrival, falsely interpreted ultrasounds have been the cause of many unnecessary and even harmful or fatal procedures due to incorrect diagnoses.

When a woman feels strongly that the benefits of using ultrasound, in any of its forms, outweigh the risks involved for her and her baby for whatever reason, she should be allowed to have the father or a support person to accompany her. She should be able to see the screen throughout the procedure and be given the results of any of the tests upon request. Only skilled technicians of ultrasound should be authorized to use the equipment and to interpret it. The woman has the right, as well as the responsibility, to ask and receive acceptable answers about the technician's training.

Public health organizations have a duty to advertise information on the effects of ultrasound, the known risks, as well as the territory of uncertainty. They should also make accessible the specifications for ultrasound operation.

Women need to know that the **electronic fetal monitor** used during labor in many hospitals, and the **Doppler/Doptone used especially during prenatal visits, use ultrasound.**

Lawrence D. Platt, M.D., president of the International Society of Ultrasound in Obstetrics and Gynecology and a practicing obstetrician in Los Angeles, says that although he encourages sensitivity to mothers' feelings, "We have to go beyond emotions in this case. We have to do the right thing. Ultrasound is a form of energy and it must be respected."

The FDA asks, "Why take a chance with your baby's health for a [keepsake] video?"

Once again, do the benefits outweigh the possible risks?

Information used with permission from Cohen, Nancy Wainer, *Open Season* and Wagner, Marsden. *Ultrasound: More Harm Than Good. Mothering.* Winter, 1995.

For more information, see websites in the resource section.

Books:

Ultrasound Unsound? by Beverley Lawrence Beech
Understanding Obstetrical Ultrasound by Jean Proud

When faced with a decision regarding your baby or yourself ask, "Do the benefits outweigh the possible risks?

Episiotomies

An episiotomy is a procedure of making a cut into the vagina to enlarge the birth opening.

While midwives almost never administer episiotomies, that number is much higher for doctors. The number of women who receive episiotomies is declining. Whether or not you will be given one is very much a matter of what your caregiver's rates are. **The American College of Obstetricians and Gynecologists has stated that "the routine use of episiotomy is not now recommended as a standard practice."** But, once again, *old habits die hard.*

There may be a small decrease in the length of the actual birthing stage when an episiotomy is used, and at times this surgical incision into the perineum (the flesh between the rectum and the birth opening) may be necessary for delivering a baby quickly if it is experiencing low heart tones. But too many women are receiving episiotomies as a matter of routine.

One argument that is used to defend the routine cutting of episiotomies is that it prevents tearing of the perineum as the baby is born. However, others refute this with the example of a piece of fabric. It is difficult to tear as is, but if you put a cut into it, it isn't hard at all to tear.

Physicians are frequently taught that neat, straight cuts will give them a better command over any injury, that it will make stitching easier.

Research indicates, however, that "tears occurring naturally in an unmedicated mother happen when the perineum is at its maximum stretch, thereby creating a tear that is not jagged, but straight. Often this type of tear requires a maximum of three to five quick-healing stitches if it needs any at all. Frequently, women who birth naturally report no tear at all or perhaps a little 'skid mark' that can't even be considered a tear and heals very quickly.

On the other hand, tearing can be severe for a mother who has had an epidural or an extremely rapid birth or for someone who is tearing at the top of the vagina, near the urethra. In these cases, an episiotomy may very well be necessary. In other cases, a mother receiving an episiotomy is put at risk for a severe tear, exacerbated by the incision itself." (Griffin 1995)

In an unmedicated birth, episiotomy is rarely needed.

No study has ever shown that cutting is better than tearing. In fact just the opposite is true. Episiotomies are cut into thick tissue and sometimes result, under pressure, in a third and fourth degree tear that extends into the rectum.

Tears started without an episiotomy are more minor and superficial because they happen, if they do happen at all (think of fabric), when the perineum is stretched to its thinnest.

A piece of fabric is difficult to tear as is, but if you put a cut into it, it isn't hard at all to tear.

"[O]utcomes with spontaneous tears, if they happen, are better than with episiotomy," says Katherine Hartmann, M.D., Ph.D., et al., in the *Journal of the American Medical Association*. She adds that women are more likely to experience the most severe tearing, from the vagina to the rectum, if they have been given an episiotomy. (Hartmann and Viswanathan 2005)

A large number of women who receive an episiotomy experience severe postpartum pain. A large number actually develop an infection. Some even experience problems with intercourse after having an episiotomy. Vaginal swelling is also common. What a miserable way to begin this new stage of mothering! Who wouldn't love to eliminate recovery from perineal injury?

What must be remembered is that **women's perineums were created to *stretch*—just as their uteruses were created to expand to many times their pre-pregnancy dimensions and just as vaginas were made to easily accommodate even a good-sized baby.** Something that some people don't realize is that hormonal changes during pregnancy cause the cervix and perineum to become extremely thick, supple, pliant, and stretchable.

Important to this process is **good nutrition** including vitamin E, Omega 3, and Omega 6 fats. These "good" fats are found in beans, nuts and seeds, cold-pressed oils, and fish. Fish oils are thought to also be great for the baby's brain development which is growing in leaps and bounds. Be sure to get a good source that is free of mercury.

Perineal Massage during pregnancy and right before birth is a procedure used to help prepare the perineal muscle for the crowning of the baby's head. K-Y jelly or vitamin E oil (such as wheat germ oil) can be used. During later pregnancy, the mother or dad (or their caregiver at the birth) can gradually stretch the perineum using two fingers, and by making a slow, stretching U-shaped motion inside the mother's vagina, from the top down and up the opposite side.

Kegel exercises are used to condition the perineum. The Kegel muscle is the same one you use to deliberately stop the flow of urine. These exercises can help to strengthen this muscle by contracting and releasing it. These exercises can also help to prevent and stop urinary incontinence and enhance lovemaking.

Another *very* helpful thing that your caregiver can do is to use his/her hands as a splint to **support the perineum** when the baby's head is on the perineum. This alleviates some of the pressure and allows time for the vaginal opening to stretch and give. Some caregivers are trained to do this and others are not.

Position of the mother is also important. Many caregivers believe that an upright position where the baby's head is fully down on the birth outlet, supported equally by all of the surrounding area, is important. The position you want to avoid is lying on your back with your feet in stirrups. In this position, the force of the weight of the baby

Women's perineums were created to stretch. By ingenious design, hormonal changes during pregnancy cause the cervix and perineum to become extremely thick, supple, pliant, and stretchable.

is mainly against the perineum. If a woman has had an epidural that hasn't worn off for the birth, however, she will probably not be able to support herself in an upright position.

Whether or not a woman will tear also depends on how she pushes. By listening to her body and allowing time for the vagina to stretch, she is working with, rather than against, muscles and flesh that are already yielding and stretching. If a woman is pushing as hard as she can under the direction of misguided people around her, she has a very good chance of tearing.

Of foremost importance, if you want to avoid an episiotomy, choose a caregiver that has very low rates of episiotomies, who uses them only a small percentage of the time, when truly necessary.

An episiotomy must be used when forceps or vacuum are employed for the birth of a baby. These are often used when a woman has been given epidural anesthesia. One important way you can avoid an episiotomy is to avoid having an epidural.

Birthing Your Baby

Using upright positions for giving birth has been the choice of many women/cultures throughout history.

A great number of women today give birth in positions that are more accommodating for the *caregiver*, but which are usually neither the most comfortable nor the easiest positions for the mother or the baby.

As we've seen in various earlier examples, change within a society or birthing system takes a long time and unfortunately we still have not fully recovered from the days of Twilight Sleep when women were "delivered" on their backs while under anesthesia.

As discussed in **chapter 4**, during early modern U.S. obstetrical care, women gave birth while unconscious, flat on their backs, and supposedly unaware. Physicians did most of the work with an episiotomy and forceps. While Twilight Sleep was ultimately abandoned, not all parts of it were. Valuable information concerning normal birth was lost. Too many medical schools are still not training students about the importance of upright positions. Too many caregivers are not practiced at assisting in any other way than with the woman propped-up or lying on the bed. Caregivers that know, however, are adamant about how advantageous the upright position is for helping a woman to give birth. (See Positions... in **chapter 13**.)

Medical scientists have listed many benefits for using upright positions for birth. (McKay 1978)

Think about it. If a mother is forced to birth her baby while lying on her back, she must birth the baby *uphill* through the birth passage. It makes a lot of sense that upright positions are the most effective because they utilize the force of gravity to assist the baby as he moves downward.

Blood and oxygen flow are stronger to the uterine muscle and to the baby in upright positions. When the woman is on her back, the heavy weight of the pregnant uterus compresses the vena cava, a major vein whose responsibility it is to return blood to the heart. In fact, women are advised to not lie on their backs for extended periods during the last months of pregnancy, as this can cause lowered blood pressure and decrease oxygen to the baby! (Humphrey, M. et al. 1973)

If a woman employs any of these positions, and if her body has not been numbed with medication, it is very rare for a baby to need to be pulled out with forceps or vacuum extraction.

Consequently, tearing is usually very minimal in women who use upright positions, partly because of the weight of the baby now being equally dispersed around the entire birth opening.

There are not only physiological advantages to upright positions, but psychological ones too. The mother naturally feels more in control when upright, **she can see better what is going on, and caregivers are now dealing with the *whole woman* and not just the birth outlet with everything else draped off.**

The upright position of squatting is thought to actually open the pelvic outlet *almost 30 percent* more than when lying flat!

You can use flat-footed squatting as you pick things up or work in your garden. This can help to prepare you to more easily hold this position during birth. You only need to be able to hold it for the duration

Unfortunately our culture has still not fully recovered from the days of Twilight Sleep when women were "delivered" on their backs while under anesthesia.

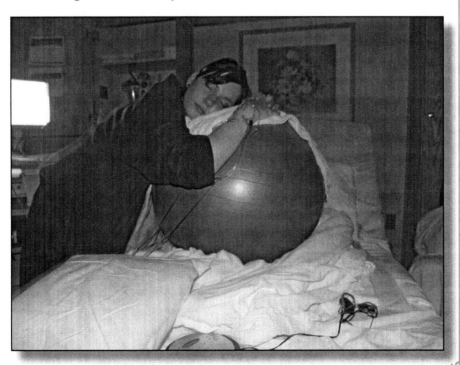

of a contraction; about forty-five to ninety seconds. At the birth, others can also help support you as you squat. Squatting for long periods can be fatiguing and not conducive to relaxation for women not used to it, though. Some laboring women find that they prefer using a **birthing chair/stool or birth ball** to any other position for labor, for the same reasons listed for squatting.

Birthing stools were used historically, long before modern obstetrics. Today's birthing stools may look like low wooden chairs with the middle of the seat cut out. Or they may be a metal frame that supports the mother in a sitting position. Both have room for the baby to descend and be received by the mother, father, or caregiver. One website has birthing stools that are rocking chairs. The middle part of the seat can be removed for the baby's birth. It can be put back together and used as a regular rocking chair after the birth of the baby. A matching stool for the caregiver is also sold. Your hospital may or may not have a birthing stool. Check out the resources in the website section of the book.

Practicing upright positions beforehand, in class or at home, is wonderful for helping you in labor to know what might be most helpful to you.

Is your caregiver unfamiliar with how to assist a woman in upright positions? Would she be willing to let you give birth in a side-lying position on the bed or at least without the use of the stirrups? These are things to discuss with her *before* the birth. If you are planning to be the first woman in this physician's experience to ever give birth upright, however, be sure that she is very comfortable with the idea—better yet, enthusiastic about it—or as with other things you may be disappointed when she is not as agreeable at the time of birth!

A word about "sounding" during labor—far too often women who are in labor or who are birthing, are discouraged from and shushed for being "too verbal." Is making any kind of natural noises perhaps a culturally "unladylike" thing for a woman to do? We hear men grunting naturally as they lift heavy things. Sounding is something that is very helpful to athletes, whether man or woman. Imagine tournaments and games in which no one was allowed to make sounds. Would anyone play very well at all? It is perfectly natural for a woman to meet the surges of labor by sounding. It does not necessarily mean she is feeling discomfort. It can actually be very helpful. **A birthing woman needs to feel free to moan, groan, grunt, sigh, hum, and yell; whatever she needs to do.** Really, if supervisors of birthing facilities were concerned about noises disturbing other women in nearby rooms, perhaps they might have thought of putting in thicker walls.

For a picture of what typically happens at a hospital birth when the woman gets ready for the actual birthing stage, the staff will probably break down the bed so that her bottom is right on the edge—just like

Some experts believe that hard, directed pushing does not shorten the birthing stage significantly, and that it can be extremely tiring and stressful for both mother and baby.

pelvic exams that are performed in the office. They will likely have her put her feet into stirrups. Nurses (others who are around may be encouraged to help too) will most likely pull the woman's bent legs back toward her, encouraging her to hold her chin down and push as hard as she can while the nurse counts. This is called Valsalva pushing or "purple pushing" by some (and it's the scene sometimes depicted on TV or in books where everyone is yelling, "Push! Push! Bear down harder! Hold your breath!" and counting while the woman is getting purple in the face).

Yet research has shown that it isn't necessary or helpful to strain with all your might. While purple pushing may make the birth *slightly* shorter, it also tires the mother, can break skin and eye blood vessels, disrupt the baby's oxygen supply, and could actually work against contractions. It also strains and tears perineal tissues that have not had time yet to stretch, encouraging an episiotomy and/or tearing.

It must be understood, that most physicians and nurses have been taught to "manage" births rather than patiently "attend" them.

In truth, many have never personally seen a woman give birth on her own as she was physically designed to do.

Direction from hospital staff may be necessary if a woman has an epidural and can't feel what is going on. But otherwise, what has applied all along, still applies. Listen to your body and do what it tells you to do!

If a burning sensation occurs as the baby descends, this is a signal to the mother to protect the perineum by not pushing and by letting the vagina stretch and open naturally as it was made to do. Being perhaps a bit frank, there is a parallel between the kind of opening you do to let a baby through and the kind of opening you do when making love—it's usually better if the process is more gradual. We're dealing with different dimensions here of course, but a woman's body was made to accommodate a baby just as well as it was made to accommodate a penis!

Women in comas have given birth with obviously no forced pushing on their part. Their uteruses and vaginas knew how to birth their babies without any thought on their part and without any outside instruction.

There are experts in the field of childbirth that have asserted for many years that women do not need to be coached in pushing. It is even thought that pushing may be a *conditioned* response for many women.

This is not to say that a woman does not feel the descent of the baby through the birth path or her uterus nudging the baby from her body. In normal, natural birth many women don't even ever voice the need to push.

Without pushing, a number of mothers, of *varying sizes of babies*, announce the eminent birth of their baby only when the baby is ready to slide out into the world.

Actually "breathing" the baby out instead of pushing can help to avoid tearing.

"...there is no evidence that bearing down during contractions helps either the mother or the child."
—American Journal of Obstetrics & Gynecology

In 2006 the *New York Times* published an article citing the current issue of the *American Journal of Obstetrics & Gynecology*. The study said, "...there is no evidence that bearing down during contractions helps either the mother or the child. They also suggest that women who are encouraged to push may be at higher risk for urinary problems after delivery...." The Times concluded, "While it is unclear how the practice of encouraging women to push came about (the researchers say it was not in the medical literature before 1950), [Dr. Steven L. Bloom of the University of Texas Southwestern Medical Center] said part of the goal might have been to decrease the amount of time women were in discomfort. The question, he said, is whether it is worth it." (Nagourney 2006)

If things are taken gradually, there is less chance for tearing, the mother's energy is conserved, contractions are enhanced, blood chemistry has more of a chance to stabilize, there is oxygen for the baby, and there is a lowered risk of tearing or episiotomy.

Research by Caldeyro-Barcia and by Barnett and Humenick shows that when a mother begins to hold her breath for Valsalva ("purple") pushing, blood pressure initially increases and then as she bears down, her blood pressure continues to drop. When she stops pushing, blood pressure gradually returns to normal. This pushing results in a decreased amount of oxygen reaching the fetus which causes fetal distress and lower Apgar scores. Some believe that hard, directed pushing does not really shorten the birthing stage significantly at all. Furthermore, several studies have indicated that even with pushing for over three hours, there was no significant increase in perinatal or neonatal deaths compared with shorter births. (Holland, R. and Smith, D. 1989)

Of course, more strenuous pushing may also be helpful in uncommon circumstances when self-guided bearing down is for some reason not working or in an emergency when the baby needs to be born hastily.

Otherwise, unless a woman has had an epidural or for some other reason cannot feel her body, a woman does not need someone coaching her to "puuush!"

Sometimes a woman will experience a resting period of perhaps half an hour once she is fully dilated, before the baby begins to descend. She should be allowed to rest and do as her body tells her to do. A woman can become easily fatigued and make little progress moving her baby down if she pushes before she feels the need—*even if she is fully dilated.* **Trust your body!** Save your energy!

Breathing down through the center of your body, down on top of your baby, can help your baby to gently descend while avoiding swelling of the cervix—something that can easily occur when the baby is pushed against a cervix that is not yet fully open.

Many mothers that have given birth to babies that have not been drugged could attest to the fact that their babies wriggled, pushed, and otherwise helped themselves to be born.

We stress once again the importance of having a caregiver that believes in your body and what it tells you!

Every woman's experience will be different, with its own blessings and challenges. There are different ways that women experience the birthing stage. Some say that it is difficult. Others describe it as easy or even orgasmic. Some are refreshed and excited to know that they are on the last lap and that they will soon meet their baby.

Birthing the Placenta and Clamping the Cord

The expelling of the placenta, the baby's life support while in the womb, is considered the third stage of labor. Uterine surges continue after the birth of the baby to help the placenta separate from the wall of the uterus and come out. Then the contractions continue to control bleeding from the placental site.

Usually in medical school, doctors are taught to deliver the placenta by tugging it off of the uterine wall. This makes a quicker delivery, but it also can cause hemorrhage! Fear of hemorrhage is the reason Pitocin is routinely given through IV or intramuscularly through a shot.

If you desire to deliver your placenta on its own time, the way it was created to do, be sure to specify this in your birth wishes and choose a caregiver that does not administer this procedure routinely. A placenta usually takes less than an hour to detach on its own. By standing or squatting, the placenta can be helped to be expelled by the use of gravity.

Another procedure often performed routinely at birth, is that of **early cord clamping**. If the cord hasn't been clamped yet, delivery of the placenta may actually be quicker. Immediate cord clamping has been shown to prolong delivery of the placenta, and

There are less respiratory problems in infants who are given time before their cords are clamped. A baby whose cord is clamped right away must use his lungs immediately, as he can no longer depend on oxygen from his mother through the placenta.

This baby enjoys a warm bath with his mother with the cord still attached to the placenta, which floats in a bowl next to him. After a bit, the cord is cut by his father.

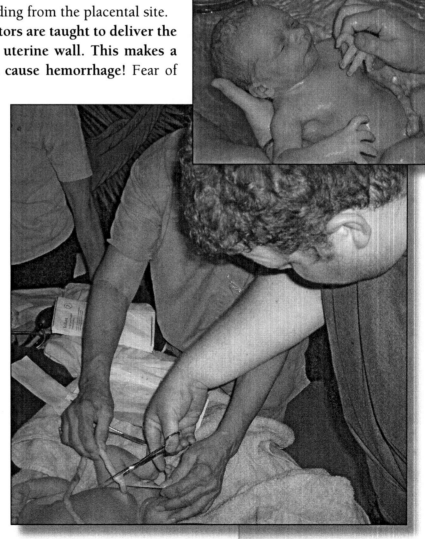

to also greatly increase blood loss in the mother. When the cord, which connects the baby to the placenta, is left uncut until after it has finished pulsing (about five minutes), the baby continues to receive necessary blood and oxygen from the placenta. But **if the cord is severed soon after birth, the blood in the placenta belonging to the infant does not get to her, and the amount of blood that is taken from the baby is said to actually equal a rather severe hemorrhage!** (*Scientific American 1969*) The systemic pressure is higher in babies whose cords were clamped later. (Butler 1986) Those infants whose cords have been cut early have a notable increase in occurrences of heart murmurs during the first fourteen days. (Buckle et al. 1965) Premature cord clamping also results in a significant deprivation of iron to the infant. (De Marsh et al. 1941) Iron's primary function is to move oxygen through the body. When the cord is left unclamped, with the placenta still attached to the uterine wall, the cord can continue to transport oxygen to the baby until he can breathe on his own more fully. Thus, **there are less respiratory problems in infants who are given time before their cords are clamped. A baby whose cord is clamped right away must use her lungs immediately, as she can no longer depend on oxygen through the placenta.** This can be a bit of a shock for an infant. In some circumstances the cord must be clamped early, such as when it is wrapped too tightly around the neck for the midwife or doctor to be able to slip it off and allow the baby to continue descending from the womb. Yet under ordinary circumstances, it appears that **the infant whose cord is clamped early does not function at the truly optimal levels that he could if his cord were simply left intact.** Finding the cord around the neck is a rather common occurrence that is not often a cause for concern, despite the scores of horror stories that float around. If the cord is actually long enough for the baby to be born, it can be unwrapped from the baby's body during or after the birth.

This homebirth midwife holds the placenta for the new mother to see. By magnificent design, the placenta, on our right, was just attached to the uterine wall. The sack held out to our left, housed the baby in amniotic fluid.

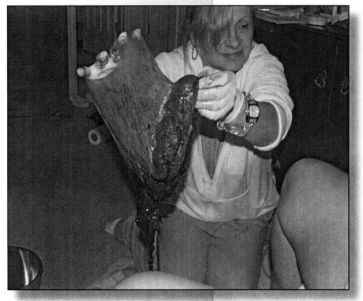

Mothers who are Rh-negative who have babies that are Rh-positive develop less contamination when the cord is left unclamped and the placenta detaches by itself. When the placenta separates *after* cord clamping, the baby's blood, which is still in the placenta, can mix with the mother's blood infecting the mother. (Doolittle and Moritz 1996)

Some people don't even want to look at the placenta—the fluids and membranes can seem a bit repugnant to them. Those who feel this way might think about *why* these life-giving and sustaining parts of a woman's body and her baby's pre-birth environment are repulsive to them.

After all, the placenta that has imparted food, oxygen, and more for the baby has literally provided for his/her healthy development. We presently do not understand all about how the placenta works and about all of the functions it performs. If you have the opportunity to look at the placenta, acknowledge it for what it is, a wondrous, *ingenious*, life-sustaining source, formed within your own body.

Some people plant a tree or bush in their baby's honor, burying the placenta under the tree to give the tree sustenance and life, just as it has given so remarkably to the child in the womb all of those months. Children can enjoy watching their very own trees or plants grow with them. Whether or not the idea of saving the placenta for this purpose appeals to you, planting a tree in honor of your child's birth can be a fun idea.

Breech Birth, and Exercises to Help Your Baby Turn

Although a small percentage of babies are in a breech position (head up) at the end of pregnancy, breech births aren't allowed in most hospitals in the United States unless it happens to be an unexpected incident. The skills for assisting with breech birth and those for External Cephalic Version have, of the recent past, been severely under-taught in medical schools.

Ironically, cesarean birth holds *greater* risks than vaginal breech birth.

The National Institute of Health Task Force on Cesarean Childbirth recommends that "vaginal delivery of the term breech should remain an acceptable obstetrical choice for delivery with an anticipated fetal weight of less than eight pounds, with normal maternal pelvic dimensions, with a frank breech without a hyperextended head, and with a physician experienced in vaginal breech delivery."

The *American Journal of Obstetrics & Gynecology* published an article in their January 2006 issue stating that the "'Term Breech Trial' recommendations to [mandate cesarean section for all breech births] are withdrawn... analysis of outcome after 2 years has shown no difference between vaginal and abdominal deliveries of breech babies.... Conclusion: The original term breech trial recommendations should be withdrawn." (Glezerman 2006)

The study basically stated that recommendations to deliver all breech position babies by cesarean section were made on a trial basis. In the end it was not proven to be in the best interest of the woman and baby. They concluded that vaginal birth should again be an option.

Ironically, cesarean birth holds greater risks than vaginal breech birth.

Where breech birth carries much less inherent risk than does cesarean birth (See Cesarean Birth…**chapter 7.**), one would think that change would be forthcoming.

But with cesarean section being long enough established for breech births in most hospitals as the only "safe" way for babies in a breech position to be born, we will probably only see a change, at least in the near future, in the most progressive of caregiver practices.

So unless her caregiver is trained and willing to assist a woman in a vaginal breech birth, a woman has a compulsory cesarean section to look forward to unless she changes to a caregiver and birth place that will assist her. While most physicians and nurse midwives have not been trained in this skill, many homebirth midwives are well-trained in breech birth and there may still be a few older doctors who have retained this skill.

Below are some things that have been successful at assisting a baby into a head-down position before the birth:

- *Breech Tilt.* At about thirty to thirty-six weeks, a couple of times a day for ten minutes or so at a time, lie on the floor with your pelvis resting on pillows a foot higher than your head. A large percentage of babies have turned within a few weeks. In this position you might try firm but gentle exercises of rotating your hips to move the baby out of your pelvis, giving him more room to rotate.
- *Talking to and Visualizing Your Baby.* Many mothers strongly believe that their babies are very in-tune with them. Sometimes mothers who have been experiencing a great deal of fear or negative feelings about their births or even about seemingly unrelated aspects of their lives, have their babies turn up into a breech position. Resolving these concerns and communicating with their babies has been found to be very useful for getting a baby to switch into a head-down position on his own. Some mothers have found it very helpful to at the same time visualizing their babies facing their back with the baby's head down on their cervix.
- *Coaxing.* Sometimes babies will turn downward toward their father's voice, to music, or to light from a flashlight held at the lower end of the mother's abdomen.
- *Hypnosis.* A study conducted by Dr. Lewis Mehl showed that with hypnosis, 81 percent of the breech babies in the study turned spontaneously from breech to vertex (head down), with half of the successful turns taking only one session! HypnoBirthing® practitioners have a script they can use to assist mothers in helping their babies to turn.
- *Pulsatilla.* This is a homeopathic remedy that can be bought in health food stores and which can assist a baby in moving into position.

Believe it or not, resolving her own emotional concerns, whatever they may be, has been found to be a very useful way for a mother to get her baby to switch to a head-down position. Some mothers find visualization to also be very helpful.

- *Acupuncture or Acupressure.* Consult an acupuncturist about points on the body that have proven helpful for encouraging babies to turn. Acupuncture is said to be highly effective!
- *The Webster Technique.* Find a chiropractor that has been trained in the Webster Technique. This is one of the most helpful ways of getting the baby into the head-down, rear-facing position.
- *Foot Zoning.* Seeing a Foot Zoner may be beneficial for helping a baby to get into an optimal position. Both physical and emotional difficulties related to pregnancy can be effectively treated with zoning.
- *External Cephalic Version.* This exercise is used to turn a baby from the outside. It can be performed at about thirty to thirty-six weeks. If the breech position is not discovered until early labor, this exercise can also be done then if the water around the baby has not released. It should be performed by a trained caregiver. Anesthesia is not necessary or recommended. For the baby's well-being, the mother needs to be able to guide the caregiver on the amount of pressure both she and the baby are comfortable with, and anesthesia does not allow for this. The process usually doesn't take very long. Relaxation of the mother during the procedure is particularly important to its success and to the comfort of the mother.

Some babies actually turn from a breech to head-down position during labor.

It should also be stressed that a cesarean is not the only option for a twin/multiple pregnancy where the first baby is in the breech position, any more than a cesarean is the only option for a breech singleton pregnancy. (See Classification of Risk…**chapter 9**.)

Too, some women's babies actually turn from breech to head-down during labor. And whether their babies are born vaginally or by cesarean section in the end, allowing their bodies to go into and through labor, may be a very good choice for some mothers of breech-positioned babies for at least two reasons, beyond the possibility that a baby can turn head-down in the process. First, the stimulation of labor helps to prepare babies for life on the outside, producing better outcomes (such as better respiratory Apgar scores in the infant) at birth. (See Apgar…in **chapter 18**.) Second, the baby has been allowed to finish his time in the womb. (See To Be or Not to Be…in **chapter 8**.)

For most births, the preferred and probably most comfortable fetal position—for both mother and baby—is indeed a head-down position with the baby facing toward the mother's back. But in Africa, it has actually been considered good luck to be born feet-first—having something to do with the child having their feet planted firmly on the ground!

Group B Strep

You may have heard that Strep B (also known as GBS or Group B Strep-tococcus) is one of the most prevalent threats to newborn babies in the United States, and that it may cause blindness, deafness, mental disabilities, and even death.

You will most likely be tested for Group B Strep late in pregnancy. Testing in *early* pregnancy is not of much use as GBS can reoccur following treatment. Ideally, testing is done around thirty-six weeks of gestation. This is when vaginal and rectal culture testing will be the most effective for determining whether treatment is necessary during labor. Both vaginal and rectal culture testing is more accurate when the two tests are performed in conjunction with one another.

While it's believed that approximately one-third of women carry Strep B, most are treated in labor before they give birth and only one to two per 333 babies that are actually exposed to GBS will end up getting sick. This is a very small number, and **infection is lethal in only a minor percentage of this number. Proper treatment almost eliminates chances of infection in newborns.**

Experts do not recommend either an induction or a cesarean for mothers simply because they have Group B Strep. A woman is also not considered "high risk" if the Group B is being adequately treated.

However, artificial rupture of the membranes (AROM), the use of the IFM (internal fetal monitor), and frequent vaginal exams are all especially and strongly discouraged for mothers who have GBS for obvious reasons of infection!

Unfortunately while the baby may contract GBS from the mother at birth, it is more likely derived from *the community or hospital delivery and nursery contact.* If you have chosen the hospital, seriously consider minimal nursery contact, avoidance of AROM, IFM, and frequent exams. (See **chapter 5**.)

As a side note, keep the baby away from community germs for the first few weeks (or months, if it is winter). Other dangerous communicable germs that appear benign in a healthy adult could put a baby in the hospital. As a side note, it's also a good idea to keep siblings healthy so that they won't be sneezing and coughing on the baby.

Treatment of Group B Strep

In the hospital during labor an IV is usually used to administer antibiotics to mothers who have tested positive for Group B Strep. Group B strep infections are commonly treated with antibiotics such as penicillin, ampicillin, and erythromycin. It is generally recommended that administration occur at the onset of labor, and be given for about four hours. However, for those wishing to avoid an IV, a woman can wear a heparin or saline lock through which antibiotics can be given for just a few minutes every four hours. This allows a woman to move around much more easily the rest of the time.

An **injectable dose of ampicillin** is an equally effective option for women who wish to avoid an IV during their labors, including those who are birthing at home. If the shot can be administered at least two hours before the actual birth this can be a very effective method.

There are some drawbacks to antibiotic use, even for GBS, which need to be carefully considered before making a decision as to treatment. The effects of antibiotics on women and babies (particularly on babies' immune systems) when taken during pregnancy and/or during labor and birth, still require further study. Another question that remains yet unanswered is what the eventual effects will be of administering antibiotics to so many women and babies, considering the fact that bacterias are now widely known to develop resistance against antibiotics in certain circumstances.

One body of research found that there was no decrease in infection or deaths among newborns whose mothers received IV antibiotics. (D.P. Ascher et al. 1994)

Contrarily, other studies showed that giving antibiotics in labor to women *did* decrease rates of GBS infection in newborns, but that the babies' resistance to bacteria such as E. coli was decreased as well.

Numerous women and babies could attest to having problems with yeast following antibiotics, such as thrush which can cause difficulties with breastfeeding.

Overall, giving general attention to health boosts natural immunity against Strep B.

Alternatives to Antibiotics

Conclusions of a study of 108 women treated with the antibiotic ampicillin and 109 that were treated with *vaginal washes of chlorhexadine* indicated that chlorhexadine was proportionately as effectual as the antibiotic treatment. Furthermore, E. coli colonization in the newborn was actually reduced with chlorhexadine use. (Facchinetti F. et al)

What other things can you do to fight Strep B in your body and obtain a negative Strep B test before the onset of labor?

Overall, good nutrition, sleep (especially sleep before midnight), lowering stress, slowing down, meditating, and giving general attention to health all help to boost natural immunity against Strep B.

Remarkably, **large doses of fresh garlic**, taken orally for a period during pregnancy, has also been found to be very effective for reducing and eliminating Strep B bacteria—as is, strangely enough, a clove of garlic used intra-vaginally (threaded on sewing thread for easy removal). Garlic has been carefully studied and shown to have powerful antibacterial properties.

An alternative-medicine specialist treats with **homeopathic nosode streptococcin**. A success rate of 100 percent was reported when it was administered regularly.

Taking **Echinacea** in tea or capsule form (two a day) has been helpful for many women for eliminating Strep B, as has taking extra **Vitamin C**. There are other powerful immunity builders that are compatible with pregnancy and which are easily found with a bit of personal research.

To aid your baby's immunity against potentially harmful illnesses, of which there can be many in a hospital, reduce stress as much as possible during and after the birth, and make sure that you and your baby are kept warm, especially with **skin-to-skin contact (with a blanket over both of you)**. Forget the man-made warming bed that is pulled from the closet at the time of birth. Keep your baby "velcroed" to you! Babies still very much need their mothers in that first while after birth!

Remember that **colostrum**, available in your breasts for your baby as soon as he/she is born, is a very powerful antibiotic with absolutely no negative side-effects!

If the mother is treated during pregnancy, her partner should most likely also be treated.

Treating Yeast Resulting from Antibiotic Use

In babies whose mothers received antibiotics in labor, you might see a small red-bump diaper rash in the diaper area and/or a white coating in the baby's mouth called "thrush". (See Caring for... in **chapter 20**.) This is from yeast that naturally occurs in the body. When antibiotics are used, the yeast grows out of control because beneficial bacteria have also been done away with.

Thrush may cause extreme breast soreness when yeast is passed from the baby to the mother during breastfeeding. Mother and baby can pass it back and forth. The mother may also experience an internal breast infection indicated by shooting, "toe curling" pain during the let-down phase of nursing. The sooner you can rid it from both your systems the better. **Your baby does not need to be weaned because of thrush**.

Very helpful for restoring natural flora after the effects of antibiotics is a high grade, pure coconut oil (not that used as a part of a cosmetic or other product). Garlic oil capsules can also be most helpful as can a magnesium supplement. Some women also swear by acidophilus capsules. Most commercial yogurts probably do not contain enough acidophilus to get the job done. It is also important to eliminate sugar intake to help the body's pH to become more alkaline, as yeast thrives in an acidic environment.

Forget the man-made warming bed that is pulled from the closet at the time of birth. Keep your baby "velcroed" to you! Babies still very much need their mothers in that first while after birth!

Cesarean Birth and Vaginal Birth after Cesarean Birth

Although the risks from giving birth by cesarean section are much higher than those associated with vaginal birth, even cesareans without medical reasons are now fully encouraged by many caregivers.

One reason for this is our lawsuit-happy culture.

Individuals who have been taught that cesarean is the save-all procedure for every endangered mother and baby are disillusioned when things go awry and they have not been "delivered" the perfect baby. Reactive to the present situation of increasing lawsuits, the cost of obstetricians' liability insurance has skyrocketed to the point that many doctors are changing the way they practice. Others choose to discontinue practicing obstetrics altogether. This is unfortunate when we are losing good doctors who could otherwise be practicing evidence-based care (such as showing a very low rate of cesareans for women under their care).

The fact is that no caregiver and no "miracle" procedure, including cesarean section, can promise a perfectly healthy baby!

It simply is *not true* that cesareans are safer than vaginal birth in the majority of cases. The physician that is honest and forthcoming will educate the families in his/her care about the reasons that so many doctors are now making this recommendation.

What are those reasons? The truth is that many hospitals are now refusing women a vaginal birth after a previous cesarean (VBAC), *not because of safety issues*, but because of the recommendation by the American College of Obstetricians and Gynecologists (ACOG). ACOG has cautioned that only hospitals with 24-hour immediate availability of the physician, anesthesia service, and an operating room should care for women wishing a VBAC. **ACOG cites lawsuits as a primary factor in their counsel to doctors to discourage VBAC. So all across the country in hundreds of hospitals, in which administrators are weighing their own profitability and malpractice exposure, birthing women are being denied the significantly safer option of a vaginal birth!**

Doctors are put between a rock and a hard place. Physicians, especially those in independent practice, simply cannot afford to cancel an entire day of office visits to attend a long VBAC labor. The way the current system is set up, attending an entire labor is not part of the services doctors are normally *able* to provide. Under regular circumstances nurses attend several women at a time, largely by EFM monitors until each is ready for the actual delivery. At this time she calls in the woman's doctor who has been given a limited amount of time to be in and out of the labor room and on to other things.

In the United States cesareans are performed close to 33 percent of the time! Before 1970, the United States' cesarean rate was 5.5 percent.

Experts and consumers are speaking out! **The countries with the lowest rates of cesarean births and infant deaths are those in which midwives serve as the primary caregivers for women with normal pregnancies.** Midwifery care is becoming more popular in the United States lately as well, though it still must be sought out rather than being a normal part of expected care. Studies show that midwives do indeed have more positive outcomes statistically. Midwives can offer more personalized, one-on-one care that is so needed at such a fundamental time in a woman's life and in that of her baby's. Midwives practices are set-up so that they can also attend a much greater part of a woman's labor than can a doctor.

Wouldn't we all agree that doctor-care is for true problems and illnesses? According to Marsden Wagner, MD, former head of the Women's and Children's Health for the World Health Organization, having a highly-trained obstetrician surgeon attend a normal birth is comparable to having a pediatric surgeon baby-sit a healthy two year old baby! It's preposterous.

Likewise, midwifery care focuses not on the chance for abnormalities, but instead on the tried-and-true, age-old processes of pregnancy and birth. It stands to reason, when one steps back to take another look, why it is so that cesarean rates are much lower when it is midwives that attend births. Part of the art of midwifery is the knowledge of how to assist babies into the world, very seldom having to resort to cesareans or even forceps and vacuum extraction.

It would make much more sense to have midwives, who spend hours getting to know and caring for the woman throughout her pregnancy, care for that same woman *continually* throughout her labor—as opposed to only the *intermittent* care that nurses (perhaps different shifts of nurses) are able to provide—and in contrast to the brief attention provided only at the time of the actual birth by a physician, who by nature of her job does not have time to really get to know a woman in any depth during her pregnancy.

Outrageous Cesarean Rates

Obstetrician Dr. Josie Muscat, who is the director of the St. James Natural Childbirth Center on the island of Malta, reported that **98 percent of the births there proceeded without complications when** medical procedures were avoided during labor and when women were instead encouraged with love and support. (Harper 1994)

The Farm Midwifery Center in Tennessee, operated by a group of leading U.S. midwives, reported that from 1970 to 2000, along with other phenomenal outcomes, only a 1.4 percent cesarean rate and a high vaginal birth after cesarean rate (106 out of 108 who attempted VBAC). (Gaskin, Ina May's Guide 2003)

In light of these and other statistics from similar birth places, it is ironic that in the United States cesareans are performed close to *33 percent of the time*! Before 1970, the United States' cesarean rate was *5.5 percent*!

In larger teaching hospitals and in some rural hospitals, the cesarean rate can be much higher. One might wonder, nevertheless, if a low cesarean rate at a particular hospital is simply being replaced with high rates of forceps and vacuum extraction births—not at all ideal either.

With that spectacular leap in numbers, one would think that at least some good should have come from it. Yet disappointingly, while the best technology devised by man is used routinely at births in the United States, **fetal death and injury rates show very little change since 1970, before cesarean section became a popular means of "saving lives."**

Ironically, **the World Health Organization (WHO) cites cesarean section as causing increased maternal and neonatal deaths and has called for a much reduced rate of no more than 10 percent per year. They say that those hospitals that intervene more are doing so too often!**

Former head of Women's and Children's Health for WHO Marsden Wagner further states, "For whatever reasons women choose CS [cesarean section], very few are clearly informed about fetal risks.... In an elective CS where the baby is [not] in trouble, the risks to the baby of doing a CS still exist, meaning the woman who chooses CS puts her baby in unnecessary danger. That some women are choosing CS strongly suggests women are not told this scientific fact. It is only logical that eventually a point is reached at which CS kills almost as many babies as it saves." (Wagner, Choosing 2000)

Thank goodness that we have cesarean surgery when it is necessary, but the present rates of cesareans are *outrageous*. It should be obvious that one in every three women in our country is *not* in need of a cesarean!

Risks of Cesarean Birth

In the United States, approximately 95 percent of babies are born in high-tech (more or less) hospitals. But the death rate of babies here is still higher than *twenty-three other countries*. With all of our machines and medicine to give us better births, our rates are still far from the best in the world. The birthing practices in the United States could stand a closer look, and a few changes!

Cesarean section is *major abdominal surgery*. Death caused by complications of cesarean is double that of vaginal birth. Some of the risks of a cesarean are high rates of infection, massive hemorrhage (7.3 percent), transfusion (6.4 percent), damage to the urinary tract, placental

Fetal death and injury rates show very little change since 1970, before cesarean section became a popular means of "saving lives."

disorders, abscesses, gangrene, paralysis of bladder and bowel, injury to bowels, hysterectomy, and possibly follow up surgery with all of its risks. (MacCorkle) Injury does happen. Too, postoperative recovery from cesarean can be extremely painful.

The Journal of the American Medical Association published a 2000 study by Lydon-Rochelle et al. that stated that women who had undergone cesarean section had twice the risk, versus women who had a vaginal birth, of being *re-hospitalized* for such further related difficulties as uterine infection (2.0 relative risk), gallbladder disease (1.5 RR), urinary tract infections (1.5 RR), surgical wound complications (30.0 RR), cardiopulmonary conditions (2.4 RR), thromboembolic conditions (2.5 RR), and appendicitis (1.8 RR).

There is also a dramatic increase of risks of severe subsequent pregnancy complications including placental abruption, with great risks to the baby. Having had a previous cesarean can predispose a woman to future problems with infertility, endometriosis, ectopic pregnancy, placenta previa, and miscarriage.

In addition to the above, in 2000 the American College of Obstetricians and Gynecologists (ACOG) listed some further risks of cesarean:

Cesarean section, as opposed to normal vaginal birth, presents such risks as a 2 percent chance of the baby being cut mistakenly, a three to seven times greater risk of dying, almost twice the likelihood of being re-hospitalized postpartum, a greater likelihood of developing a uterine infection and obstetrical surgical wound complications, a five times higher chance of having persistent pulmonary hypertension, developing cardiopulmonary ethombolic conditions, and a ten times greater likelihood of having a hysterectomy for hemorrhage. Those having a cesarean are also at a 24 to 38 percent vs. 4.5 percent risk of placenta acreta. Risks are even higher with *repeat* cesareans, reports ACOG, naming increased rates of placenta previa and acreta, uterine rupture, injury to internal organs, excessive blood loss necessitating hysterectomy, and maternal death. (Also see Post-Cesarean Discomfort in Recovery in **chapter 19**.)

Are cesareans really needed for all **breech** babies? (See Breech…in **chapter 7**.)

Advantages of Normal, Vaginal Birth

Babies have better Apgars if they have been born vaginally. (See More Choices…**chapter 18**.) They generally do better in comparison to those born by cesarean, because labor is good for babies! Babies born vaginally are much more likely to be born with clear, healthy lungs. For those that choose or must have a cesarean, experiencing labor prior to delivery can be very beneficial for the baby. The stimulating effects of the labor itself, prepares the baby for post-natal life. There are some rare circumstances where laboring prior to a cesarean would be contradicted, such as when a mother is experiencing placenta previa.

Vaginal births are much **less expensive**.

When a baby is born by cesarean, the parents may only get a glimpse of their baby as she is taken away. Often more careful observation and aid is needed by a baby who does not experience the rigors and massaging of regular labor.

Babies born normally are **less likely to be born prematurely** (if they haven't been induced), and so there is much less risk of having babies in the intensive care unit for perhaps even a lengthy amount of time, even after the mother has been discharged.

Recovery for a normal, natural birth is inherently quicker and more comfortable. Transition into parenthood is therefore easier. Studies indicate that women who birth vaginally are generally more satisfied with their experience than women who give birth by cesarean. Women who are more satisfied with their birth experiences are less apt to experience postpartum depression.

Vaginal Birth after Previous Cesarean

If all women who have had unnecessary cesareans had been spared this major surgery during previous births, **think of the number of women in this country today who would not now be being forced into another cesarean**—*forced without legitimate reason*, we might add!

One reason given for compelling more women to have cesarean sections today is the very small risk of uterine rupture.

Very rarely, rupture occurs in a vaginal birth whether or not there has been a previous cesarean.

Women are reportedly at a 0.5 to a 1.0 percent risk of rupture when it comes to having a VBAC. VBAC with a low transverse incision holds almost the same level of risk as having had no previous c-section depending on the reasons for the previous cesarean. **Published reports of women dying from rupture of the uterus due to a vaginal birth after cesarean are extremely rare**, although this was evidently the main concern of doctors before VBAC was proven to be the best alternative after a previous cesarean. **The numbers of casualties due to cesarean birth are much higher (35 in 100,000).**

The term "rupture" may bring to mind frightening images of gushing blood. This is not an accurate picture and is much exaggerated. In fact some "ruptures" are not even discovered until years later when a cesarean is performed. Those so-called ruptures are actually dehiscences or windows, and are simple separations of the flesh which, though benign, were also factored in to the statistical figures of uterine ruptures, making numbers appear much higher than they really were.

Too many women schedule cesareans due to a belief that their bodies somehow just don't work.

There are women who have never had a cesarean who also have uterine ruptures. This number is also very small.

The risk of fetal death among VBACs in one study was 0.038 percent. Considering the fact that no amount of medical intervention can reduce the number to zero percent, this number is small. The chance of a baby dying of causes that do not include rupture is actually twelve times higher. (MacCorkle 2002) Why then are women being forced into risky major surgery against their will?

Do keep in mind, though, that **women who are having a VBAC *are* at a much greater risk of rupture *if* they are being induced, especially with a prostaglandin such as Cytotec!** (see Risks of Inducing...).

Too many women schedule cesareans due to a belief that their bodies do not dilate or just don't work. They fear that because they had difficulty last time, that somehow something must be broken. Again, **women's bodies work!** What actually went wrong last time, anyway? Was the mother by any chance induced far before her body had the hormones and other necessities in place to actually prepare to do the natural work of dilating? What positions were used? Did she have proper nutrition and hydration during labor? Was she "on the clock"? What were her fears during labor that could have caused her to stop progressing? What is the whole story? (See Women's Bodies...in **chapter 3.**)

Those desiring a VBAC can **contact the nearest International Cesarean Awareness Network (ICAN) group** near them. This organization strives to lower the cesarean rate through education and to provide a forum where women and men can express their thoughts and concerns about birth. They assist with healing from past birth experiences, and help parents prepare for future births. Visit their website to find important recommendations for getting the VBAC you wish. To contact ICAN, call 310-542-6400. See resources for other websites on this subject.

Silent Knife and *Open Season* by author **Nancy Wainer Cohen** are both excellent books about vaginal birth after cesarean. Wainer coined the term VBAC years ago and did much for the cesarean prevention movement.

Caregivers and Avoiding a Cesarean

Your choices of caregiver and birthplace are probably the most significant factors in whether you will succeed with your wishes to give birth vaginally after a previous cesarean! If your doctor doesn't support VBAC for normally healthy women and babies, if he/she has the mind frame of, "We'll see, but don't expect anything," or if you are going to be treated like a disaster waiting to happen (IV in place, on the electronic fetal monitor, the timer set, etc.), find someone else—no

Your choices of caregiver and birthplace are probably the most significant factors in whether you will succeed with your wishes to give birth vaginally after a previous cesarean.

matter how wonderful she might seem in every other way. RUN! Forget about walking!

In *Mothering Magazine*, MacCorkle wisely urged, "Given the current political climate regarding VBAC, it is critical that women select their caregivers with caution. Find a caregiver who practices the midwifery model of care. Many healthcare providers pay lip service to a woman's desire for VBAC to gain her business, only to reverse their position as the woman approaches the end of pregnancy. Having a caregiver who truly believes in birth and in VBAC is a major factor in planning for success. Also remember that it is never too late to change caregivers or the planned place of birth. Women have walked out of hospitals mid-labor and changed caregivers even while pushing." (MacCorkle 2002)

There have been women who have actually reported that their doctors have told them that their babies will die unless they agree to a cesarean! Women deserve the *real* answers from physicians who are honest and forthcoming about why they will not aid a woman in a VBAC.

Having a caregiver who truly and emphatically believes in a woman's ability to birth and in VBAC is a major factor in planning for success. Furthermore, all of that extra fear—both theirs and yours—is not conducive to easy birthing. If you haven't found what you are looking for, you can request a file transfer to your new caregiver, and of course it is beneficial to let the former caregiver know, in writing, why you have changed.

Countless women who have had previous cesareans for reasons such as "failure to progress" and "inadequate pelvic dimension" have gone on to have one VBAC after another for *larger* babies than the one they were sectioned for! *Silent Knife* and many other wonderful books and Internet sites contain a multitude of triumphant VBAC birth stories that are worth reading by anyone preparing for a VBAC. Women are standing up and saying, "Hey, enough is enough!"

A VBAC birth isn't much different than any other vaginal birth. Still, a great deal of support is recommended for the woman having a VBAC. Especially—but not only if—you will be birthing in the hospital, get a doula that has all confidence in a woman's ability to give birth vaginally after a cesarean and who will be an encouraging voice throughout your birth.

There are places that are better than others, caregivers that are better than others, choices that are better than others if you want a vaginal birth.

Many women have opted for and *loved* their VBACs at home. When a woman gives birth at home it is called an HBAC (homebirth after cesarean), called HBA2C for her second homebirth and so forth. With the climate the way that it is in the hospital at this time for women wanting to avoid another cesarean, this option is one that is well worth considering. (See At Home... in **chapter 5**.)

Countless women who have had previous cesareans have gone on to have one VBAC after another for larger babies than the one they were sectioned for!

Economic Incentives for High Cesarean Rates

Nancy Wainer Cohen asserts, "*Economic Incentives* are involved: increased earnings for obstetricians—more money for less time, a predictable expenditure of physician time, added length of hospital stay with increased hospital earnings, and greater reimbursement by third-party payment for a cesarean—provide little incentive to support vaginal birth or to adopt a 'wait and see' attitude that could culminate in a vaginal delivery. Several physicians stated that they simply 'couldn't afford not to do cesareans' (Marieskind, 1979) because of fear of malpractice suits or because of time constraints involved in attending deliveries and keeping office hours. Marieskind suggests that a policy of accommodating deliveries to the 'working day' also contributes to the cesarean increase." (Cohen, Silent 1983)

One doctor voiced his opinion that scheduled cesareans would optimize the use of the operating room, allowing the staff to be ready and prepped for their next patient. This time and labor saving technique, the scheduled cesarean, can only be convenient for the hospital and physician.

Thankfully there are those doctors who still have low cesarean rates and who have not instead traded them for high forceps and vacuum extraction rates either!

Scheduled Cesarean Surgery

Many doctors today offer the option to women of electing to give birth by cesarean.

One advantage of a scheduled cesarean is the convenience of knowing when your baby will be born. Another benefit of scheduling a c-section is the avoidance of the work of labor. But when it's all said and done, is a cesarean actually the easy way out?

Most women, however, do not choose a cesarean because of the above reasons. Many are simply doing what their caregiver recommends—without the information necessary to make a wise decision.

Important to consider is that **although elective cesarean section has been touted by some professionals as "the way to go," there are some grave risks involved.** Babies born by elective repeat cesarean are at a 3.55 percent risk of respiratory distress syndrome (a serious, life threatening condition often necessitating NICU time and possibly mechanical ventilation and drug therapy) or/and transient tachypnoea of the newborn, putting them at a seven-fold risk over newborns that are born vaginally. They are also at a five-fold increase for persistent pulmonary hypertension. Prematurity, a grave problem in our hospitals today for which physicians have long been searching for answers is also a well-known risk of elective cesarean section. Though believed to

Babies born by elective repeat cesarean are at a much higher risk for a variety of serious problems.

be under-reported, the incidence of a baby being accidentally cut during a cesarean is reportedly 2 percent overall, and 6 percent in breech babies. Even with all of the risks of forceps, vacuum extraction, and episiotomy, etc., there is still statistically greater risk in choosing an elective cesarean. (MacCorkle 2002)

Beware of those suggesting that cesareans are perfectly safe and healthier than vaginal birth! Cesarean section is *major, abdominal* surgery.

One of the excuses that have been used to encourage women to give birth by elective cesarean section is that it will allow her to avoid pelvic, rectal, and urinary tract damage. This implies that women should sustain all of the risks of major abdominal surgery in order to prevent dysfunctions that are reported by many women who have not even given birth before! What about all of those mothers around us today that have given birth and whose pelvic floors function well? Most women have given birth. To say that most of the women who have urinary incontinence have given birth is like saying that most of the women who have urinary incontinence eat lunch every day!

In fact, one study of a group of nuns, who presumably had never given birth, showed comparable numbers in pelvic floor dysfunction to women who had previously given birth. (Buchsbaum)

ACOG states that pelvic floor injury does not offer sufficient evidence to mandate a change in the standard clinical management of labor and birth, except for women who have had reconstructive pelvic floor surgery, damage, or vaginal prolapse.

There are many factors that are suggested as to why women have urinary incontinence—including such things as being an athlete, obesity, and even having neurological deficiencies. There are certainly things to do to avoid injury during birth. Reports suggest avoiding such things as vacuum extraction and forceps. Avoiding pudendal anesthesia and passing up episiotomy are also advised. (Newman, Diane) Other rough, routine procedures are also discouraged. Strengthening and preparing the pelvic floor muscles with Kegel exercises can be helpful for conditioning the pelvic floor muscles in preparation for and following the birth (the sooner after birth the better).

Cesarean is major abdominal surgery.

Unplanned Cesarean

If, for whatever reason, you do give birth by unplanned cesarean birth, you can still find wonderful reasons to rejoice. This may not be the birth you wanted for you and your baby. But if you will allow yourself to experience the joys of this birth, as you birth in the awareness of the moment and everything around you, continuing to make the best decisions possible in the place where you now find yourself, you will be doing the very best you possibly can for you and your precious baby.

Progressive hospitals may soon allow babies to stay with their parents directly after a cesarean birth.

You will also have a far better chance of being happy with the memory of the way you handled the situation.

Following the suggestions from the birth wish list section in this book about options available for women giving birth by cesarean can help to create a better experience. See Birth Wishes...in **chapter 6**.)

One more word—a great many hospitals routinely insist that you and the baby be away from each other for some time, "for observation" following a cesarean birth. Hopefully there will be a change in this common policy in the future. This is *such a crucial time* for that initial connection with your child. We wouldn't remove newly-born animal babies from their mothers in this way! **A child and her parents need this time together—Apgars go up when babies are held by their mothers after birth!** However, if you find that no one will budge on this, fathers are encouraged to go to the nursery with the baby and bond with her there as much as possible.

Last, but not least, mothers who have given birth by cesarean can still breastfeed! Contact La Leche League with any questions you may have. www.lalecheleague.org

8

To Be or Not to Be Induced

"**I** ALWAYS HAVE TO BE INDUCED. My body just doesn't go into labor by itself." It's a common enough statement in our culture today, but logically how many of our grandmothers and their grandmothers before them had the same problem? Have the bodies of modern women suddenly quit working like they should? If so, maybe we ought to be more concerned. After all, think of all of the women who are conceiving and growing babies within their bodies right now who will in the end get to the point where they will not be able to go into labor on their own! What if medicine suddenly became unavailable and we had all of these women who were "eternally pregnant"? Talk about misery for everyone involved! Seriously, how many women in history have finally died or had their babies die because they just never went into labor?

Labeling Babies "Overdue"

Too many babies are labeled "overdue" or "late." A woman's body does not miraculously conceive, nourish, and grow her baby to a healthy and full maturity only to forget how to get the baby out! **A woman's body was designed to go into labor when the baby and her body are ready—on her *true* "due date."**

It is completely normal especially for first-time mothers to give birth even *weeks after* her *estimated* (estimated by those who *surely* must know) due date. Too many inductions have been initiated unnecessarily only to bring forth a premature baby.

Seven out of ten babies are, by our less than perfect calculations, late. How dare they!

But it's true. Very few babies are born on their estimated date of arrival. Babies can come within a thirty-six to forty-three week time frame, and still be considered within the "normal" range. One woman, who is an example of "normal, though not average," knew her date of conception but gave birth to a healthy nine pound-plus baby *five* weeks after her due date.

Very few babies truly need to be induced! Why not let a woman's body and baby tell her when her true due date really is?

Nature works within its own time frame—but in the end it *does* happen. Likewise, human babies have their own timing! And pregnancy and labor times vary from woman-to-woman and baby-to-baby.

Just as you read about in **chapter 7**, a woman should not be rushed through labor and birth on the Friedman Curve just because someone else behind her needs the room. Neither should a woman be rushed into labor for the convenience of someone else. Even the same cake recipe takes different lengths of time to bake in two different ovens! Babies take different amounts of time to be fully ready for life outside the womb.

Premature and low birth weight babies often carry health problems with them throughout their lives. The March of Dimes has been a leader in working to lower numbers of premature births. Sadly, too many babies have been born prematurely by inductions that have been due to simple lack of patience and a incorrectly calculated due date. Research is showing that babies *need* those final days and hours in the womb.

Why Hurry Babies?

We are a society that does not have a lot of patience; it is true.

To boot, Americans have grown up with a distrust in the ability of women's bodies to give birth. We might fear that the baby is getting too big, or again, that we may never actually go into labor. Another thing that may worry us about an "overdue" baby is that the placenta, the baby's life source, may not still be functioning to capacity. An induction might also be suggested if a woman has a history of short labors and lives a distance from the hospital. Inductions may be demanded by women themselves, because of impatience and discomfort in late pregnancy. Most women are led to believe that induction is safe.

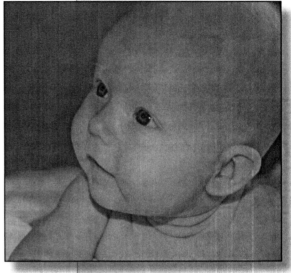

There are times when it truly is necessary to medically induce labor such as when toxemia or diabetes becomes a threat to the mother and baby. And when there is true concern, mothers and babies must receive necessary intervention.

Unfortunately, believe it or not, **one *very* common reason that inductions are performed is for the convenience of an overworked practitioner.** If a woman can be induced in the morning, for example, a busy physician can hope to accomplish office work and visits, go back to the hospital to finish the birth, and be home at a reasonable hour that day. He can also avoid being called at night, on weekends, or on his day off by making sure that a woman has delivered prior to these times. Many hospitals have an induction schedule. In fact, about *44 percent* of all babies are now induced! Just observe the number of babies in a hospital nursery just before the weekend or a holiday. Compare that to how few there are during the actual holiday! **Good caregivers do not put a healthy woman and her baby on a clock**, telling her that her baby must be born by a certain time—or else something terrible will happen.

Unfortunately, too many hospitals still use an assortment of technology and drugs, including those for induction, *routinely*. While most of us are very thankful for technology when it is needed, when it is not needed and it is used to intervene into *natural birth processes*, grave and serious problems can result. **Before long, a woman who has simply been induced may need a whole long list of interventions** with a scene that goes something like the following: Someone decides to simply release the

Trust your body.
Your body knows what to do!
Believe that it will accomplish the task at hand in its own time.

bag of amniotic fluid surrounding the baby "to see if that will get things going." At that moment, a whole series of events are set into motion. It is not uncommon that when this procedure is done, that perhaps—because there is no longer a cushion for the baby's head—the baby will start to show signs of stress. The baby's heart rate goes down, requiring more monitoring (with of course more time in bed for the mother), rather than allowing for much more comfortable, upright, labor-conducive positions. Because of the broken amniotic sac, there are now also dangers of infection and fever if labor is prolonged, particularly if vaginal exams are frequent. The mother is now "on the clock." If labor is not progressing as quickly as caregivers would like, Pitocin is started through an IV. A bit later, if things still are not moving along in a consistent manner, the suggestion of a cesarean comes up. And now, what was once a normal labor has become a medical situation. At this point, major surgery is in the works. Unfortunately, **this type of scene is *not rare at all* when labor is induced** and when interventions into natural processes are initiated.

The above scenario is of course not always the case—many times Birth carries on about her business undaunted, interventions or no interventions, and the baby is soon born safely and soundly to a healthy mother. But we must stop and ask ourselves, when so much is at stake: How smart is it to play with fire?

Parents would do well to search out what is best for their situation, carefully weighing the pros and cons concerning their specific needs. **Synthetic induction can truly be like putting your labor onto a runaway train.**

Induction can be like riding on a runaway train.

Tips for Waiting Peacefully

Aside from the fact that many women can become quite uncomfortable and feel that their patience is being pushed to its absolute limits toward the end of pregnancy, there is a very good case for letting our wise bodies go into labor when they are *ready*. Following are some things that can put our minds at ease:

1. It is a good idea to start a **fetal movement chart** early in the third trimester of pregnancy. If the baby begins to slow down in the amount of movements counted as time goes on, the efficiency of the placenta may be decreasing and the baby may be trying to conserve energy. This is rare, however. Still, your caregiver will be able to compare the earlier counts with the ones closer to your *estimated* due date. It can mainly be used as a source of reassuring any doubts. There is also the "non-stress test," a currently popular test used by doctors that records the baby's heart rate in relation to the baby's movements. The results from the non-stress test when used alone have been known at times to be

wrong. A simple fetal-movement count chart can give an overall picture of how the baby is doing at present.

2. **One of the most important things to do is to be especially careful to eat well.** The placenta, and thus the baby and your birth experience, depend on it. As far as your baby becoming too big, this is a fear that unfortunately has been passed down from the early nineteenth century. (See Women's Bodies…in **chapter 3**.)

3. If you have any reason to question a diagnosis that would result in an induction, you might do well to **get a second opinion**. Sometimes, for example, a woman is told that her amniotic fluid is extremely low only to find out that it is normal from another caregiver. This sort of thing happens often enough that it must be brought to the reader's attention as a possibility to be aware of.

4. It is imperative that you **trust that your body really does know what it is doing**, and that you *will* eventually go into labor. *Your patience is a gift to your baby.*

Inducing Labor with Drugs

There are risks of inducing labor with Pitocin, Cytotec, or other labor-stimulating drugs as well as other procedures.

Pitocin

Pitocin is a synthetic form of the hormone Oxytocin which is naturally made by the body. **As many women who have experienced a birth started or augmented with Pitocin will tell you, Pitocin is not the same as its natural counterpart!** Too many families have learned this the hard way. It often becomes hard to wait at the end of pregnancy. Mothers may become physically uncomfortable, even miserable. The husband is going on a business trip. Or perhaps it's the doctor who is going on vacation—or does not want to be called in the middle of the night. The waiting game isn't an easy one.

Yet **medications that stimulate contractions of the uterus have been well known to over-stimulate the uterus** in a large number of women causing titanic, painful contractions and placing them at risk for placental abruption, uterine rupture, and deprivation of oxygen to the baby.

An epidural is often one of the next steps following the administration of Pitocin or AROM (Artificial Rupture of Membranes) because of the discomfort of the forceful contractions that generally follow these interventions. **Births started synthetically often end in an instrumental delivery of the baby by forceps, vacuum extractor, or c-section**

There is a very good case for letting our wise bodies go into labor when they are ready.

because the baby and mother's body are just not ready, and because the mother is frequently unable to participate in the birth of her own baby due to the epidural.

The use of Oxytocic drugs in labor is also associated with a dangerous pressure on the baby's head (and, though not often, occasionally creating a cranial hemorrhage in the baby). Pitocin-induced babies often have jaundice, and other problems as well due to unhealthy, low birth weights.

Recent studies link Pitocin use in labor with ADHD. (Haussmann and Kurth 2011)

Because of the increased danger of using Pitocin in labor, hospitals insist that a fetal monitor be used—with all of the increased risks of doing so, including the necessity of being stationary during its use. This adds unnecessary risks as well as discomforts.

Unless there is a good reason for these procedures, such as toxemia or diabetes, many caregivers wisely *discourage* medical induction.

Pitocin can be a valuable drug for use with postpartum hemorrhage. However, it is usually *routinely* employed to correct a hemorrhage after the *routine* use of traction (tugging) has been used on the cord to hurry the detachment of the placenta. These hemorrhages would generally not otherwise have occurred if the woman's body was allowed to release the placenta on its own. This though, requires time—something that a hospital staff does not have a large supply of. Sometimes, even if the placenta has been left alone, there is still bleeding that needs attention—and for which Pitocin is usually quite effective. If a woman has chosen not to have an IV, Pitocin is easily given by injection. As a precautionary measure, the uterus is often massaged through the abdominal wall by caregivers or the woman herself to keep the uterus contracting and to encourage closing of the placental site.

Cytotec

Although not approved by the Food and Drug Administration (FDA) for use in childbirth, Cytotec (pronounced Si-to-tec), also known as Misoprostol, is one of the main drugs used to jump-start labor today. What's more, most women are not made aware of the fact that it has not been approved by the FDA.

Cytotec has been connected to many cases of emergency hysterectomies, cervical and perineal tearing, brain-damaged babies, stillbirths, newborn deaths, and deaths of mothers. However, because single reports have not been compiled into one study, most practitioners are probably not fully aware of the dangers of Cytotec.

For the greatest number of women whose labors are stimulated with Cytotec, live birth usually results within 24 hours. It is quite effective and very inexpensive. Nevertheless, because of its known risks,

Your patience is a gift to your baby.

Cytotec administration requires a woman to stay in the hospital for observation once it has been given.

While Cytotec has been approved by the FDA for *peptic ulcers*, the drug's manufacturer, Searle, prints the following clear warning on its label: "A major adverse effect of the obstetrical use of Cytotec is hyperstimulation of the uterus which may progress to uterine tetany with marked impairment of uteroplacental blood flow, uterine rupture (requiring surgical repair, hysterectomy, and/or salpingo-oophorectomy), or amniotic fluid embolism. Pelvic pain, retained placenta, severe genital bleeding, shock, fetal bradycardia, and fetal and maternal death have been reported. There may be an increased risk of uterine tachysystole, uterine rupture, meconium passage, meconium staining of the amniotic fluid, and cesarean delivery due to uterine hyperstimulation with the use of higher doses of Cytotec; including the manufactured 100 mcg tablet. The risk of uterine rupture increases with advancing gestational age and with prior uterine surgery, including Cesarean delivery. Grand multiparity also appears to be a risk factor for uterine rupture. The effects of Cytotec on later growth, development, and functional maturation of the child, when Cytotec is used for cervical ripening or induction of labor, have not been established." (Cullen 2002)

What warning could be clearer than that? Well then, why is it being used in large numbers of women today? Even though **Cytotec has never been approved by Searle or the FDA for obstetrical use**, when a drug is approved for one use, it can be prescribed for any other indication. This is legal, and *no additional testing needs to be done*! Women are usually not warned of these possibilities. Today's women are the guinea pigs of years of experimentation from which findings will very likely (and often do), go unreported and unpublished. We do know that **women attempting VBAC (vaginal birth after cesarean) have a 5.6 percent risk of uterine rupture when they are given Cytotec, which is a *28 fold* increase in risk of uterine rupture!** Still, even though its use has clearly been shown to cause injury and death to women, the use of Cytotec only continues to climb.

There is also a disagreement about the way Cytotec should be administered. Some caregivers insert it vaginally inside the cervix, some behind the cervix, some rectally, and some by mouth. It is usually given in inaccurately sliced tablets, as the pills are not scored. In the past a whole tablet was given. But when problems began surfacing, the dosage was decreased. There is no agreement as to what amount is appropriate. **When the tablet has been absorbed by the woman's body, it is no longer possible to remove it in the event of a negative reaction.**

In 2000, the manufacturer of Cytotec sent letters to 200,000 caregivers warning that its off-label use had caused death in mothers and babies, uterine rupture, hysterectomy, retained placenta, severe vaginal bleeding, shock and pelvic pain. **One-third of hospitals have reportedly forbidden any further use of Cytotec to induce labor—yet many hospitals still do use it.**

Cervidil is another drug that is similar to Cytotec. Although it can be removed when complications begin to appear, the risks are still great.

Numerous studies show that women who have had a previous cesarean are *not* at a significantly increased risk of uterine rupture in comparison with their non-cesarean counterparts. Giving birth vaginally is much safer than a subsequent cesarean—*but* a woman who is having a VBAC is at greatly increased risk for uterine rupture when induced by Cytotec and Pitocin—particularly Cytotec. **In fact, the American College of Obstetricians and Gynecologists, itself, specified in 1999 that Cytotec should no longer be used in women who have had a previous cesarean.**

Induction usually does not work well if a woman's body is not already on the verge of labor. Once started, the woman is "on the clock" and if she hasn't had her baby within a certain amount of time, she is likely headed for a cesarean for "failure to progress."

Stripping the Membranes

Stripping the membranes is a procedure sometimes performed by a caregiver during a late pregnancy prenatal vaginal exam. This may encourage labor to begin, but often it only produces an uncomfortable (some say extremely uncomfortable) exam, perhaps some bleeding, and a few hours of cramps. **Too many times, though, this procedure is performed without permission from, or explanation to, the pregnant mother—as if there is no reason for either.** If the woman has not consented to this—and too often she has not, prior to its being done—it is certainly a violation of her body!

Rupturing the Bag of Waters Artificially

Artificial rupture of membranes (AROM) is one intervention that is routinely and frequently performed. It may be used to induce labor, establish a more effectual labor pattern, or to hurry a labor along.

The procedure is done by tearing the bag that holds the amniotic fluid that surrounds the baby. The instrument that is used resembles a crochet hook. The breaking of the bag is not painful in itself to either mother or baby, but soon afterward, **contractions often become extremely intense.**

AROM may also cause trauma to the baby's head because of the loss of the cushion that the fluid provides. This can cause a baby's heart rate to begin to decelerate. Now, without the cushion of the water, the baby's weight rests at the bottom of the uterus, with the possibility of compressing the cord if it lies beneath the baby. This is dangerous because oxygen to the baby is therefore decreased. **Before long, the mother and baby may be on the road to more and more invasive interventions.**

Artificially breaking the bag of waters also comes with the serious risk of cord prolapse, where the umbilical cord drops into the vagina along with the amniotic fluid, and the baby rests on the cord and constricts oxygen flow to the baby. An emergency cesarean is usually performed.

Yet another drawback to allowing the bag of waters to be artificially released is that it puts more of a time limit on the labor. If a baby hasn't been born within a certain amount of time, some caregivers feel that infection may become an issue. **Once the bag is released, labor is "on the clock."**

There can also be a decrease in the pH of newborns when an early amniotomy is performed.

Of lesser consequence, but nevertheless worth bearing in mind, after having their bag of waters ruptured some women dislike the feeling of continuously dripping into a pad.

Some other advantages to keeping the bag of waters intact if they have not released naturally on their own, are that **amniotic fluid provides warmth, a cushion, and a lubricant so that injury may be prevented to both mother and baby during movement.**

Many practitioners believe that the labor process should only be hastened when there is good reason to do so and never out of mere convenience for their own schedule.

Women facing induction by AROM or any other method would do well to consider being tested for fetal maturity, amount of amniotic fluid, possible intrauterine conditions, heart rate, position, and station of the baby to assess whether induction would be successful.

The fewer the vaginal checks during labor the better, as this prevents the accidental (or intentional—without first seeking the woman's permission) breaking of the waters during the examination.

Trust your body and, unless there is very good reason not to, allow your water to release on its own, in the way and in the time it was meant to!

Amniotic fluid provides warmth, a cushion, and a lubricant for both mother and baby during labor.

Inducing Labor Naturally

Remember that probably no form of induction (even by synthetic means) will work very well unless you are on the verge of labor anyway. This is one reason that if you are induced medically before your body is ready you might be on the road for a cesarean due to "failure to progress."

But if you are facing an induction, trying natural induction methods first may help you avoid medical induction.

At the least, natural methods can help to give you a bit of a head start and help to soften and perhaps thin out the cervix a bit so that the induction has more of a chance of being effective.

Be sure to ask your caregiver before using any of the following. There are some things Dad can help with.

- Nipple stimulation releases labor-starting hormones. (Tug and/or twirl—one side at a time only. When a contraction starts, continue stimulation for only a minute into contraction and stop. Wait 5 minutes and start again.)
- Walking
- Orgasm
- Semen on the cervix
- Use Clary Sage essential oil. (Put a few drops on a cotton ball and put it near your pillow, or use it in massage on acupressure points.)
- Get your baby into the right position, especially if you are having a lot of ineffective contractions. This can work wonders. (See Back Labor…in **chapter 13.**)
- Stimulate foot, leg, and ankle acupressure points.
- Talk, write, or draw about fears and issues that might be bothering you. (See Mind/Body…in **chapter 15.**)
- Try herbs and homeopathic remedies (consult an Herbalist/Homeopath).
- You can try castor oil, but it can cause terrible cramps, nausea, vomiting, and spastic uterine contractions on top of tasting awful—consider whether you want to deal with all of that in labor.
- Use acupuncture. This is reportedly *very* effective especially if you are nearing your due date. You might consult a chiropractor to find someone who offers this service.
- Go in for Foot Zoning or Craniosacral therapy.

Most important, as long as you and the baby are doing fine (if fetal movement counts are good), remember that the majority of babies go past their due dates and that "**estimated due dates**" are only guesses. **Each mom and baby is different.** Mothers with longer menstruation cycles may actually have a later than calculated due-time and so forth. If her mother had longer pregnancies, she may also. Every woman is different and every pregnancy is different. Too many babies are born prematurely. Although it is hard at the end of pregnancy (when you may be so uncomfortable, and others continually ask if you are "ever going to have that baby?"), *patience is truly a gift of love for your baby!*

Keeping Track of Your Baby's Activity

It is to your advantage to keep a record of your unborn baby's activity because if he/she is remaining active, the placenta is most likely functioning as well as ever. Then, even if you pass your *estimated* due date, you and your caregiver can be reassured that the baby is doing well and that you do not need to be induced with any of the inherent risks and discomforts of doing so.

This could be one of the best things you do to ensure a normal and easier labor.

Use the chart here. Begin about three weeks before your estimated due date.

	Mon	Tues	Wed	Thur	Fri	Sat	Sun
Week 1							
Week 2							
Week 3							
Week 4							
Week 5							
Week 6							

1. Each evening, on a separate piece of paper, write the time you begin counting movements (for example, 8:15 PM).
2. When you have counted ten movements, write that time down (for example, 8:45 PM).
3. Now figure out how long it took to get ten movements (in this case, 30 minutes) and record it in the appropriate box in the chart.

Keep this record *every* night until your baby is born.

If it takes more than two hours to reach ten movements, call your caregiver.

If each night it takes longer and longer to get ten movements, call your caregiver.

9

Procedures and Tests

BLOOD PRESSURE TESTS, amniocentesis, ultrasound, gestational diabetes screening, electronic fetal monitoring, prenatal vaginal examinations, GBS testing, blood sampling from you and/or your baby, abdominal examinations, newborn tests, and more. How can you know which procedures and tests will be helpful to you and your baby and which will be potentially harmful?

We have covered the basic and common procedures for labor and birth in this book. But we have chosen not to include a whole assortment of prenatal tests. And new procedures are continually introduced.

In your future probably lies a great many decisions concerning dentistry, nutrition, surgery, medications, house and car buying, and on and on. Before making any important decision, it is wise to turn to trustworthy sources for further information as you weigh the pros and cons.

You will probably have a number of tests and procedures suggested to you throughout the pregnancy, labor and birth, and postpartum.

Questions to Ask

The following are questions to assist you in finding answers now and in the future:

1. How common is the abnormality that you would be tested for?

   _____

   _____

   _____

   _____

2. If an abnormality is found, what can be done to correct it? If nothing, will the results of the test serve only to create worry for you?

   _____

   _____

   _____

3. How accurate is the test? Many have a wide range of error, so rather than stilling your qualms, could the test actually cause more (often unnecessary) fears?

   _____

   _____

   _____

4. While testing might lead to a sense of security, what is the possibility that the test will tell you that everything is fine when really it is not?

   _____

   _____

   _____

5. What is the range of normal for this procedure? Some people normally have lower blood pressure than the average person. What is normal for you? And do you agree with your caregiver's definition of what is normal?

   _____

   _____

   _____

6. What will be the psychological impact of agreeing to the test? Many women find that waiting for results can be extremely stressful.

_____

_____

_____

7. Why has this test or procedure been ordered? Is there truly cause for concern or is it a test that everyone receives? Is it conducted routinely for liability purposes—primarily to cover your caregiver?

_____

_____

_____

8. Is the procedure used for all women "just in case" even though only a very few people experience the abnormality? Just a few examples are requiring all birthing women to be on an IV, and withholding food and fluids in labor. For babies, the Vitamin K, eye ointment, the PKU test, and routine antibiotics for all are a few interventions given to the mass to protect a small few. Say that a particular hospital, or perhaps your doctor or midwife, has just had a bad experience. Their fear that this rare event will happen again may lead them to feel particularly strongly that all women should have a particular intervention. Too, most caregivers are very busy people and a great many do not stay up on current research. Some feel an urgency to do what fellow practitioners are doing for a variety of reasons. Others cling to what they were taught when they were trained, despite recent information. This does an undeniable disservice to birthing women and their babies.

_____

_____

_____

9. What are the physical risks of this test or procedure? Do the benefits outweigh the risks?

_____

_____

_____

10. Will a particular test serve only to medicalize your birth? Will the outcome of a test affect future choices? One example is agreeing to electronic fetal monitoring during your labor. Countless women have been given cesarean sections because it appeared that the baby might be in distress—only to discover later that the baby was fine.

_____

_____

_____

11. If you agree to a procedure, might it lead to another intervention and yet another? Just one illustration of "the intervention cascade" might start with induction of labor which necessitates monitoring. Monitoring leads to more time in bed. More time in bed can lead to a less comfortable labor. A less comfortable labor might lead to a desire for medication for discomfort. Medication might cause distress in the baby and can make it difficult for a woman to feel when and how to push. Forceps may be required. An episiotomy must be cut. It is possible that the baby or mother might be injured due to a forceps delivery. The risks of needing a cesarean section are increased. Tests might also lead to further interventions.

_____

_____

_____

12. What sort of possibilities might occur if you decide against this intervention? How likely is each of these? If this possibility did occur, what could be done to deal with the situation?

_____

_____

_____

13. Has the intervention actually been shown to work? What percentage of the time does it do what it was designed to do?

_____

_____

_____

14. What would happen if you decided to wait awhile and then re-evaluate the situation?

_____

_____

Which tests are right/not right for you and your baby?

Some caregivers believe that it is safest for all women to undergo all routine interventions.

Other caregivers believe that individual women have the right to make these decisions themselves, based on their own circumstances. They are happy to discuss each of these procedures with the woman. You may be requested to sign a release form if you wish to refuse a test or procedure. This again is simply to protect the caregiver or birth place. But it could be the best trade-off for being able to avoid an unnecessary intervention that is only in place to protect the facility or caregiver.

Please note that we are certainly not encouraging you *not* to have *any* tests. Some could be very valuable. The bottom line is, which tests are right, or not right, for you? Don't let anyone pressure you. **It is you, and quite possibly your baby, that will deal with the end results of your choices, whatever they may be.**

"High Risk"

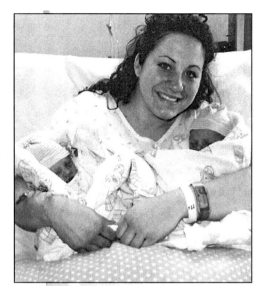

In today's obstetrics, it is common to classify women into the categories of "high risk" and "low risk."

Some factors for classification into the groups "high risk" and "low risk" are more objective and evidence-based than others.

Before clumping everyone into the same ball of wax, one must ask what the contingencies for being placed within a certain division are, and whether they are accurate for evaluating a woman's *specific, individual* needs.

For example, what about expecting twins, being obese, having had a previous cesarean? Should these be reasons for categorizing a woman as "high-risk"—even if she has no other true complications that would represent a true problem?

Should a woman having her first baby at, or over the age of, thirty-five be considered "high risk"? Further questioning might give us a better picture. Does she have a regular exercise program and a wholesome diet? Is she otherwise healthy? Life expectancy and general health is better now than in our grandmothers' day.

What about a woman who is overweight? Better indications of potential trouble would be whether her blood pressure and blood sugar levels are abnormal. Does she exercise regularly and follow good nutrition? Is she otherwise healthy?

If a mother is expecting twins, does she really need to be treated as "high risk" if her pregnancy is normal in other ways? Sometimes when babies are multiples, one or more of them will be breech. Some multiple pregnancies are treated by a practitioner as "high risk" simply because it is a multiples pregnancy. Depending on the pregnancy itself, a multiples birth does not necessarily warrant its being placed directly into the "high risk" category. Women have been giving birth to multiples for ages. It is simply a variation of normal (meaning that there are a variety of circumstances in which birth can still be normal and safe). Lots of breech multiples have been born safely at home over the centuries to the present time. Since the alternative would be a cesarean (which holds greater risks than does breech birth), and since most homebirth midwives are trained at assisting at a breech birth (of course also depending on other considerations) homebirth can be a very good choice for mothers expecting multiples. (See Breech ... in **chapter 7**.)

Some conditions such as having experienced preterm labor with past pregnancies, or such things as diabetes, toxemia, etc. do indicate the necessity for more vigilant care.

But what can a woman—who is *considered* "high risk" for situations that actually would not prove to be a problem—do to avoid a birth that is filled unnecessarily with interventions?

Too many labors are tampered with simply due to protocol and without consideration for more applicable rationale.

First, lifestyle choices are important to consider. Exercise and a healthy diet can help to lower blood pressure and blood sugar levels, reduce fatigue, and improve one's state of mind. Ample rest is also essential to a healthy pregnancy. These and other healthful efforts might even eliminate a problem she has been experiencing all together.

Second, it is helpful for the mother to make mindful choices about her health care team. Finding a midwife or doctor who is watchful, but who is not overly anxious (treating her as if she will explode at any minute) is indispensable. Place of birth is also important to consider. What type of midwives or nurses is a particular birth center or hospital known to have? Hospital protocol plays a consequential part in her care as well.

Consider a woman who is having a vaginal birth after cesarean who had a low transverse incision. A VBAC holds almost the same level of risk as having had no previous c-section, depending on the reasons for the previous cesarean. Let's say that she and the baby are healthy in all ways and that there are no other indications for concern. It is important for this woman to find a midwife/doctor and birth place that use evidence-based care and who avoid the unnecessary—and even harmful—interventions imposed upon otherwise normal, healthy women in some hospitals today.

Too many labors are tampered with *simply due to protocol* and without consideration for more applicable rationale.

Interestingly, evidence shows that midwifery care can be an excellent choice for women in some types of high-risk pregnancies. As well, midwives are often better able to attend to the greater needs for support—due to emotional vulnerability and anxiety so common in women in high-risk pregnancies—than are physicians with their cramped schedules. Women who choose those midwives who provide more personalized care can increase the possibilities of having a normal birth even in high-risk cases. In fact, both normal and high-risk pregnancies benefit from midwifery care.

Visiting with a few midwives (Homebirth and/or CNM) can give you a better idea of whether midwifery care is an option for you.

10

Being a Partner in Your Care

A S A WOMAN HOLDING GENERATIONS within her body, you have certain rights and responsibilities. If something you have been told just doesn't seem right, do some study about it. If what is being suggested isn't based on facts and if it is not in your best interests, seek elsewhere until you find the answers to your questions. Is each policy in *your* best interest, or is it in place only to cover the caregiver and/or birthplace?

If something you have been told just doesn't seem right, be sure to study it out.

Understanding Your Rights and Responsibilities

It is your **right** to obtain honest and complete information and to ask for time to think about things. Decisions should be yours to make. You should be able to refuse **anything** (any procedures, drugs, etc.). You have the right to be with your baby and have family members with you no matter what.

It's your **responsibility** to be informed, to educate yourself, and to make conscientious decisions about your care. It is your duty to ask questions if something is unclear, and to ask for what you want. **It is also essential that you pleasantly, but** *assertively* **(as opposed to** *aggressively* **or** *passively***),** let your caregiver know that you approve or disapprove of the care they are giving. Remember, you are a team!

It is *helpful* to speak clearly and kindly with your caregivers, and to make arrangements when you schedule an appointment for extra time if you need it. It is also beneficial to have your questions written down before an appointment so you don't forget what topics you want to discuss. Be sure that there is enough time allowed for your needs. Tell your caregiver early on in the appointment that you have questions for him or her. If the list is long, you may need to discuss them over several visits.

You can be an assertive, educated partner in your care.

Finding the Power Within

How do you feel when you are meeting with your caregiver? Do you feel like you are a listened to and taken seriously? How do you feel about your relationship with those you have hired to serve you?

Being an active partner in your care involves finding the power within yourself to do what may not always be easy. **A look at the contrasts in power between caregivers and "care-receivers" is most interesting.**

Following are some insights into the overall reasons why some women have found it difficult to find the power within to birth their babies themselves:

At prenatal appointments and at the birth, the caregiver stands upright, composed, often prestigiously dressed while the woman is lying down, partly naked in a borrowed gown. If in labor, she may be without makeup or without her hair styled as usual.

The caregiver has information that the woman doesn't have and sometimes uses medical vocabulary that the woman doesn't understand. The knowledge that the woman has about what is going on within her—that which the caregiver doesn't have—is often not considered important.

The woman must rely on interpretation by the caregiver as to what is going on in her own body. The caregiver uses tools and machines.

The caregiver is primarily in control of the situation. He/she is in a position of strength and authority while the woman may not feel that she is in a particularly strong position at all. The caregiver is not in pain while the woman is most often not the most comfortable she has ever been.

And the caregiver is also not in any physical danger. The woman may feel as if she is, and is oftentimes distressed and anxious.

A woman is usually on the caregiver's turf.

This contrast in power can cause a woman to feel weak and inept without exactly knowing why. This is precisely the opposite of how a woman who is giving birth needs to feel in order to give birth joyfully and with strength!

Becoming More Powerful

Following are some tips to help you feel and become more powerful and active in your own care and that of your baby:

Consider your birthing place. How do you feel when you are there? Is this truly where you want to give birth? Research your type of birth place as to whether or not you will get the kind of birth you want in this environment.

Consider your caregiver. Do you feel powerful when you are with him/her? Do you feel as if you give your power to him/her, in a sense, when you are in his/her presence? When you are choosing your caregiver, search carefully for someone that will be a good match for you. Ask questions. Interview caregivers—this is your birth and your baby, and you should have every right to be in charge and make decisions that you feel are best for your baby and yourself. Don't be so worried about offending someone that you are afraid to ask for, and work for, what you need and want. Find your voice and use it effectively. Again, sometimes it is necessary to be assertive; not domineering, overbearing, or pushy, but to pursue what you want and to boldly speak up and work for it.

Become educated! This book is a good place to start. Find out about any proposed tests or procedures from books and resources that give you the *full* story, not merely the ones that imply, "This is a totally safe procedure. Don't worry yourself about it. We will take care of everything." You owe it to yourself and your baby to know more!

Prepare your birth wish list.

Hire a doula to support you, assist you with comfort measures, and to help you in obtaining your wishes.

> A woman can give birth joyfully and with strength!

Remember that your body was made to give birth. Generally, a woman does not need to have someone *deliver* her baby for her. The close observation and assistance of a caregiver can be invaluable. But *you are the one having the baby.* **Don't let anyone take your ability to do so away from you.**

Consider avoiding pain medications, as these can greatly decrease your abilities to deal with your labor and to birth your baby without assistance.

Choose upright positions for your labor and birth. You will have more physical power to birth your baby. This also encourages the caregiver to deal with you as a *whole* person.

Find the strength within to get what you need! Why have we let this power be taken? Why, even today, do so many women stand back, oblivious to the circumstances of our day? Why are we allowing so many cesareans and other things to be done to us without our informed consent? *Why* are we giving away the power of receiving our very children from our own bodies? Isn't it time to take back our power?

Being Informed

You deserve honest, trustworthy information.

Question everything! Look at where your information comes from. If a company is sponsoring a pamphlet, it is probably safe to assume that their first intention is to sell a product. For instance, those promotional diaper bags with ads, free formula samples, and "information" given when you check out of the hospital are not just nice little gifts after all. You can bet that they probably aren't the best place to get information on breastfeeding!

Expect more than the implied, "Of course it's safe. Don't worry. Just leave it to the professionals." You and your family deserve for you to be educated and to know the answers fully.

Don't accept everything you are told just because someone in a position of authority is saying it. Use the list under the heading "Questions to Ask" at the end of this chapter as you search for answers. Consider carefully every procedure that is routine. *Any intervention, large or small, can disturb the birth process and cause harm to you or your baby.* Be sure anything introduced is a necessity!

Find out about your caregiver's beliefs and her rates of medical intervention. If your caregiver gives episiotomies 84 percent of the time, expect an 84 percent chance of having an episiotomy! Care differs from caregiver to caregiver. Your challenge is to find a caregiver whose care matches the kind of care you want.

One way to tell what kind of philosophies your caregiver has is to look at what kind of information your caregiver supplies you with.

Some caregivers' offices offer literature that has been prepared in a manner so as not to scare you. Therefore, not all of the information is presented. Selecting a caregiver that supports your involvement in the process of information gathering is important. For example, does the literature you were given on amniocentesis, the early pregnancy test, state that this procedure has resulted in 14,000 fetal losses to miscarriage per year? Does it tell you that The American Diabetes Association does not recommend screening of all women for gestational diabetes and that this test can actually be harmful?

You are not a child after all. Always remember that, while your caregiver has access to certain information, **you** are the only one that has passage to the *inner* information about you! It's crucial to be active in the decision-making. So be sure your caregiver is comfortable with your active role.

Don't forget that your caregiver works for *you*. You are their *client*, and a *partner* in your care.

Does your caregiver make decisions with or without you? Some caregivers, for example, feel that it is their right to "strip the membranes" without telling the woman what they are doing. (See Stripping … in chapter 8.) Some will order tests and simply tell the woman when to go in for them, without discussing them with her—as if she really has no reason to consider the decision at all.

Caregivers, when it comes down to it, are *human*! They make mistakes too, no matter how skilled and qualified they are. With their harried schedules it can be easy to miss details that are obvious to a woman. **She must feel comfortable being a team player. Her role is vital!**

There are times when procedures are necessary. Really understanding the procedure can help you to know more about your further options.

Here are a few questions and thoughts to ponder as you embark on obtaining further knowledge about your options:

Who is paying for this information you are reading/studying, to be produced and made available to you? Do they have an ulterior interests for providing you with this information?

What philosophies does the person who is offering this information have? When you inquire of them **are they willing to expound upon their beliefs** or do they quickly dismiss the issue?

If your caregiver or someone else is offering information, are they **willing to talk about where it comes from**? If not, how open will they be when it comes to discussing and making decisions with you—especially in the "thick of things"?

How balanced is the information? Does your source rely on statistics that seem frightening (but which are actually in your favor), knowing that most people will picture themselves as one of the one percent of those that this rare event will happen to? Do they leave out the facts about the other side of the coin? Do they give you the whole picture?

You are the only one who has passage to the inner information about you!

Can the information be verified? If the information (perhaps from TV, newspapers, the Internet, and even parenting magazines) cannot be supported by evidence, studies, long term results, etc., it might simply be the opinion or agenda of the writer—nothing more.

Does the book, magazine, handout, childbirth educator, caregiver **offer further resources** for more information on the subject?

Even if your source seems to be very trustworthy, does the information **feel like it's correct?** Does it fit with what you already believe deep within yourself?

Does this information seem to imply that "everyone" is making this choice? Does it insinuate that you should do likewise (whether or not you want to, or it is right for you)? What historical events can you think of where large groups of people followed something or someone who led them into disastrous circumstances? Each of these followers was his own individual. It would surely have served them well to stop and think on their own for a moment.

Throughout life in other various avenues, you will be given opportunities to learn more about your family's health. Getting into the habit of taking charge and learning all you can about something gives you the chance to make educated choices about many things that will impact those you care about the most. **You can and should be allowed the opportunity to be the major player in this, *your birth*, and in all aspects of *your health* and that of *your family's*. In reality, you simply cannot afford to do otherwise.**

You deserve to be treated with respect, whether you decide to accept or decline a course of action.

Questions to Ask

The following questions are helpful for finding out about any testing or procedures that are suggested during your pregnancy, labor, and after the baby is born and for deciding whether or not you will accept them.

You do not need to ask all these questions; you may choose one or a few from the list.

You do have the right to *be informed* and to *give—or not give—consent* to *any* intervention. No one, not even an authority figure, has the entitlement to do anything to you that you have not agreed to and/or do not fully understand, except perhaps in an emergency situation or when you are unable to make a decision for yourself. Though strongly stated, it is something to keep in mind. This is *your* body and *your* baby and *you* are the one who is responsible for making the decisions.

Remember, you deserve to be treated with respect—whether you decide to accept or decline a course of action.

Select those questions appropriate to your circumstances:

What are the *benefits* of this procedure, and what are the *risks*?

Do the *advantages* outweigh the *disadvantages*?

How accurate is this procedure/test?

What other procedures might we end up needing, and what would we do differently, as a result?

What are some alternatives that we could try first or instead?

What would happen if we decided not to do it?

What would happen if we waited an hour or two before doing it?

Some tips for getting answers

After receiving answers to the above questions, it can be extremely helpful to ask, "Can I think about it for a little while?" While helping to prevent an awkward situation and giving you time and freedom to think, it can also provide time to study and seek out further information to help you assess what you really want to do. Your doula is one source who can offer additional insights and explanations about the procedures. Only in the most urgent of circumstances (which are rare) will there not be time to talk or think about a certain intervention that has been suggested.

Again, it is important to speak clearly and good-naturedly with your caregivers. Sometimes it is necessary to be assertive—not domineering, overbearing, or pushy—but to pursue what you want and to boldly speak out and work for what you want.

When you schedule an appointment with your midwife/doctor, make arrangements for extra time if you are going to need it for any questions you have for him/her. Tell your caregiver early on in the appointment that you have questions. Write your questions down so you don't forget what you need to discuss. And if the list is long, you may need to discuss your questions over several visits.

The above questions are also helpful to keep handy to be used throughout your life and the life of your family as issues for other kinds of care present themselves!

Be sure to slip this book into your bag before you leave for the hospital so that you can use it as a reference as necessary.

Adapted with permission from Penny Simkin.

11

Choosing a Caregiver

THERE ARE SOME outstanding caregivers in both midwifery and obstetrics who devote their lives to making sure women and babies receive safe, evidence-based, gentle, and respectful care. Perhaps one of them introduced you to this book. Women are wise to seek out these practitioners.

Types of Caregivers

Caregivers for birthing families may be divided into several categories: homebirth midwives, certified nurse midwives, obstetricians, and family physicians.

Homebirth Midwives

If you believe that women were made to give birth, and if you have the desire to birth with as few interventions as possible, a direct-entry midwife could be your best choice. Homebirth midwives are caregivers that attend families with low-risk pregnancies at home. Midwives are the only professionals whose credentials and qualifications are based solely on serving the childbearing woman. They are trained in both normal birth and emergencies. A midwife often spends time educating a woman about her *own* ability to give birth. Midwives care for women prenatally, generally allowing an hour or so per appointment. Because of this, she comes to know well the needs of the family. She serves the birthing family exclusively throughout their labor and birth. Often one or more midwives work together as a team.

Certified Nurse Midwives

A CNM most often works in the hospital. Usually women, these caregivers work with a back-up doctor. Often they provide a bit more time at prenatal visits than do doctors, and usually attend a woman throughout a larger portion of her labor in the hospital, rather than arriving just for the delivery of the baby as most physicians do. As with all types of caregivers, there are varying philosophies between nurse midwives, some being more midwife, others being more nurse. In a few states, certified nurse midwives and/or doctors are allowed to assist families at homebirths.

Obstetricians and Family Physicians

If you have a truly high-risk pregnancy, your best choice may be an obstetrician who specializes in high-risk pregnancies.

A family physician becomes familiar with the needs of your family, and ideally he/she will be interested in all aspects of your health, not just your pregnancy. A family doctor continues to care for you and the baby after the birth, as the child's pediatrician. A family doctor can serve as your doctor at your birth. If complications occur, an obstetrician or other specialist may be called in, but your family doctor will still be in charge of your case.

Because of restrictions on time, doctors are usually unable to spend more than ten minutes with their clients at a prenatal visit, and may feel pressured to expedite a birth. With the way that doctors must practice, a woman typically only sees her doctor briefly during her labor and then again only when it comes time to actually give birth.

Importance of a Good Match

When it comes to the kind of experience you and your baby will have, the decision of who your caregiver will be is as essential a choice to make wisely as is where you give birth.

Some people choose a caregiver simply because he has a beautiful office, goes to their church, was their mother's doctor, or because he is kind or even handsome, though they don't know much about him/her beyond that. Sometimes the only qualification is that the doctor is a woman.

But it is important to find a professional whose philosophies match yours *closely*. You want to be sure that decisions are made in a way that you will feel are best for you and your family. You deserve the best!

Interviewing caregivers can help you to decide whom you want to hire. Some caregivers want you to schedule a prenatal appointment just to talk to them. You should at least be able to make an appointment to talk while fully dressed. A physical examination and anything else can wait until you've made your choice!

See **Appendix D** for questions to consider when choosing your caregiver.

Hopefully you will easily find, or have already found, a satisfactory match! There are a lot of wonderful caregivers in the United States.

If you are having qualms, it is important to know that it's really never too late to find a good match until after your baby is born.

You, of course, want the very best care—even if it will mean a bit of sacrifice and creativity in figuring out how to change to another caregiver mid-pregnancy.

It might also be wise to look within yourself. Are you too picky? Sometimes you may find that a caregiver may not be *everything* you would want, but he/she *is* the best around that matches your philosophy. If he/she is willing to work with you and serve you to the best of his/her conscience, he/she may be your best choice.

If you find yourself changing from caregiver to caregiver, the reason may lie in the fact that you are choosing the wrong *type* of caregiver all together. If you can obtain your wishes better in another *place* or with a *different kind* of caregiver, why not make it easier on everyone, including yourself, and seek out whatever option will best meet your desires and needs—and those of your baby?

Who your caregiver will be, is one of the most crucial decisions you will make.

You do not need to stay with a caregiver just because you started there or because she was your doctor at your last birth. What you needed previously may not be what you need now.

If you do have to pay some cash out of pocket and you don't have a lot of money, is it still impossible? Most of the choices or options are financially available to you in some way.

Some women realize after their birth that they knew deep within that something was not right in their relationship with their caregiver but for the sake of saving face, or money, or in order not to hurt feelings, they stayed.

You can be one of those that prepare the way for others who think like you. What you tactfully ask for may influence what caregivers will be willing to provide. You can help people that come after you by writing a letter and telling the caregiver what you liked or what you would have changed.

Do, of course, make sure the caregiver you would choose will be able to take you as a client before bidding your previous one goodbye. And unless you are sure there will be no hard feelings, it might be a good idea to check and see if the two caregivers are closely acquainted before making a decision.

It might seem like something that would take a great deal of courage, but just as women withdraw their business from a store or a home construction contractor who is not meeting their expectations, you have the right to do so in this situation as well. Women have even changed caregivers during labor because they weren't happy! The sooner the better, though. We deserve to have people around us who will give the best service.

12

Taking Care of Yourself and Your Baby

RESPONSIBILITY FOR THIS new human being starts long before you give birth. Right now she is depending on you to do what she cannot do for herself. It is up to you to prepare a safe and nurturing pregnancy and birth. You and your baby are worth the effort.

Diet and Exercise

Do not underestimate the importance that nutrition plays in your pregnancy and labor. **You have only one chance to produce the body that your child will occupy for a lifetime, and the fuel you give your body can have a huge impact on the health of your baby, yourself, and your birth.** Dieting, which some caregivers still recommend to a degree, is not a good idea. Good nutrition is common sense.

A good diet helps with the formation, implantation, and growth of the placenta, muscular development of the uterus, expansion of blood volume, and in dealing with increased stress on the liver. Wise food intake can also go a long way in preventing intrauterine growth retardation, preeclampsia (first signs of toxemia), preterm birth, fetal distress during labor, low birth weight, retardation, and learning disabilities in the child, stillbirth, anemia, maternal postpartum hemorrhage, and much more.

Why in the past, have women been told to diet during pregnancy? In the nineteenth century, it was advised that expectant women should not gain much weight during their pregnancies so that babies would not grow to their normal size. This, it was believed, would be the answer to avoiding problems at birth that were stemming from child labor practices of the day. During this time period in Europe many children grew up working many hours in dark, stuffy factories without adequate nutrition. This resulted in deficiencies in nutrients needed for normal bone growth. A pelvis narrowed by poor nourishment as a child often made birth more difficult and sometimes life-threatening (so of course this only added to common fears originally formed during those days, about babies not fitting through women's *now very adequate* bodies). The phenomenon of babies not fitting because of a malformed pelvis due to rickets is extemely rare in this present time in the history of the United States. Nonetheless, weight-restriction has prevailed without further questioning until just a short while ago.

Now it is being shown that mothers with inadequate diets and poor weight gain are more likely to have complications, including babies with problems!

The benefits of a daily diet that contains mainly whole foods cannot be overestimated. This means that foods remain as unprocessed and as close to their natural state as possible, and that they are prepared simply. Eliminate white flour and sugar as much as you can. Whole food also means real eggs, cheese, and butter—not fakes, substitutes, or highly-processed varieties.

Whole grains, as opposed to food made with nutrient-stripped white flour, is the way to go. Try making your own muffins, substituting white flour for a mix of several whole grain flours such as oats, millet, wheat, rice, and more. Results and flavors vary with different types of grains and you may be surprised at how much better baked goods can taste as

Wise food intake can go a long way in preventing a variety of problems.

you learn about whole grain baking. Even better, experiment with using grains soaked overnight (make muffin or pancake batter and place in fridge until morning for example), or sprouted, in various recipes.

It is also very important to eat a variety of **fresh fruits and vegetables** in all the colors of the rainbow.

Do take caution not to eat your dark, leafy green vegetables raw as it is thought that this can actually bind iron. Lightly cooking them, as is done in Asian cultures, is best. Greens are, of course, also rich in minerals and vitamins. While greens do have some calcium, it is not in great amounts. Dairy sources remain some of the best for providing much needed calcium. However, dark leafy greens are also rich in **magnesium, an important precursor for taking calcium into the body.** It is also thought by some that magnesium may play a significant role in the baby's ability to tuck his head, facilitating an optimal positioning of the crown of his head on the mother's cervix for a more efficient, more comfortable birth! Magnesium is also found in walnuts and almonds and would you believe chocolate? Craving chocolate lately? The darker the chocolate the better the source of magnesium, and the kind with almonds is a good choice because they also have magnesium.

Listen to your body!

Listen to your body! If you only know how to interpret your cravings and aversions, you will learn much about what your body needs. The body really is smart and will communicate what it needs to you! You just need to know how to listen to it. For example, pregnant women often crave things like ice cream, chocolate, pickles, salty foods, and potatoes. These seem like strange things for a pregnant woman's body to be asking for, until we begin to comprehend more about her needs!

Something important to understand is that *calcium* is dependent on *potassium* and *sodium* as escorts into the body. Sodium and potassium are important electrolytes. Previous bouts with diarrhea, vomiting, perspiration, and loss of blood lead to loss of electrolytes in the body. If these are not replaced, a woman can be in for a hard time in pregnancy and following birth. Highly sweet, strangely colored commercial electrolyte drinks are not good substitutes, though.

Calcium deficiency shows itself in such ways as being unable to sleep and having charley horses or aching muscles. Believe it or not, ice cream is actually not a bad way to get calcium as calcium is also dependant on carbohydrates/sugars as escorts! It is not just your bones that need calcium. There are different systems in your body, and those in your growing baby, that require calcium. If there isn't adequate calcium to go around, it will be drawn from the mother's bones and teeth. Pregnant women who do not get adequate calcium can also suffer from morning sickness. **Morning sickness, brain fog, and fatigue could all be greatly alleviated with *calcium, potassium, sodium, and iron.***

Potassium is found in orange juice (fresh orange juice that is not from concentrate is key), and in fruits, potatoes, beef, legumes, and other foods. The body is dependent upon salt to take in potassium. Of interest to some pregnant women, is that potassium and sodium play an important role in avoiding constipation.

The myth about pregnant women needing to avoid salt during pregnancy is one that has met its time. **Salt is crucial for a normal pregnancy.** Mothers on no-salt diets have been shown to have more preeclampsia than women who had as much salt as they wished. Sea salt is suggested because of the important minerals it contains. Getting too much is not an issue as the body will eliminate excess. It is also important to understand that the body is dependent on salt to eliminate unneeded water from the tissues. Be aware, though, that pregnant women's bodies do naturally and wisely carry some extra fluid, particularly toward the end of pregnancy and most women experience a bit of swelling.

Pregnant and nursing mothers' needs for iron can also not be overestimated. The form of iron in iron supplements is not a good source of iron at all. Iron is also necessary for taking in calcium. Interestingly, while iron supplements can be the *cause* of constipation, iron from sources such as red meat can help to *solve* the problem. Not a popular food, but very much worth mentioning, is liver. Mom was right. Liver is extremely beneficial, and probably the very best source of iron you will find, particularly for pregnant women and women who have just given birth. It helps prevent depression and low energy—just a couple of the many reasons to seek out ways to prepare this excellent food at least once a week (teriyaki meatballs of a mix of beef and liver served perhaps with mushrooms over rice, or in a pasta sauce, etc.)

Getting adequate iodine is crucial in pregnancy and when breastfeeding too. Babies get their iodine from the mother's valuable stores. Maternal problems with hair loss, memory, cysts, and a score of other problems can occur when mothers become low on iodine. Babies that do not have sufficient amounts of iodine to draw from are also at risk for a variety of serious problems. Sea salt does not contain adequate iodine, nor does standard table salt contain a quality type of it. Taking a proper source of iodine, such as kelp is probably a good idea.

Protein is also extremely important during pregnancy, and is believed to greatly decrease the risk of preeclampsia, because it is so essential for the body to have. It is recommended that pregnant women consume eighty-plus grams of protein daily. Protein can be found in eggs, cottage cheese, meat, and a variety of other sources. Beef, in particular, is a wonderful source of both protein and iron. If you do not normally eat meat, pregnancy and breastfeeding are times of greatly increased needs for the nutrients, including vitamins and minerals, contained in meat. You will need to be particularly vigilant and creative in seeking out other foods with these necessities. Many mothers feel remarkably better and find health issues resolve themselves when they

It is essential to supply your baby and your body with proper nutrients during your pregnancy.

add meat, beef in particular, to their diets during pregnancy and when nursing.

Fatty acids are beginning to receive more attention as nutritionists realize how essential they are. Fats received a bad rap, especially in the 80s and 90s. Researchers are discovering that fats are important components of foods that normally contain them and that some of the nutrients in those foods cannot be absorbed without the fat that naturally accompanies them if left whole. Women who are pregnant and breastfeeding, and babies too, have a greater need of good fats in their diets. Fats are important for placental attachment to the uterus and then detachment at the time of birth, for the umbilical cord, suppleness and stretching abilities of the vagina and birth opening, and for avoiding stretch marks.

Now, during pregnancy and breastfeeding, are excellent times to buy organic or better yet, grow your own organic garden if possible.

It is essential that you do not starve your baby! Don't let anyone discourage you from supplying your baby and body with proper foods!

Exercise is very important as well. Although you will probably want to avoid high impact exercises that might put you or your baby in danger, many caregivers agree that it is fine to continue most exercises you were used to before pregnancy. Myriad benefits can come from simply *walking* daily. Walking has even been found to be a remedy for preeclampsia.

Practicing strengthening exercises is especially helpful. **Prenatal yoga** can be a wonderful option. There are many benefits to this low-impact form of exercise including increased strength and energy, better balance and control of the body, greater flexibility, breathing capacity, a sense of well-being, stress reduction, a greater sense of confidence, and an increased level of pain management.

When exercising, be sure not to become overheated or exhausted. If you are becoming exhausted or if you feel any pain, it is best to stop and take it easier. Babies can be put into a hazardous situation when the mother becomes overheated by exercise or by taking baths that are too hot, because the baby cannot cool off as easily as the mother can afterwards.

Be careful of household cleaning products and other chemicals. With such natural products as baking soda, table salt, distilled white vinegar, lemon juice, trisodium phosphate (TSP, which doesn't emit fumes), and a plunger, it is possible to clean drains, wash windows, degrease, prevent mold and mildew, disinfect, and scour.

Drinking, drugs, and smoking are also very dangerous for your baby. It is imperative if you have any of these habits that you stop immediately! Avoid caffeine intake too, and switch to decaf or herbal teas.

There are some superb resources on the subjects of nutrition and exercise for pregnancy that are available. Of course be sure to consult your caregiver with any questions you have about dietary changes, or before beginning a new exercise program.

Many are the benefits of regular exercise during pregnancy.

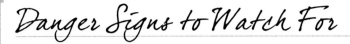

Danger Signs to Watch For

Many different changes can occur during pregnancy. Sometimes it is difficult to determine whether what you are experiencing is normal or if there may be cause for concern.

Swelling, increased urination and discharge, ligament discomfort, occasional dizziness, backache, gas pains, pressure from the baby's weight, contractions, and even spotting can all occur normally in pregnancy.

Contact your doctor or midwife—*immediately*, in some cases—if you experience any of the following symptoms:

- **Sharp or continuous abdominal pain, vaginal bleeding, fluid leaking from the vagina, severe or continuing nausea, chills, fever, persistent vomiting, or a nagging feeling that something is wrong.**
- **Blood during pregnancy or labor**—especially if discharge is heavier than a light period, and particularly if you have a sudden or persistent pain that is different than contractions. If you feel faint, if you feel that something is not right, go *right* to the hospital. It's better to be safe than sorry.
- **If you feel something come down into your vagina when your water releases**—this may be the cord. Get on your hands and knees with your bottom up, and get to the hospital *fast*. This is a prolapsed cord; oxygen to the baby can be cut off when the cord comes down first. This doesn't happen very often, but it is dangerous.

   The presence of meconium when your water releases—If fluid is yellow, green, or dark or has pieces of refuse in it, this indicates that the baby has already had a bowel movement. This isn't rare; it happens fairly often. It could mean that your baby has had some distress. But if your baby seems fine and you are feeling normal movements from the baby, there is probably no need to worry at all. Meconium can be expelled long before labor even starts.

   "The presence of meconium in the amniotic fluid without signs of fetal asphyxia is not a sign of fetal distress and need not be an indication for active intervention." (Miller 1975)

   The meconium *itself* isn't something to be concerned about until the time of the actual birth or emergence of the baby. Your caregiver will probably be very cautious that the baby doesn't inhale some of the fluid as he begins to breathe, and will probably carefully suction out the baby's mouth and nose before his body is fully delivered.

- **Infection**—Chills, fever, vaginal discharge with a foul odor, pain or burning when urinating, decreased amount of urine.
- **Signs of shock**—Fast, weak pulse; low blood pressure; feeling faint or dizzy; perspiration; paleness; convulsions.

- **Possible preterm labor**—Four or more contractions per hour *prior to thirty-six to thirty-eight weeks*; dull lower backache; menstrual-like cramps; intestinal cramps and/or diarrhea; unusual pressure in pelvis, lower back, abdomen, or thighs; water or large amounts of "birth gel" leaking from vagina; red, pink, or brown discharge; bag of waters releasing; or other signs of labor require attention.

   If signs of preterm labor begin, you will probably wish to take the course of least regret. Stop what you're doing, call your caregiver immediately, empty your bladder, drink a quart of water, lie down on your left side for an hour, palpate your uterus to feel for contractions (your uterus feels a bit like the firmness of your forehead when contracting). If nothing drastic seems to be happening, and your caregiver does not seem too concerned, but you've had a few of these signs, it may be best to take it easy the next few days.

- **Decreased activity of the baby**—Less than one kick an hour after the fifth month, or a change in usual pattern of the baby's movements (See Keeping Track... in **chapter 8**.)

- **Preeclampsia**—Persistent or severe headaches, dizziness, blurred vision, spots before the eyes, excessive swelling, sudden and rapid weight gain, protein in urine, increased blood pressure.

Preeclampsia

Preeclampsia usually doesn't occur until after twenty weeks of pregnancy. Diagnosis includes elevated blood pressure plus at least one of the following: *excessive* edema (although some retention of fluid is normal and purposeful in pregnancy), rapid weight gain, headaches, dizziness, visual disturbances, or protein in the urine (protein accompanied by edema may indicate kidney impairment).

The exact cause of preeclampsia is not known, but there are several theories. **It is thought that low protein levels can cause fluid to leak from the cells, causing edema.**

Too, the liver may be experiencing difficulty handling the extra workload of pregnancy.

Overdoing it may be a contributor. Resting and taking it easier for even just a day can help greatly.

There are a variety of things that can be done to prevent or overcome preeclampsia.

Dangers of Preeclampsia:

- Reduced blood flow to the kidneys, which produces a rise in blood pressure for compensation. Reduced blood flow to the uterus can cause fetal growth retardation and fetal distress during labor.
- A premature separation of the placenta (which occurs about 8 percent of the time) may result in fetal death and maternal hemorrhage.
- If preeclampsia progresses to eclampsia, convulsions and coma may occur in the mother and death may come to both mother and baby.
- Be sure to report any of the following to your caregiver:
  - Severe headache
  - Upper abdominal pain under rib cage
  - Visual disturbances
  - Decreased urine output
  - Extreme nervous irritability
  - Elevation of the bottom number (140/<u>90</u>) when blood pressure is taken
  - If you have **an intense headache or pain under the right rib cage, go right to the hospital.**

Keep in mind that just because someone is showing signs of preeclampsia it does not mean that she has toxemia and needs to be rushed right in for induction!

Often the following tips can be helpful for keeping preeclampsia in check until the woman goes into labor on her own. (See Labeling "Overdue" Babies, Inducing Labor with Drugs, and Inducing Labor Naturally in **chapter 8**.)

If you have signs of preeclampsia, the following can be helpful:

- Sometimes bed rest, on the left side, for a day or two is all that is needed. Mothers experiencing preeclampsia sometimes find they have simply been overdoing it in their activities, putting too much stress on their bodies.
- Be cautious not to stress the body.
- If lying in bed is more stressful than not, carry out some low-stress activities that give satisfaction and contentment.
- Massage under right rib cage where the liver is located.
- Daily immersion in deep water to neck level may help.
- Walk every day.
- Elevate and massage your feet.
- Don't use heat on swollen ankles as this can aggravate the symptoms.
- Talk positively to, and think positively about, your body. Doing so can actually help things to normalize.

Just because someone is showing signs of preeclampsia, it does not mean that she has toxemia or that she needs to be induced.

In addition, these dietary tips can help:

- Take in **80 grams of protein** daily and eat a healthful diet.
- Cut out processed foods high in salt. Many caregivers recommend continuing to salt to taste. For more information see Diet and Nutrition in this section.
- Eat raw vegetables and fruit, especially watermelon, cucumbers, celery, beets, and carrots.
- Take dandelion supplements (two capsules at breakfast and two at dinner).
- Drink lemon juice in water first thing in the morning.
- Take a multiple B vitamin at lunch.
- These have been found to be very effective:
    - One large vitamin E three times a day
    - Herbs marshmallow and gravel weed
    - Bananas and lemon juice

Does your blood pressure seem to rise just before or during appointments with your caregiver? If so, you might examine why this might be so. For example, is your body telling you something that you need to know about your relationship with your midwife/doctor? Deep breathing and relaxation can be helpful for lowering blood pressure to a more accurate number.

Of course confer with your caregiver concerning your specific needs before following any of the above suggestions.

Craniosacral therapy offers a variety of benefits to mother and baby.

Craniosacral Therapy

Craniosacral therapy (also spelled Cranial Sacral) is beneficial from pre-conception to postpartum for the well-being of both mother and baby. It may encourage optimal health, a gentler birth for both mother and baby, and a better, faster postpartum recovery for both mother and baby. Traditional midwives have used hands-on body work for centuries. Body work is a time-honored way of supporting women through pregnancy, labor, and postpartum.

Prenatal Craniosacral therapy is therapeutic and relaxing physically and emotionally and is done fully clothed. Craniosacral therapy helps release restrictions in the body and pelvis for a better birthing experience. It has been known to ease low back, hip, and ligament discomfort, improve pelvic health, relieve muscle cramps, promote relaxation, and decrease stress. It also helps to prepare your body for an optimal, more efficient and comfortable labor and birth by promoting **optimal fetal positioning, an important factor in the efficiency of your birth.**

Additionally Craniosacral bodywork can be used for the **baby within the womb** for optimal labor, birth, and bonding. Moms have reported that their babies in the uterus responded happily to the session as if they were enjoying it as well.

After your birth, Craniosacral therapy can nurture the new mother by enhancing post-birth physical healing and by helping to regulate her emotions.

Craniosacral therapy is for babies too! Particularly helpful after their birth, a newborn baby can be helped tremendously physically, mentally, and emotionally with Craniosacral therapy. It can help a baby who is fussy or who might have different issues caused at either the birth itself or by birth procedures. Parents have reported a marked difference, even when the birth was easy and straightforward. Babies seem to enjoy the visit and find it relaxing.

Craniosacral therapists are also sometimes massage therapists, so you might begin your search for one in your area by calling massage therapists. Find someone who has had experience working with pregnant women and newborns.

Celebrations for Entering Parenthood

In some cultures, women will take part in ceremonies that acknowledge and celebrate the transition into motherhood. Other cultures may have rituals for men entering fatherhood. You might be interested in having your own celebration. These can be made to fit the individual woman.

Unlike baby showers, which may be given at a separate time, this ceremony focuses on celebrating the *mother* during this intensely significant time in her life.

Some women enjoy being pampered, massaged, sung to, having their hair braided, or other such things. Throughout a ceremony, friends may wish to form an intimate circle around the mother, where she is the center of attention. Be creative. Read about celebrations in other cultures, pick out music that fits your theme or message, have a potluck or prepare a special dinner. You might use natural materials, candles, incense, bubble or herbal baths, massage oils, flowers for her hair. You may want to share inspiring birthing stories and poetry together, having everyone bring something to contribute.

At one ceremony, each friend brought a bead to put on a necklace. The cord was passed in turn to the giver of each bead. The giver spoke to the woman about why she had chosen to present this bead to the honored woman, what it signified, and expressed her hopes and wishes for this woman and for her transition into motherhood. A page was also passed around so that the messages could be recorded and later placed in the baby's book. The necklace was worn by the woman during her birth. A bracelet is another idea. Those giving the ceremony might want to bring extra beads to choose from if someone forgets. Also be sure to remind friends to choose a bead with a large enough hole, and be sure to have a string that while strong, like fishing line, is not too thick.

There are many different ways this ritual could be carried out.

It is most helpful when stories and talk are kept positive, uplifting, and encouraging.

What about dads? What might fathers have done in ages past? What could be done to celebrate this voyage into a whole new world for him?

(See *Blessing the Way* in the media section of **Appendix E**.)

13

Comfort Measures for Labor

Whether or not you decide to have medication, you will most likely have quite a bit of opportunity to put comfort measures to use. Wise caregivers advise holding off on an epidural at least until active labor (about five centimeters dilation). This is to prevent, as much as possible, your labor from stalling or stopping. Also, the medication sometimes does not work at all or only gives patchy relief. Comfort techniques are very valuable to know, whether or not you think you will use medication. The good news is that labor is normally quite doable.

Personalized Comfort Techniques

There are a myriad of comfort techniques and most of them are simple to use if you are prepared. Here we name some of the most helpful.

What is important to *you*? What kinds of things do you think would make *you* feel more comfortable? What helps you to relax? A doula is a great asset for helping to personalize comfort techniques for *your own* specific needs.

Having proper support and being prepared with comfort techniques can make all the difference!

1. Your **environment** is one of the most important things to consider. The place where you will give birth should be one in which you will feel comfortable. It should be a place where you feel confident in your ability to birth your baby, and that not only feels safe, but is safe. It is helpful to have some space where you are able to move around and experiment with different positions. Some little things that can mean a lot to a woman in labor are lighting, her own pillows, the bed, even scents. All of these can play a role in how she feels, how she relaxes, and how her birth will go.

2. **Relaxation** is an extremely important element of a comfortable birth.

3. **Deep breathing** is one of the most important tools you can have with you in labor that can help you to stay relaxed enough to be able to go within and let your body more easily birth your baby. Be warned that "hee-hee-haw" type breathing is *not* a very effective coping technique for most women!

   Find a comfortable place, and as you use your deep abdominal breathing techniques, practice **going within**. Your breathing can help you to be able to stay there. This is a good place to use **imagery**.

4. Relaxing **music** can also be very helpful for setting the mood and helping the laboring woman to relax and be comfortable. At other times, simple **quiet** is found to be invaluable. During pushing, energetic music can prove to be very helpful.

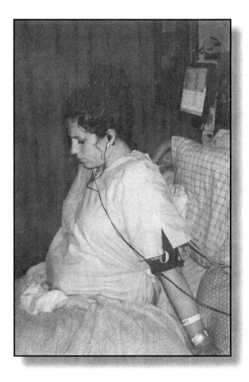

5. **Massage** can be a very effective comfort technique for many women. Others do not want to be touched during labor. Holding the mother's hand during surges and during cervical exams can be comforting to her. Some will find strength in being held in their husband's arms. Others find a doula's hands to be her most important tool.

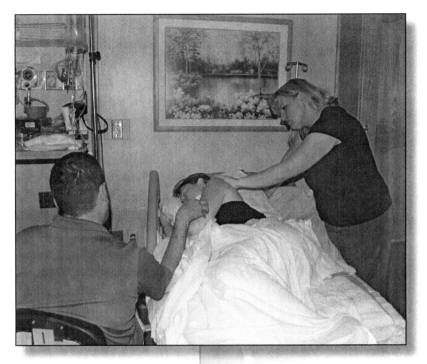

A wonderful way to enjoy the benefits of aromatherapy along with massage is to prepare a small bottle (perhaps a half ounce bottle) with a carrier-oil from your health food store such as sweet almond, apricot kernel, jojoba, or olive. Fill your bottle about ¾ full and then add your essential oil. Peppermint, clary sage, and lavender are favorites in labor (but should be used cautiously in pregnancy). Some women like their oil to be more strongly scented; others, less. Check with your labor companion to be sure this scent is agreeable with him/her as well. Doulas often bring oils with them for massage.

6. Helping the mother to keep **a positive attitude** is so important!

England and Horowitz, the authors of *Birthing from Within*, introduce the following demonstration to illustrate how powerful your attitude about labor is: Hold an ice-cube in your hand for one minute. This is not the easiest thing to do, but don't let go for the entire sixty seconds. As you do, express your discomfort, be whiny; complain as much as you want about how much it hurts. Now, do it one more time for sixty seconds. Hold the ice in your other hand. Use your deep abdominal breathing this time. Go within your body and just notice how the ice really feels in your hand. Pay attention to the sensation. How does the center of the sensation feel? How about the edges? Be curious. It's interesting how much faster the second minute passes merely because of the fact that you aren't complaining about how much it hurts! The discomfort of holding ice in your hand is not the same sensation that labor is, but it does show how enormously important your attitude is! If you are thinking, "I hate this, I can't do it," it will probably be a lot

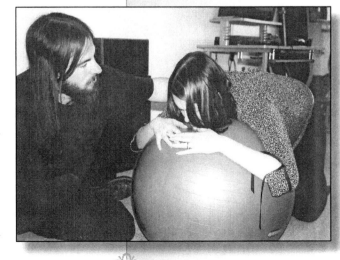

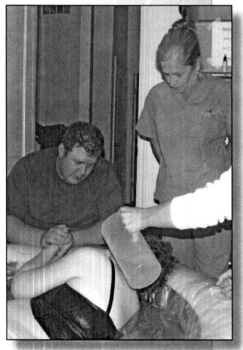

Inviting only those who will be able to serve and assist in some way is wise.

harder than if you go in and meet it with curiosity, and just deal with it. The same is true in other aspects of life as well. A positive attitude really does make it easier.

Ina May Gaskin teaches how imperative it is for a woman to be kind to those around her in labor, to have good feelings and connection between her and her husband and their birth attendants. Gaskin tells her readers that lots of endorphins (a laboring mother's best friend) are released when good feelings are encouraged from the very beginning.

7. It is helpful for a laboring woman to hear such things as this: "Melt away, letting your body grow soft. Make space for your baby to be born easily. Just fall away, release…let it happen. Open and make room for your baby to be born."

8. Appropriate **humor** is part of this. Tactful wit about the present situation can help a woman to relax and to dilate faster.

9. **Vocalization** in deep, humming tones is one way that women have naturally been managing labor for ages.

10. Don't forget that one of the biggest ways to obtain comfort is by using body **positions** that feel right to you. (See Positions…in this chapter.)

11. An essential question to consider is who you will invite to the birth. Having too many people, especially those that are just there to watch and not to help in some way, can be draining to the energy in the room and to that of the mother. Inviting only those who will be able to serve and assist in some way is wise. Make sure **support people** share your beliefs and that they will be able to remain calm throughout. Laboring women can pick up on the emotions of those around them.

12. **Water** is a wonderful comfort measure. (See Using Water…in this chapter.)

13. **Hot and cold packs** can feel great! A clean sock filled with rice, tied at the top, and heated in the microwave does wonders for achy discomfort (back, lower abdomen, etc.) Another form of a hot pack is a hot, wet cloth on the perineum prior to the birth. This can help prepare the area for the birth.

    Ice in a rubber glove can feel great on a sore back, as can alternating hot and cold. A cool wash cloth on the forehead is refreshing, particularly when she starts becoming rosy and flushed as labor progresses, and while giving birth. Ice can also feel good on the perineum after the birth.

14. Keep in mind that around the end of your labor, unless you are using hypnobirthing, many women find that they get to a place where nothing works any more. **Don't give up! You are probably almost there!** Having those to help you at this time is really important.

15. **Be able to step out of the way** and let your body just do what it was made to do! (See The Body/Mind…in **chapter 15**.)

Natural Comfort Measures For Labor

Aromatherapy	Visualization	Fresh Air
Hot and Cold Packs	Massage	Relaxation
Shower/Jacuzzi!	Birth Ball	Cool Cloths
Upright Positions	Environment	Walking
Eat and Drink	Acupressure	Appropriate humor

Be alone as a couple together.   Touch Relaxation

Remind her, "There's a baby!"   Go within

TENS   Kissing and Loving!

Remind her to feel the ecstasy within herself.

Hypnobirthing!   Quiet

Massage tools—paint roller, tennis balls, etc.

Consider whether each of those you have there will be a help or a hindrance.

Release tension from the mind.   Bean Bag Chair

Counter Pressure   Keep a positive attitude.

Practice Relaxation Skills!   Stay home as long as possible!

Positions   Save some techniques for the right moment.

Support! A doula!!

Perception of Sensations
(Examples: "rushes" or "ecstasy" or "pressure" instead of "pain" or "contractions")

Music   Deep Breathing   Let Go!

Vocalize (deep low tones)   Don't give up! (birth companions too!)

Other ideas:

Slow, Deep, Abdominal Breathing

What have you heard your friends say about the "prepared" breathing they learned in classes? Did any of them actually totally get through with breathing techniques only? How many women have you heard say that she became really upset with her husband for counting incorrectly or for trying to make her count? What a stressful thing to ask a couple to do—to try to pattern-breathe during labor!

The truth is that **classes that teach prepared breathing techniques usually don't have high rates of women going without medication.** Why is that? "Hee-hee-haw" type of breathing is prepared to make a woman focus on something outside of herself and to take her out of her laboring mind. However, if a woman is able to naturally go to this place in her mind (some call it Labor Land), she can meet the contractions and work *together with* her labor.

Now it's important to say here, that the sensations of labor are much different than stubbing your toe. If you stub your toe, distractive activities like "Hee-hee-haw" breathing or focusing on something external can be helpful, and we instinctively do some panting at those times! But *labor is different.*

You will probably be surprised at how helpful, and how simple, that deep abdominal breathing really is at helping you to be very relaxed and labor with very little, if any, discomfort. In fact, deep abdominal breathing is a very natural type of breathing that is used instinctively by many laboring women.

This is the type of breathing that is used by hypnobirthing methods. These methods have their own, specific forms of slow, abdominal breathing *as well as other techniques for labor.*

Are you ready to try it out? Having someone read this to you the first few times can be helpful. **You can do this exercise mentally after that, or tape it for your labor.**

And by the way, while some people say these kinds of exercises seem a bit corny, others find the imagery to be extremely helpful. If you are one of those that find it a little corny, don't let yourself be thrown off by it. This is only one form of this exercise. Make up your own imagery, using the basics here that you know will be able to help you during your labor (You might imagine actually seeing your cervix opening instead of a rose, for example).

This breathing is used mainly *during* contractions. By practicing it each day you can be assured that it will be with you during labor.

Make yourself comfortable. Lightly let your eyelids close. Take a deep, cleansing breath through your nose. Take it all the way down to your toes. Let it out through your mouth with a long "whooo." Continue to breathe

---

A trained support person can help you to stay on top of your deep-breathing techniques and on top of each contraction.

in through your nose, imagining breathing in a cool, golden light that is all around you. Let it be a healing light; natural endorphins that you can actually breathe right in. With a slow "whooo," breathe out all of the tension, any negative thoughts, any fear. Breathe in the golden light. Take it to your baby and see it surrounding your baby and your uterus. Hold the light within. Breathe out anything negative with a "whooo," and continue to breathe at this pace. See your uterus working smoothly to bring your baby into the world. See your cervix, the opening at the bottom of your uterus. Continue to breathe in and out at this pace. You may want to imagine your cervix as a flower, the most beautiful flower you have ever seen, opening, petal by petal, outward. At the center of the flower, see your baby, softly, easily descending from the center of the flower, being gently released. Breathe in the cool, golden healing light. Breathe out any tension or fear, anything negative. See all of this being breathed out. Breathe in the golden light, right now to any part of your body. See it surrounding that area, massaging, healing, and eliminating the discomfort with each "whooo" that you push out. In and out—continue this breathing for as long as you want or need to. Then, when you are ready, you may open your eyes.

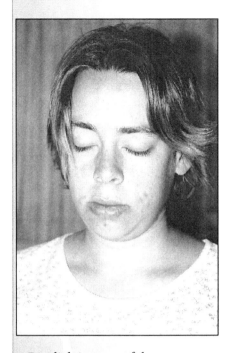

Dim lighting, peaceful surroundings, and deep breathing help a woman to go within herself and find that place where she can work with her labor. She may look as if she is asleep or even a little spaced-out. Time becomes irrelevant to her. She lets her body do what it was made to do.

NOTE: Although deep abdominal breathing is one of the most helpful tools you can take with you to your birth, the other element that makes the most difference seems to be continuous support. A trained support person can help you to stay on top of your breathing and on top of each contraction.

Hypnobirthing

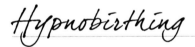

Almost everyone seems to have heard about hypnosis-for-birth by now. The obsession of hypnobirthing has spread across the country—and with very good reasons! There are different methods to choose from, including Marie Mongan's HypnoBirthing® and Hypnobabies, to name just two.

Hypnobirthing families are reporting **shorter labors with no frenzied pushing stage, that they are better able to bond after the birth without exhaustion on the part of either the mother or the baby, that they have quicker recoveries, less postpartum depression, greater breastfeeding success, and babies with higher Apgar scores.** Those **benefits alone are amazing.**

Some other things that many moms really enjoy are that they are **awake and aware during their labors. They can talk, think, move, and are full participants in their own births.** During contractions, the birthing mother may look as if she is asleep, but really she is merely in a very relaxed state. She is using easy-to-learn techniques including imagery and special kinds of deep abdominal breathing, mentioned above. Moms often happily converse with others in between the surges. In fact, it is not uncommon for a hypnobirthing mom not to be taken seriously upon arrival at the birth place because of how comfortable she appears!

So how does hypnobirthing work? In part, women learn how to eliminate the fear-tension-pain cycle that is often experienced at birth. And **although the goal of a program may not be to make labor "pain free," many women have reported having a totally pain-free birth!** Those that have had a particularly trying birth experience in the past can especially benefit by learning how to eliminate the fears they have

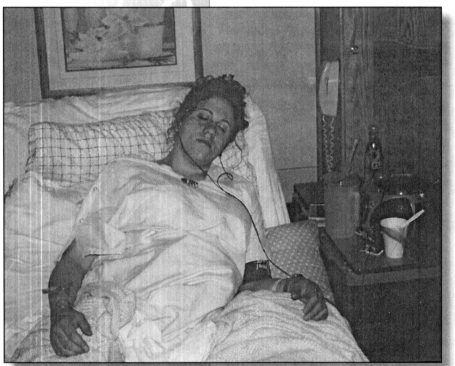

for this birth. Fear is an integral part of a common cycle: Fear creates tension. Tension creates pain. Pain creates more fear, and on and on. Getting rid of fears she may have of giving birth is one of the most important ways a woman can prepare for a more comfortable birthing. Instructors help participants in the class to deal with fears so that they don't come up to haunt a woman during her actual birth.

Is using hypnosis-for-birth **a morally acceptable option?** The Catholic Church has long approved of the use of hypnosis in obstetrics, and it has also been a very useful tool in the medical field for some time, adopted formally in 1958.

Through our minds, so much more than we ever imagined is possible. Women have been provided with the ability to give birth comfortably and joyfully. Childbirth does not have to be a dreaded experience to be endured for the privilege of bringing children into the world!

Why are women in other countries reported to have given birth with so much more ease than many of their American counterparts? Are they simply better made for birthing? Of course not—our bodies were made to birth just as theirs were. Hypnobirthing teaches women how their birthing can be as comfortable as women who are birthing in other cultures.

Some common, unfounded fears that might keep couples from investigating hypnobirthing are that they will get stuck in hypnosis, that they will not be able to control what they do and say, that someone else will be in control of their mind, or that they will enter some other realm. They might also fear that they could never become hypnotized. None of these things need to be worried about. They can be asked of the instructor over the phone before signing up for a class.

Women have also had much success with using hypnosis to turn a breech (head up) baby into the head-down position, preparatory for birth.

Although a woman can use the skills she has learned from her hypnobirthing class on her own, ideally with her partner, we still enthusiastically encourage couples to seriously consider also having a doula as a part of their birth team.

Be careful, since some programs may profess to be teaching hypnosis-for-birth when they are not.

For more information see the Resource section in this book.

Positions for Labor and Birth

The positions that you employ during labor will truly make a difference in your level of comfort.

Many Amish women, known for their "easy" homebirth labors, naturally continue on with their household chores throughout early and active labor, just as many women of other cultures have done throughout time. Only when heading into the more intense period of labor, just before birth, do they began to really get down to the business of birthing their babies. Continuing their chores generally requires upright, mobile activity. This helps the baby to find the right position to descend. And it prepares the woman's body to give birth.

This woman is sitting in an upright position on a birth ball while her husband uses a hypnobirthing massage technique.

Interestingly, the positions you find your body moving into naturally as you labor are often the very ones that will best help you to get the baby out. Listen to your body and do what it tells you to do. Lying down is *usually* not what you'll find is most comfortable.

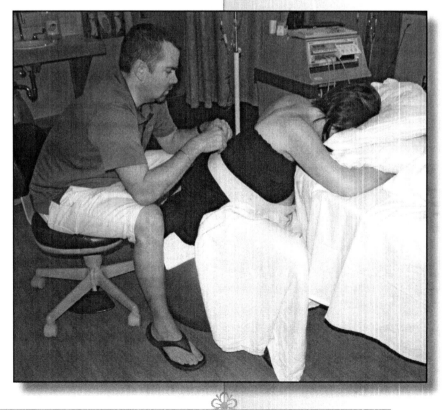

Risks of Staying in Bed for Labor

1. **Labor can be a great deal more uncomfortable lying down.** Ask a woman who has had to lie in bed to be electronically monitored (See Electronic Fetal Monitor...chapter 7.) or for some other reason during early and labor, how much better it felt to have someone just help her sit up for each contraction!

2. **Labor can slow.** Though, if a woman is able to develop a deep state of relaxation, this could be a good position for her at least for awhile. Position changes every half hour or so, can be helpful.

3. **A woman is given, and gives, the impression that she is a patient, that something is wrong.** After all, here she is in a patient's uniform, in a hospital gown, in a hospital bed, and she is hooked up to an assortment of machines. Women's bodies were *designed* to give birth—just as they were designed to breathe, digest food, pump blood, and everything else a body does naturally, without difficulty and with no thought required! Birth is a normal, bodily function. Babies' heads and bodies were designed to be born. Women's bodies were designed to give birth. There is no reason, unless something is actually wrong, that a birthing mother needs to be considered a "patient."

4. **It puts a woman in less of a powerful position, giving the impression to others around her that she can't do this on her own.** In fact, it doesn't help a woman to have much confidence in her own ability, either. Everyone else seems to think she is sick and needs to be helped. She is surrounded by people in upright positions and uniforms that cry, "The person wearing me is powerful!" All of these things, intentional or not, are not conducive to allowing a woman to find the power within herself to believe that *she can birth her baby*. (See The Body/Mind...chapter 15.)

5. **Most importantly, do what your body tells you to do.** Particularly toward the *end* of labor many women do often choose to lie down. Do what feels right.

Following are two lists. One is a list of positions for labor and the other is a list of positions for the actual birth of your baby. Some of these choices may be more attractive to you than others. This is by no means all of the possible positions you might find comfortable, but they are ones that are quite commonly used.

Try each of these now, before you are actually in labor. Note which positions you like best, but keep an open mind. In labor you may be surprised at just how much you are drawn to particular positions according to the needs of your body and your baby. And they may not be the ones you think they will be!

Laboring women often instinctively choose upright positions.

Positions for Labor

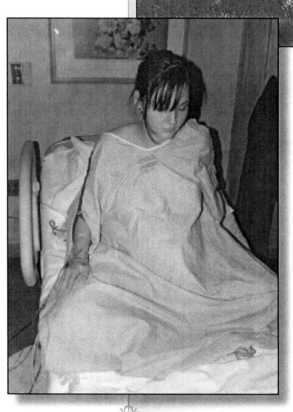

1. **Standing**, like other upright positions, uses gravity. It is one of the more comfortable positions, and contractions can be more effective. Upright positions are good for helping the baby move into proper alignment. Leaning can be more restful and feels so much better than simply standing. A woman often finds that leaning into her husband or doula is extremely helpful. If a contraction starts and he/she is not nearby, leaning into the side of a doorway is a nice alternative, but not as nice as a support person. Walking, then leaning in for a contraction, followed by more walking, has been a favorite pastime and technique of many a laboring couple.

2. **Walking**—Gravity is used. Walking helps the baby move into an optimal position. It can help the uterus in its work and may speed up labor. It can reduce backache. It can't be used by a mother that has very high blood pressure or one that has continuous fetal monitoring unless she has permission to walk around her room a bit during monitoring—this being "iffy" for a variety of reasons. For homebirth families, taking a walk in the fresh air around your neighborhood can be rejuvenating.

3. **Stair climbing**—This exercise can help to "shake things up a bit," and even turn a posterior baby into a rear-facing position. It uses gravity, and by helping to move the baby down onto your cervix, it may help you to dilate more quickly.

4. **Squatting**—It is helpful if this position is practiced often during the months you are preparing for labor so that you will be able to hold it during contractions. It is one of the most effective for helping the baby to move easily through your body and out. It utilizes gravity and spreads the pelvis open even more, allowing more room for the baby. It can aid in an easier pushing stage. If used for a long length of time, though, it can be tiring to the mother. Birth companions can help the mother with supported-squat positions. The birthing stool/chair offers many of the benefits of the squatting position while allowing for an easy way to rest at the same time. The **birth ball**, a tool used often by doulas, is wonderful for these same reasons, and is so wonderfully comfortable.

5. **On toilet**—The toilet is a natural place to relax and to open. Gravity and privacy are both utilized.

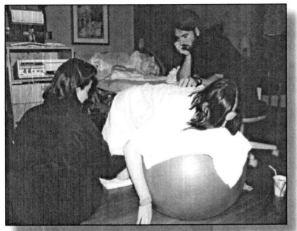

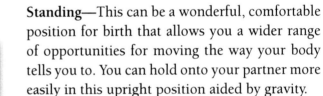

6. **Sitting**—This one is good when a rest is needed. Sitting uses gravity and can be employed with use of an electronic fetal monitor. Sitting on the birth ball is a favorite of many moms. Hip rotations on the birth ball can be great for helping the baby to maneuver down.

7. **Hands and knees**—This can be great for back labor; exercises can be used in this position to help a posterior-positioned baby to turn. An added plus is that it can take pressure off hemorrhoids for women that are suffering from them. Another option when using this position is leaning over the birth ball.

8. **Rocking chair**—Some mothers have found using the rocking chair to be helpful. The simple ritualistic and *rhythmic motion might be very helpful to some mothers.* It is possible that this position might hinder rotation of the baby, or allow the baby to fall back into a posterior position which can cause back labor and a longer labor.

9. **Belly dancing** (See **Belly Dancing** in this chapter.)

10. **In bed throughout labor**—As you've read above, while you may find that being in bed during the latter stages of labor is the most comfortable, during early/active labor confinement to a bed is usually is not what is most comfortable. You need the freedom to move as desired.

Rather than requiring this woman to leave the position that is presently most helpful to her (kneeling over a birth ball) to lay on the bed for another round of intermittent electronic fetal monitoring, this hospital caregiver sits next to the mother on the floor to monitor the baby. This is one example of willingness to find creative solutions that accommodate the mother and baby foremost.

Positions for Birth

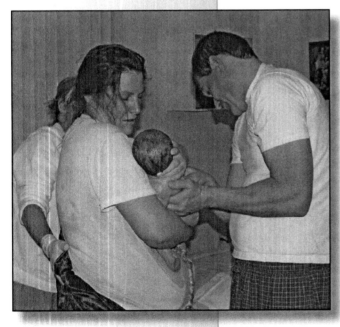

1. **Standing**—This can be a wonderful, comfortable position for birth that allows you a wider range of opportunities for moving the way your body tells you to. You can hold onto your partner more easily in this upright position aided by gravity.

2. **Lithotomy**—This is the term used to describe the mother lying flat on her back. Unless the mother's instincts have guided her into this position, which would be a rare occurrence, this is one of the least favorable positions. Mothers who are in labor seldom choose this position on their own. When a pregnant woman lies on her back, the pressure of the baby compresses the vena cava, one of the major blood vessels of the mother's body. This can cause oxygen deprivation to both the mother and the baby. Episiotomy and tearing are more likely in this position and there is no use of gravity to assist the mother and baby.

3. **Side-lying**—This position is good if the mother has high blood pressure. It can be used with an epidural. It allows good visibility for the mother and those present. Access to the perineum is not as easy for the caregiver but this may also help to avoid an episiotomy! There may be some added stress on the perineum, but not as much so as with semi-sitting. This can be a good compromise if a doctor insists upon having the woman up on the bed.

4. **Squatting alone or using a squatting bar**—Squatting can shorten the birth outlet slightly and expand the pelvis by about 30 percent! Gravity is utilized and this can shorten pushing time. Again, practice this during your pregnancy so that you will be used to holding the position for the length of a contraction. You can use it in your everyday chores. Keep in mind that the pelvis isn't just bony and rigid. It was made to expand to huge proportions if given the chance. Squatting allows good access to the perineum. One way to use the supported squat is to have the partner sit on the bed with the mother's back toward him as he holds her under her arms in a hanging supported squat. Another form of the supported squat is where two companions stand on either side of the woman and hold her under her arms as she sinks down into their support in a squat during contractions. If a mother knows that using squatting would cause too much tension in her body, it may be best to choose a different position that would better aid relaxation.

5. **Sitting on the birthing stool**—The use of this handy device offers many of the benefits that the squatting position does, while allowing for an easy way to rest at the same time. The woman's partner has better access from behind the stool for holding her, and lending her strength while she pushes. There is good visibility for the mother and caregivers.

6. **Hands and knees**—This one is a great position for avoiding episiotomy and tearing, good for birthing a large baby, and a wonderful position for birthing a baby that has shoulder dystocia. It can be good for back labor and it can help a posterior-positioned baby to turn as well as taking the pressure off of hemorrhoids. The baby has to be born between mother's legs and it may be difficult for her to see the birth. The mother can also kneel while leaning over the birth ball. This may be a good choice for a waterbirth.

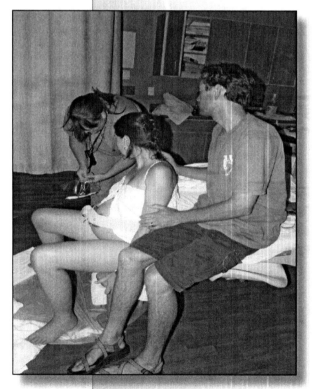

This father sits on the bed next to his wife who is using a birthing stool and resting between contractions.

7. **Sitting on the bed, curled into a C**—This position is the most frequently-used position in hospitals today. This and the side-lying position are both options for a woman who has an epidural. The staff will break down the lower portion of the bed so that the woman's bottom will be on the edge of the bed, her feet up in stirrups. Nurses may encourage those around to help pull the woman's bent legs back to her. She is encouraged to hold her chin down and push as hard as she can. This is probably the most

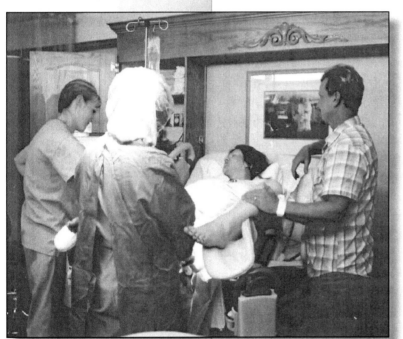

convenient position for the doctor, but is it the most convenient for the woman? Perhaps it is if she is birthing with an epidural. Otherwise, this may only be the easiest of positions for everyone else *but you and your baby*. This position provides good visibility for the mother and others present, yet there is a decrease in the proportion to which the pelvis can open. If you are having your baby without medication, it is certainly not the most comfortable position. It is harder to push a baby upward against gravity. Access to give an episiotomy, to use forceps, vacuum, and perform other different procedures is the best in this position—those wishing to steer clear of these procedures might do well to choose a different position for birth altogether anyway. Tears from an episiotomy are also more likely in this position. Backache may be a problem because of the pressure of the baby on your back, though adjusting the bed may help. Also, a woman's blood pressure sometimes decreases in this position. So what if this is not the position you would choose? Is kneeling beside a woman, in a more comfortable position for *her*, beneath some caregivers? Some American caregivers have never assisted a woman in any of the more comfortable positions for giving birth. A good caregiver will not mind sacrificing a bit of his/her own comfort for the greatly increased comfort of the mother and the baby.

Used in waterbirth, sitting in a C might actually be one of the best positions with the normal cons and risks of using it removed. A benefit to using water in labor is that one can much more easily change from one desired position to another in the buoyancy of the water as needed.

Using Water for Labor and Birth

Many women are drawn to water during pregnancy and labor. Water has even been referred to by some as, "Mother Nature's Epidural." Numerous women have reported that laboring in water seemed to help make contractions seem less intense. Water is especially helpful for bearing weight and it therefore helps the mother to not become as physically tired. It promotes deeper relaxation which is of course very helpful, sometimes causes labor to progress rapidly once a woman is in, can lower blood pressure, and even seems to help soften the perineum to help reduce injury to the tissues. In fact, Michel Odent a well-respected and well-known doctor who assisted many women in waterbirths at his birth center in Pithiviers, France, reports that in 100 waterbirths, no episiotomies were performed and only 29 women had tears—*all* of which were minor surface tears. (Giles 1999)

The time length of the birthing stage may also be greatly reduced.

For the baby, being born into water is certainly more comfortable as he or she comes from the warm, dark, amniotic fluid-filled space that has been home for the last nine months. Still unaccustomed to her own weight and to the surprises of the outside world, she glides into warm water and unfolds gradually into her new surroundings. The relaxing essence of water is indeed a soothing element for a **gentle welcome**.

How safe is water birth? Dr. Odent stated that they had encountered no risks with either underwater labor or birth. Dr. Rosenthal, another well-respected doctor, who has also assisted a large number of women in waterbirths at The Family Birthing Center in Upland, California, reported that by the summer of 1993, almost a thousand women had given birth in water at the center. There were *no* complications or infections in either the mothers or the babies. (Harper 1994)

If the water is clean, the risk of infection from birthing in it is nonexistent. Some advise expectant mothers to avoid tub baths once her bag of waters has released for fear of bacteria entering the vagina and causing an infection. Realistically, when a woman is actually in active labor, there is not time for an infection to develop, especially if vaginal checks are kept to a minimum. Dr. Rosenthal points out that everything is headed downstream when labor is in progress, inhibiting the passage of bacteria up the vagina and into the uterus— even if there were time to develop an

This laboring mother utilizes deep relaxation techniques and floating in a tub of warm water. She welcomes offers from her small support team for frequent sips of water and fresh cool cloths for her forehead.

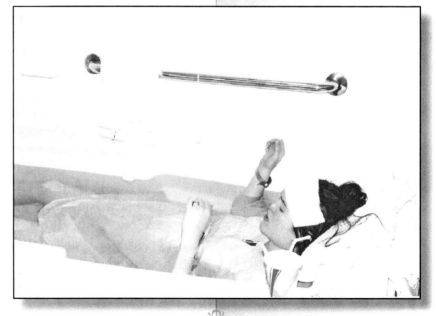

infection. Dr. Igor Charkovsky, from the Soviet Union, who first made waterbirths popular in the 1960s said too, that there are no risks implicated with the husband being in the water with his wife, since they share the same bacterial flora.

Having as few cervical checks as possible in labor is important for preventing infection. There are few medical reasons that a woman needs to be checked often throughout labor. In fact, some caregivers might check only once, just before the baby begins to descend, to make sure the cervix is fully dilated. Some don't require cervical checks *at all.* It depends on your caregiver and on you. There are other ways to know just how far a woman is progressing. Women have physical and emotional signposts that are easy for an experienced assistant to read. These signs tell you which stage a woman is in without even needing to check.

Presently, it may be the protocol in your hospital that once a woman's water has released that she is not allowed into the water except with her caregiver's permission. If you plan to labor and/ or birth in the water, be sure to get your caregiver's signature or initial of authorization at the top of the birth wishes that you will give to your nurse! If you are choosing to have a doctor, he/ she will probably not come to attend you until you are ready to actually give birth, so you need to discuss this with him/her at a prenatal appointment.

Some believe it is best not to get into the water until into active labor. As mentioned above, for some reason labor actually seems to increase in length when a woman gets in before she is five centimeters dilated and in active labor. Some theorize that this is because oxytocin can be diluted in the tissues when a woman gets into the water prior to active labor, and that it can slow her labor to get in too early. However, after that, labor can actually be shortened in length. Once in awhile when a woman gets into water, she progresses through transition in as little as ten minutes.

Make sure that the water temperature is comfortable but not hot. Water that is too hot can zap a woman's strength. In fact, German midwives are proponents of cooler, room-temperature water for facilitating labor.

Can the baby continue to receive oxygen underwater? Waterbirth experts have said that there is virtually no danger of the newborn drowning, that there need not be a rush to bring the baby to the surface. But they also stress that keeping the baby under the water for more than a few moments isn't recommended. For a short time, *while the placenta is still attached to the uterine wall,* the baby continues to breathe through the umbilical cord, and usually does not began to breathe until thermoreceptors in the skin are stimulated by air contact. Even if the baby were to gasp underwater, an automatic reflex would shut off the windpipe as soon as water entered the throat. Why not prolong the

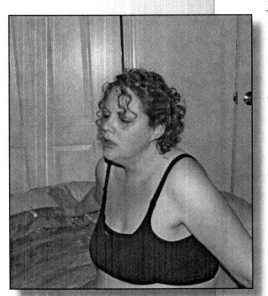

Many women find various forms of hydrotherapy invaluable during their births, making water a favorite tool for doulas.

conditions so beneficial to the baby? Living in the water is totally natural for a newborn. He's never done anything else. It's a more peaceful beginning. The baby should be slowly and gently raised to the surface.

Dr. Odent declared that they never needed to clear breathing passages after a waterbirth, and that women seem to perceive that it is not risky at all to give birth in water. He points out that there is no danger to the newborn who to this point has known only a watery environment.

Some women enjoy laboring in water and then just feel better about getting out for the birth. Be able to be open to the situation.

Parent-infant bonding can begin in the birthing tub. Breastfeeding can also be started. Once the mother gets out, the father can continue to hold the baby in the tub. If a birth attendant is less experienced with waterbirth, it may be wise for a woman to get out not too long after the birth, because it may be difficult to gauge blood content in the water if he/she has not done so before.

Waterbirth can also help eliminate medical interventions. Heart tones can be found with an underwater Doppler (Doptone). If using a regular Doppler, the mother would need to put her hips out of the water. It may be possible to put the Doptone in a zip-locked bag, or

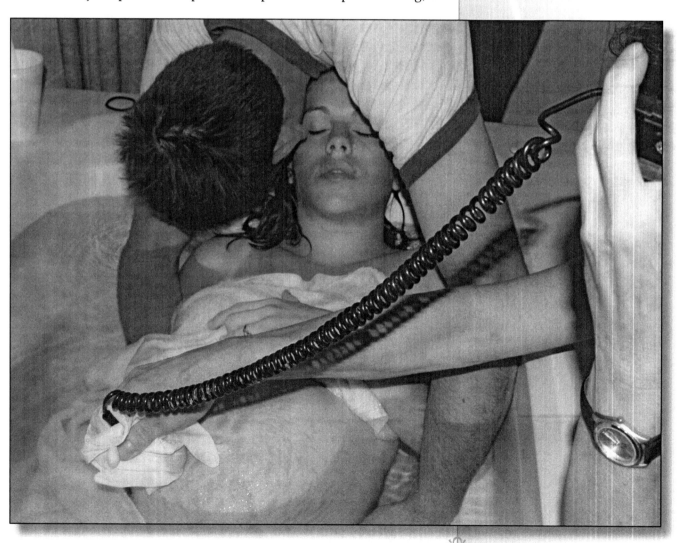

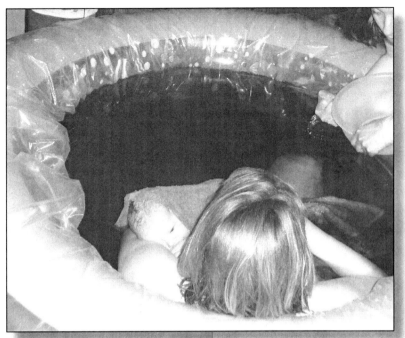

She glides into warm water and unfolds gradually into her new surroundings. The relaxing essence of water is indeed a soothing element for a gentle welcome.

perhaps better yet, to use a fetoscope if your midwife is able to hear with it.

Mothers can give birth in different positions including sitting, squatting, and on hands and knees.

Some people make their own birthing tub. Garden ponds or even brand new animal troughs that are long, wide, and deep enough are options. How to fill, empty and heat these *safely and easily* would take some thought. Keeping them heated with waterbed heaters is a possibility. Brainstorm if you think this might be an option you are interested in. Kiddie pools, with the air-filled rings that make up the walls of them, are comfortable pools to use. You can ask your childbirth educator or midwife for someone that rents waterbirth tubs, or refer to the website sources in this book. Prices for renting tubs might range around $250. To buy one might cost around $250 to 1,200 with equipment for the tub not included in that price. Some midwives have tubs they will loan to their clients.

Certainly you would want your caregiver to be confident with assisting at a waterbirth. Although not impossible, waterbirth may not be a simple option for you. Depending on your area, home may be the only place that waterbirth is available right now, although the hospital might have Jacuzzis for laboring only. But some hospitals and caregivers might allow you to bring and set up a birthing tub in your room.

Many women find various forms of hydrotherapy invaluable during their births, making water a favorite tool for doulas. Showers, using the Jacuzzi (even if the hospital allows use only for labor and not birth), and hot wet towel compresses are all very helpful.

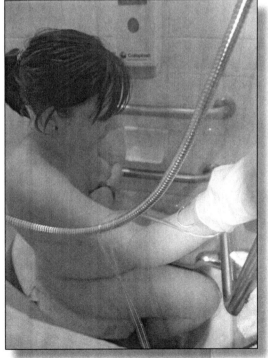

Sitting on the birth ball in the shower can feel great in labor. A nurse has wrapped this mother's IV site so that she can still use hydrotherapy. This can be done as well for a woman that wishes to labor in the tub.

Back Labor

It is most common (and comfortable) for a woman to birth her baby when it is in a rear facing, head down position. But it is not an uncommon occurrence for a mother to be carrying her baby in a posterior position (with baby facing the mother's front instead of her back) at the time of birth. With the baby in this position, the mother can generally expect back pressure and discomfort during labor. Labors in which the baby is posterior often result in longer labors, with contractions being short and mild. Instead of a regularly progressing labor there might, for example, be an hour of strong, long contractions, and then an hour of short, weak contractions. A long pre-labor may occur due to the fact that the pressure of the baby's head is not being applied directly onto the cervix in the same way it would be if the baby was in an anterior position.

Think about it. *It is easier to move straight like an arrow* through a snug tunnel, especially if assisted by gravity, than to try to squeeze through while aiming off to the side. Likewise, when the baby's chin is tucked to his chest, with the crown of his head down on the cervix and the baby facing the mother's back, descent is easier for both the mother and the baby. The crown of the head puts equal pressure over the cervix, helping it to dilate efficiently and allowing the baby to move through more easily.

An experienced caregiver can feel what position your baby is in and teach you what to feel for so you can also recognize your baby's position. A baby may feel to someone on the outside like he is all arms and legs when in a posterior position. You don't feel a lot of arms and legs when the baby is in the rear-facing position.

Avoiding bucket-shaped seats and chairs that cause you to lean back is a good idea.

Theorized Reasons for Posterior Position

There are various reasons why babies may rest in the posterior position. It is reported that babies are carried in a posterior position most often during the winter months. Wearing a warm coat over your belly when it is chilly may help.

A mother may often sit with her hips lower than her knees. When a woman leans backwards during later pregnancy, perhaps in a couch or at a desk, the baby will probably have a tendency to follow gravity and naturally slide back from the optimal position— with the baby facing her back, to his back resting against her backbone. Leaning forward with her hips higher than her knees, perhaps with legs apart, is a good position for the mother to practice so that the baby stays in a better position. Avoiding bucket-shaped seats and chairs that cause her to lean back is a good idea.

The mother's pelvis may not be aligned well with the rest of her body.

Measures to Help a Baby Turn

Making sure your baby and body are aligned with one another can help you to have a much shorter and more comfortable labor and birth. The following are some things you can do to help your birth be easier and more efficient:

Making sure your baby and body are aligned with one another can help you to have a much shorter and more comfortable labor and birth.

1. **Visit a chiropractor who is familiar with the Webster Technique** (which is also very helpful for turning a breech baby) if your baby seems to be turned in a posterior position a great deal of the time during the latter part of pregnancy. If your pelvis is out of alignment, one of your legs may seem to be shorter than the other when lying down. A chiropractor (a wonderful resource for a more comfortable pregnancy, as well as labor) can help to determine this and can use the Webster Technique to fix this. If the baby turns back again, you may need to return for another visit.

   You can also do the following at home: Lie on the floor with a paperback book (perhaps two or three inches thick) under the sacrum on the side of the shorter leg for twenty minutes. This can help to align your pelvis and turn your baby into an anterior position. This may not be very comfortable, but it is one of the best techniques we know of for helping to turn a baby from a posterior position. It is usually recommended that you do not lie on your back during pregnancy. As always, listen to your body during this exercise.

2. **Use the Polar Bear position.** *This is a very valuable position to take note of.* Kneel with *open* knees to chest for about thirty to forty-five minutes—especially at the *beginning* of labor if contractions are not regular (seven to 10 minutes apart, 30 seconds long, felt mostly in the lower abdomen, and progressively getting longer, stronger, closer together, and remaining regular.)

   This can quiet contractions down in the days prior to labor starting, when it isn't yet time, and will allow you to get some rest and be ready for when it really is. **At the beginning of active labor, it can help to get the baby into position for a much more efficient, more comfortable labor.** Although this may seem like it would be uncomfortable, it has been just the thing some women have found has helped to get their babies into a more optimal position, shaving off time and making labor easier.

3. **Try the Cat position.** On hands and knees, the mother lifts her back into an arch, resumes a normal flat-backed position (not sway-back), repeating the exercise a number of times.

4. **Do the lunge.** The mother places one foot on a chair, or on a staircase, and with a straight back, makes a forward lunging motion.

5. **Climb stairs.**

6. **Take a warm bath or shower** (during labor, remember to stay out of the water until active labor—about five centimeters dilated—as this can slow labor). Direct the **shower's spray onto the lower back.**

7. **Gently massage the abdomen from right to left.** It is said to be very effective for the mother to **visualize** the baby moving into the correct position while you **talk to him,** telling him to "roll over."

8. Have a support person **massage your abdomen from right to left while you are on your hands and knees.**

9. **Crawl backwards.**

10. If you have chosen an epidural, **try lying on your left side, with two pillows under your right knee, which is jack-knifed, the left leg straight out and toward the back.** It is best to **avoid an epidural** because while epidurals severely limit a mother's movement, babies can turn more easily if the mother is able to be up and active in various positions.

11. **Do belly-lifting.** Stand up, flex your knees, bend backwards slightly, and place your hands under your uterus and try to align the fetus with your body. A woman's partner can help to gently perform this exercise from behind.

12. **Use a birth ball and/or some belly dancing.** Kneel over or sit on a birthing ball and move your hips in a circling motion to rotate the pelvis from side to side. This can help to rotate the baby into position within the pelvis, encourage fetal descent, and relax the pelvis so that it is easier for the baby to get into position. The double-hip squeeze, massage, and hot and cold packs can all be used with the birth ball. See below for more information about birth balls and belly dancing.

13. **Avoid having your baby's bag of waters released.** It is more comfortable and effective if the baby can use the bag of water as a cushion to rotate against as he makes his way out.

14. **Use Rebozo Techniques.** Ask your doula if she uses a rebozo. Rebozo techniques for pregnancy and birth come to us from traditional Mexican midwives and are some of the most helpful for moving a baby up and out of a less effective position and giving him room to wriggle into one that is much nicer for him and for mom. (Read more in Positioning Baby Optimally For Birth in **Information on the Internet in Appendix E.**)

15. Seeing a Foot Zoner may be beneficial for helping a baby get into an optimal position. Both physical and emotional difficulties related to pregnancy can be effectively treated with zoning.

When the baby's chin is tucked to his chest, with the crown of his head down on the cervix and the baby facing the mother's back, descent is easier for both the mother and the baby. The crown of the head puts equal pressure over the cervix, helping it to dilate efficiently and allowing the baby to move through more easily.

Help to Relieve Back Discomfort

Along with the above tips, which can solve the problem altogether, following are some additional helps for relieving back discomfort:

1. Have a support person do the **Double Hip Squeeze**. With the mother in a kneeling position, squeeze the mother's hips together.
2. Apply **counter pressure to the small of the mother's lower back.**
3. **Have her take a shower or bath**—but as described above, staying off her back will help her to avoid having the baby move into a posterior position. The shower spray can feel wonderful on her back.
4. **Roll a rolling pin, frozen juice can, or a massager on her back** (support people can trade off, using good body mechanics themselves).
5. Have her **sit, straddling a chair backwards.**
6. Have her **sit in a firm chair or against the wall, with a support person pressing her knees back toward her hips.** This can really feel great.
7. **Many of those things which are recommended for turning the baby into position are also helpful for relieving back labor discomfort.**
8. Ask about a **sterile water injection.** Ask your caregiver about these injections and find out if they are familiar with this technique. This can help to relieve backache without any apparent side-effects.
9. **Hang in there. Mother and support people too! Have faith! Support team can continue to help Mom to stay relaxed. They need to remember to also stay relaxed themselves!**
10. **Again, remember that while pain medication can take the pain of back labor away, it won't cure the problem and may result in a cesarean** as it is more difficult to birth effectively and it is harder (if not impossible) when using pain medication, to use positions to encourage the baby to turn. It also takes longer. The right positions help to create more effective labor patterns.

It must be stressed that **many a baby has been born vaginally while in a posterior position. A posterior position is not a good reason for cesarean section.**

Belly Dancing, Birth Balls, and Rebozos

What does belly dancing have to do with a woman who is in labor? A whole lot, as a matter of fact!

It is rumored that belly dancing actually originated as a dance for women in labor! Whether this is true or not, the motions used for belly dancing can indeed serve a woman in some very helpful ways.

Granted, a woman—even if she were a professional belly dancer—would probably not feel extremely comfortable shimmying in her no more than semi-private hospital room! And, at least in the beginning, a lot of women would not feel entirely at ease with belly dancing in private either—especially when she is fully ripe with child!

But, hey, whatever works, right? So dismiss those inhibitions, put some Middle Eastern music in the CD player, and get moving! Really, any music that you like that has a good beat is fine.

It's actually kind of fun! So how is this supposed to help? **Getting the hips moving can help the baby to find its way out, to rotate, and to move down into place.** Think of how you put on your sneakers. Do you just plunk your foot in? No, it commonly takes a little bit of wriggling and twisting to slide your foot in does it not? Your baby needs to travel down and engage deep into your pelvis. Your bones, with the help of gravity on the baby, have the chance to open, spread, and encircle your child, helping him to find his way out into your arms.

And what tool do professional labor assistants often use to help women to get their babies down and into place? The birth ball! Big, soft physical therapy balls are brought by the doula for the mom to sit on. The ball assists her in a sort of squat, helping to open the pelvis wide. She then makes circles with her

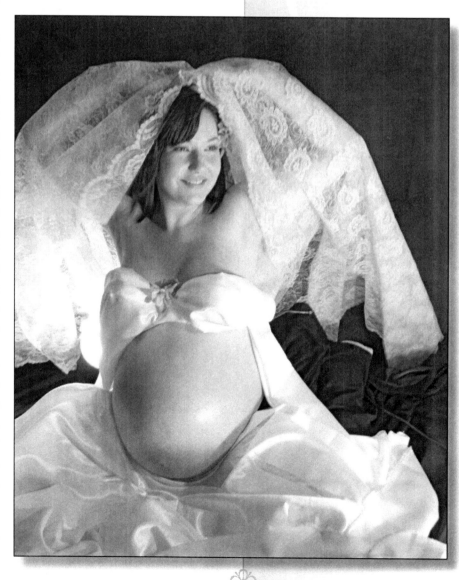

hips—comparable to belly dancing! A few laboring moms get on the ball and don't get off until it's time for the actual birth. They can also kneel over it on hands and knees and move her hips. Some caregivers are willing to perform cervical checks as the mother continues to sit on the ball.

Another extremely helpful tool for "dancing" the baby out, is the Rebozo which has been previously mentioned in Measures to Help the Baby Turn in the above section Back Labor. (See Positioning Baby Optimally For Birth in **Information on the Internet in Appendix E**.)

So why don't all childbirth classes inform their students about this amazingly helpful bit of information? Beats us!

Being able to turn the music up and work with your baby and body in the privacy of your own home is another reason to delay going to the hospital too early in labor. Once at the hospital, it can help to shut the door, or to shut yourself away in the bathroom or shower for a little while.

If it makes your labor easier, what's stopping you—especially if it helps to shave off some extra time by helping your child to move down and out?! Sooo…start shimmying! Come on!

14

Your Support Team

Inviting the right support team to be around you during your birth, can aid you in having more of the kind of birth experience you would like to have.

You will want to give some careful thought to who would be best for the job, and about your selection of those who will be able to help you to facilitate your specific wishes. Who will help you with comfort measures? Who will help you to maintain your confidence? Who will help you to increase safety for you and your baby?

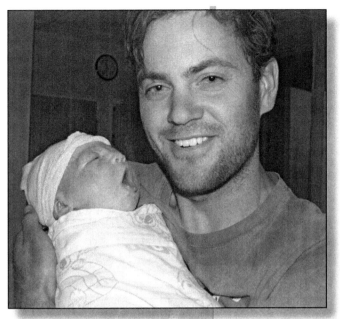

Dad's Role

Most fathers anticipate the birth of their child with excitement and warmth. This can be a stressful time for fathers too. A father may feel concerned about the safety of his wife and child, and about how life will change. It isn't unusual for dads to experience anxiety about meeting everyone's expectations at the birth. A father may even feel left out at times. Sadly, many fathers feel somewhat invisible at prenatal appointments and at the birth itself.

Most of our grandfathers, and many of our fathers, weren't invited into the birth room. Historically, birthing was "women's business."

When the birthplace shifted from home to hospital, everyone familiar to the mother was excluded from the birth scene, including the woman's female friends and relatives. But hospitals underestimated the value of having a woman's husband, familiar woman friends, and/or a doula present. Nurses usually did not have time to give this kind of support, and so the woman essentially was left alone. As you can imagine, this created a terrifying and lonely experience for many mothers.

In the 1970s, though, birthing classes sprang up. In an attempt to reduce mothers' isolation, classes promoted fathers' participation. This was a positive thing for families. Fathers were able to play an even larger role than they ever had in history. Now the father and mother were allowed to be together during this life-changing event for the family.

Perhaps this was the foundation for the greater involvement that fathers seemed to increasingly take in their children's lives.

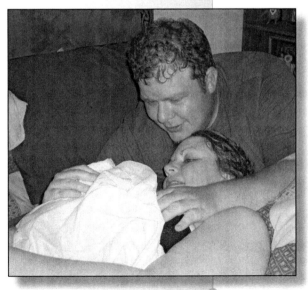

With this change, Dad was soon to learn that he was expected to be his wife's "coach" as she gave birth. Most men, being less than entirely knowledgeable about the female body and the process of birth—let alone what giving birth in that day and age meant—had probably never attended a birth before with the exception of his own.

Nevertheless, he came to understand that among other jobs, he was to manage his wife's breathing pattern, fight off medical personnel, remind his wife she really didn't want drugs (is it any wonder that laboring women are famous for yelling at their husbands?) and be in charge of the situation. And when it was all said and done and things didn't go as planned, who would be to blame? Talk about being set up!

No matter how tough a guy was, was it really fair to ask him to "coach," manage, and fight during one of the most moving and amazing passages in his life? Did a woman with her innate ability to give birth *need* a coach anyway?

Ironically, when it came down to the actual experience, **Dad still was not considered, when it was all said and done, to be a very significant figure at the birth of his own child;** sometimes he felt like he was more "in the way" than that he was one of the most important members of the couple's birth team.

Doula's Role

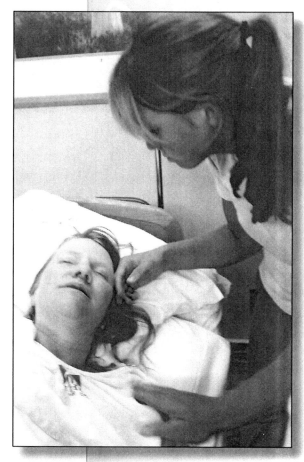

In the early 1990s some very positive **studies began to emerge showing the benefits of having the constant nurture and support of a professional labor assistant.** (Kennell 1991) A new member of the birth team, the "doula" was introduced. This professional, usually hired by the couple, sometimes provided by the hospital, acted as a guide for the laboring couple. Families who sought out a doula found that she took much of the pressure from the father's shoulders. Her training and experience were especially helpful at the birth when the couple was confronted with any unplanned circumstances.

The father was free to experience, to simply hold his wife if wished, to protect his wife and child if he saw fit, to perhaps receive his baby into his own hands if he wanted. The couple, depending on where they birthed, was allowed to define the role he would take.

With a doula to bridge the gap, he was no longer expected to "coach." Now, as they all worked as a team, the doula could offer helpful suggestions and help deal with different situations that would arise. Her presence was assuring to both the laboring woman and her husband—providing the opportunity for the father to be more involved, if he wished, than he would normally have been able to be. The doula was there to shelter the family, guiding and serving. The doula could go over the birth wishes with the family, and help them to know how they could best go about achieving those wishes, what was practical and what was not. Best of all, although not available in all areas, doulas were affordable to all families. In time, insurance companies began to see the cost-saving benefits for themselves, and it wouldn't be long before more would begin to pay for professional labor assistance.

So what *is* the best place for today's new father to fill? That is something the couple can best answer for themselves. This is the birth of *their* child. The mother usually has some great suggestions about what she knows she will need the most. What about loving support, hugs, telling her when she looks beautiful in labor (women in labor are very beautiful!), having her husband bring juice or cool cloths for her face, **having him just be there to experience this awesome event *together*, unencumbered by outside expectations.**

Having a doula at the birth allows the dad the freedom to serve as little or as much as he and his wife choose. But sometimes women express that they would like to have a doula but that they are afraid to even approach their husbands with this. A woman may be afraid that her husband would feel that she wasn't confident in his abilities or that if they hired a doula he would feel displaced or unneeded at the birth of his child. She may also fear that having a doula present might distract from couple togetherness during the birth. These fears are doubtlessly common among couples who have never worked with a doula before. Talking about these things openly, in a sensitive manner with one another, can be helpful.

It can be reassuring to know that doulas actually can provide *more* opportunity for couple intimacy. It can also be comforting to both the father and mother to know that they have an ally, someone who helps birthing families often, a woman who can help them get more of the kind of birth they are hoping for. Doulas sometimes even provide some photos and a written account of the minute-to-minute events of the labor and birth as they happened.

Frequently, couples state that they were much more satisfied with the births in which their doula was present. Couples who hire a doula once will often choose to hire a doula for the births of all of the rest of their children.

Benefits of a Doula

Doulas are guides to make this the most comfortable, manageable, and beautifully memorable experience possible.

Doulas, in their own capacity, work alongside doctors, midwives, and nurses. Although some nurses are able to offer support during labor, most are unable to stay continuously with the laboring woman due to other clinical tasks. A nurse may kindly give some comfort, if she is not rushing between labor rooms and her charting responsibilities. But this is not a nurse's job, nor has she generally had any professional training in the art of labor support. Many busy nurses would rather encourage pain medication because they are kept so busy. Doctors usually come in when a nurse calls to let them know that the baby is close to being born. If your caregiver is a midwife, she may be able to give support some of the time during your labor, but there are times when she

It can also be comforting to both the father and mother to know that they have an ally, someone who helps birthing families often, a woman who can help them get more of the kind of birth they are hoping for.

needs to focus primarily on the clinical needs at hand. If she is a Certified Nurse Midwife and is working in the hospital, she may have more than one woman laboring at the same time. Ideally, a good birth team will include a doula who is there just for the woman and her family, for their comfort, and for advocating for their personal needs and desires.

Although she cannot work miracles in less than favorable conditions, just the presence of a doula at your birth can encourage your caregivers to help you have the best experience possible.

Doulas use a variety of comfort and labor-enhancing techniques such as use of the birth ball, positions that are beneficial for both the mother and the baby, massage, walking, shower and Jacuzzi, encouragement and positive feedback, and other coping techniques.

Many couples (first-timers especially) wanting to save some money, forego having a doula, even though they see a lot of benefits. They want the birth to be an intimate, bonding experience and so they want to be alone. While it can be a wonderful bonding moment, many couples have found that in the end the birth was not exactly the way they had imagined it. **It's often the couples having a subsequent baby that choose to hire a doula because they can see how much she could have helped to facilitate that bonding experience the first time.**

A doula's help and presence are some of the best "things" you can bring with you to your labor.

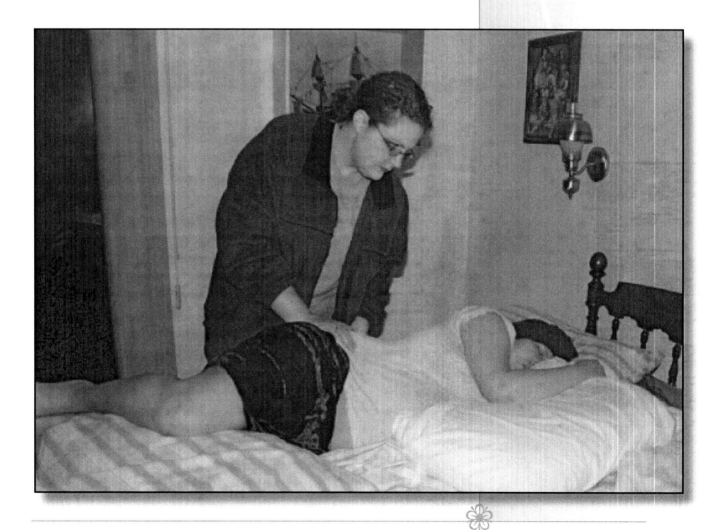

Doula fees are very reasonable, and most doulas will not withhold services from anyone desiring labor support. If you are on limited means, ask your doula what can be worked out.

Studies by Dr. Kennell and Drs. Klaus and Klaus report the following significant benefits of having support in labor:

- A 40 percent reduction in use of Pitocin
- A 50 percent reduction in cesareans
- A 30 percent decrease in analgesia (pain medication) use
- A 60 percent decrease in request for epidural (pain medication)
- A 25 percent decrease in length of labor
- A 40 percent decrease in use of forceps
- Decreased tearing and episiotomy rates
- Decreased fear and pain
- Reduction in medical costs
- Increased participation of father
- Increased breastfeeding success
- A safer, healthier birth and baby

Doulas and Pain Medication

If you've decided on an epidural or other pain medication, it is still helpful to have a doula.

1. **Usually epidurals do not take away all of the sensation.** Sometimes an epidural will only take away feeling in one area. The administration of an epidural before about 5 centimeters dilation can cause a labor to slow or stop, often necessitating other procedures including a cesarean, so many caregivers will not administer them until that point is reached. Your doula can be priceless for helping you with relaxation, position changes, and comfort techniques. Frequently there are side effects to epidurals, such as nausea, shaking, and itching. A doula can help a woman deal with these.
2. **A doula can be an advocate for your choices,** to help you to get the things you want from your birth, and to support you in your decisions.
3. **A doula can be your personal one-on-one information source** about your options in any given situation.
4. **An epidural doesn't cover the emotional aspects of labor.** The need for the emotional support that a doula can give doesn't change. Epidurals don't give massages and reassurance, suggest a change of position, or offer cold sips of water. They don't sit with you and hold your hand. They don't explain things, or give you information that can help you to make decisions.

Couples who hire a doula once will often choose to hire a doula for the births of all of the rest of their children.

If Mom Loses Her Confidence

What can a birth partner do to help a woman if she starts to feel overwhelmed during labor?

First, **help her to release tension**. Relaxation during a contraction can be very helpful. You can help her to release tension by telling her to relax wherever you touch her. With your hands, stroke the tension away. You can also talk the tension away by simply saying, "Relax," "I'll hold you," "Take a deep breath," and other such words. Music may also be helpful.

Once past five centimeters, if she doesn't have an IV, she can get in the **water**, which many women have reported was *extremely* helpful for them. Help her to hold out until then. If she does have an IV, perhaps she can ask to be disconnected from it for awhile to get into the water, keeping her arm with the needle out of the water.

Apply **counter-pressure** to her back if she is having back pressure.

Lead her in deep and slow abdominal **breathing**.

Reserve some things (such as having her use the Jacuzzi or shower) in the back of your mind, and save them for just such an occasion.

If things are becoming very difficult, she may be nearing or in transition, the time just before actual birthing. Usually it isn't too much longer. If she has desired to have no pain medication, encourage her by **telling her that she is almost there**, and that you are there with her, that you will help her, and most importantly that she can do it.

Hold her, **love her**, and allow her to cry.

Encourage the use of **sounding** if she wishes (humming, moaning, etc. but **keeping the pitch of her tones low**). This often comes naturally and helps a woman to let go and to open.

If she says, "I can't do this anymore," see this as a sign that she is asking for help, for **support**. Let her know that you know that it's difficult, but that **she can do it**. Reassure her, praise her. Try to get her to focus on staying on top of the surge. Help her to think of her cervix opening wider and wider.

Sometimes a woman really panics. This is, again, often at the time of transition when it is almost over. What to do?

- **Get her to look into your eyes, take her face firmly in your hands, and tell her to breathe with you (deep abdominal breathing).**

Help her to focus on staying on top of each wave as it comes, like she would if she were surfing the waves at the beach.

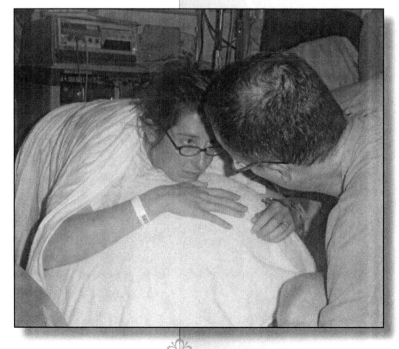

Kneeling over a birth ball, this woman depends on the much needed support of her entire birth team during a challenging time in her labor.

- Reassure her that you are there throughout each contraction and that each one is bringing the baby closer.
- Stay with her emotionally.
- Just holding her can make a big difference.

NOTE: Have a doula with you, to be there for you and the birthing mother! Coming from a woman experienced with childbirth, rather than from her husband at a point like this, some of these suggestions may be more readily accepted by the mother. A doula's help and presence really are some of the very best "things" you can bring with you to the labor—whether or not you are planning on pain medication.

Siblings at the Birth

Be sure those who will be assisting you are comfortable with your choice to have your children present. You might want to call your birth place beforehand to find out how many families have had their older children present during labor. One way to find out more about their comfort level with this option is to ask how they would suggest preparing a child for the birth. **If they are less than enthusiastic about having your children present, you may want to reconsider either your decision to have your children at the birth, or your decisions concerning caregivers and birth place.**

Prepare children for what to expect. While birth is a wonderful, awe-inspiring experience, it is helpful for children to be taught that there is blood, and that mothers make sounds (groaning, moaning, sighing, and even screaming) because they are "working hard."

You might want to show them pre-viewed birth movies (or parts of them) and explain them. There are also good children's books about birth and babies.

Children may be surprised at the appearance of the baby all red, wrinkly, sometimes with a bit of a disproportioned head or coating of vernix (a creamy substance on the baby's skin).

Siblings should also know that for the most part, babies are only interested in eating and sleeping, that they aren't a grown-up brother or sister with whom they can play right away. Educate them on how they can help you and be a part of things (such as bringing you soup or massaging your feet, etc).

You also might want to see if there are sibling classes in your area. Depending on the type, they may or may not prepare the child for the actual birth experience.

A special bonding can occur between siblings when the older children are invited to witness the birth of their brother or sister.

Children often enjoy putting a hand on their mother's abdomen and feeling the baby move within. You can **let them come with you to pre-natal appointments** and let them hear the baby's heartbeat. You might take the child to the birthplace beforehand for a tour.

Emphasizing that this is indeed your older child's baby too can help to make the postpartum time easier for him—and for you, because instead of the child feeling as if he might be being "replaced" with a new baby, this baby is for him too!

Having support people for each of the children can be an excellent idea. If the dad is trying to deal with the children at the same time he is trying to be there for the mother, it may be a bit of a disappointment to the couple that he was not able to be as involved with her as he had previously wished to be. Children may lose interest at times during labor and may need to leave the room for walks, to play, and to eat. If the child has his own doula, she/he can be sensitive to their needs of wanting to leave if, for example, the noise seems to be bothering him. The support people need to realize that they may miss the birth, as the

Many a sibling who has experienced the planned birth of a brother or sister has had wonderful, positive memories of the experience, and has developed a view of birth unlike that of individuals who have never witnessed real birth.

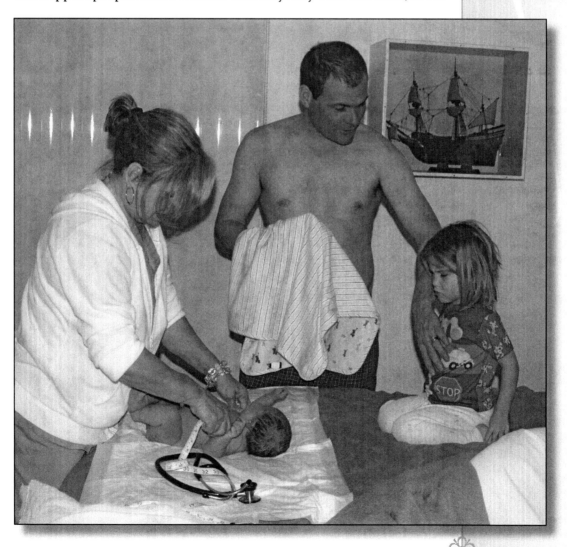

older child is their first priority, so choose this person carefully. (Would grandma mind if she missed the birth?) It can be so helpful to talk in a happy and reassuring manner with them if they seem at all concerned.

If the birth is at home, and is at nighttime, the children may be asleep in the next room until just before or after the birth, but it is good to have the bases covered and be sure there is someone there to help with them. And in the uncommon case that you should need to transfer to the hospital, someone would already be there to care for the children while you are away.

Many a sibling who has experienced the planned birth of a brother or sister has had wonderful, positive memories of the experience and has developed a view of birth unlike that of children who have never witnessed any kind of birth other than frightening, made-for-television ones. Their positive views are carried into adulthood and will likely influence their own families. In addition, a special bonding can occur between siblings when the older children are invited to witness the birth of their brother or sister.

You may wish to have support people for each of the siblings present at the birth.

15

Psychological Aspects of Labor and Birth

IMAGINE YOUR FAVORITE FOOD. See the way it looks. Smell the aroma. Taste it in your mouth. Feel the temperature and the texture. What is happening to your body as you simply *imagine* smelling and tasting it? Do you perhaps feel your mouth begin to produce saliva? This is just one example of how our thought processes influence our body.

When you experience anger, happiness, attraction, fear, or sadness, your body responds accordingly to what began only in the mind. **Our minds and bodies are inseparably connected. The mind greatly influences the body and the body's experiences.**

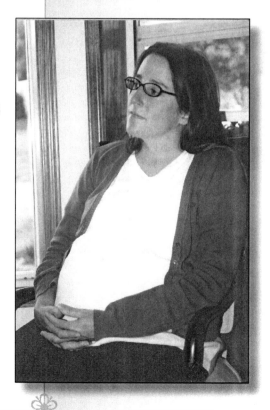

The Body/Mind Connection

Why must we consider the Body/Mind Connection?

Think about an athlete's training. What she believes is possible, and whether she can see it happening in her mind can make all the difference in whether she is successful in her goals or not. **To neglect her psychological preparation would be to put an athlete at a great disadvantage. So it does for a woman who is about to give birth!**

This is one reason why hypnobirthing programs are so successful at helping women to birth easily and comfortably. What you believe really does make a difference in what you will experience, and what your birth will be like.

Psychological issues are of such consequence, in fact, that a large number of caregivers today believe that they are *even more important* than the size of the pelvis and the size of the baby.

A pelvis was made to open and stretch, just as its counterpart the uterus was made to open and stretch to accommodate a growing baby—little by little, but surely and truly! Likewise, the vagina expands to what might seem amazing proportions, and then returns quite close to normal after the baby is born. Amazing, yes it is—impossible, not at all. It is what has been happening countless times a day for ages and ages, over and over again, for numberless women and babies! It has only been in the last few years that birth has been institutionalized—a very few, when considering the amount of time babies have been emerging from women upon the earth. From the modern United States viewpoint, we should be just amazed that the human race did not die out before it began—let alone survive until *now*!

American women have a lot of cultural intimidations to overcome. The messages to women as to what they are supposed to believe about the limitations of their bodies are loud and clear.

Many, *many* a woman has been told that there is some doubt about the size of her pelvis, as if pelvises weren't made right, weren't designed to stretch and give and open.

What is not understood is that a woman who has been unduly alarmed by well-meaning family, friends, or even a caregiver that doesn't believe in her body, can be in for a very difficult time.

What words and images will *you* bring with you to your birth? What pictures and stories do you carry in your mind? Do they empower you? Do you believe your birth can be wonderful?

Sadly, it is not uncommon for women in our culture to doubt that their bodies can actually give birth. Is it any wonder that rates of cesarean sections performed for "failure to progress" are so high in our country? A woman who is frightened, upset, preoccupied with, *and overly alert* to outside goings-on around her may soon find herself at odds with the clock for not dilating "efficiently."

What has your mind, and as a result your body, been conditioned to expect?

The Importance of Feeling Safe

How can understanding the importance of the Body/Mind Connection help you to create a better birth? **It is crucial that a woman is able to birth free of *harmful* distractions.** Laboring mammals search for a protective, warm, safe, quiet, dark place to give birth. These elements encourage the release of endorphins. Fear and stress inhibit endorphin flow and cause adrenaline to rise. If the security of a mother's birth place is meddled with, labor stops so that she can fight or take flight. If she feels safe, she births her young.

When disturbed by a predator such as a coyote or human when birthing, a female animal's labor may actually stop, and she may even draw the partly born baby back into her body! Infant animals whose mothers are disturbed and frightened during birth are sometimes born dead. How important is it then, to have greater respect for nature and to be sure that women aren't frightened or bothered with a lot of invasive exams and connected to a lot of manmade machines?

Ina May Gaskin explains, "Excretory, cervical, and vaginal sphincters function best in an atmosphere of intimacy and privacy—for example, a bathroom with a locking door or a bedroom, where interruption is unlikely or impossible.... These sphincters cannot be opened at will and do not respond well to commands.... When a person's sphincter is in the process of opening, it may suddenly close down if that person becomes upset, frightened, humiliated, or self-conscious. Why? High levels of adrenaline in the bloodstream do not favor (sometimes they actually prevent) the opening of the sphincters . . . a rough and uncompassionate pelvic exam can *reverse* [*emphasis added*] a mother's cervical dilation." (Gaskin, Ina May's Guide 2003)

What about invasive **cervical checks**? Just by observing the outward signs, someone that is experienced with this should know what stage of labor a woman is at without cervical checks needing to be performed. Outward, emotional signs can actually be a more accurate indication of where in labor a woman really is. How far open her cervix is can be deceiving. For example, if the cervix takes the time to thin out before opening, as is often the case with first time mothers, a woman's cervix may actually be 90% effaced (thinned out) but only 3 cm dilated when checked. If she is showing emotional signs of transition (see Ways Dads or Birth Partners May Be Supportive in **chapter 17.**), it would probably be wise for the caregiver not to leave to go back to the office! Women often rapidly progress once they are completely effaced. Emotional signposts will often tell more about what is going on than even cervical exams will. Why are so many of those who are assigned to the care of laboring women not trained in this simple skill? More than a couple of vaginal exams, if any at all, are usually completely unnecessary and can be very harmful to a woman's state of mind while in labor. If she is feeling as if she is nearly ready to give birth, to be told she has only progressed three

The months of pregnancy are a good time to get those things that might hinder a woman in labor worked out!

centimeters can be unduly disheartening—not to mention that it takes her out of her laboring mind, which before was only requiring her to do it moment by moment. She can better do that if she has encouragement rather than deceptive numbers to deal with. This is not even to mention the risks of infection involved with this intervention. Imagine the trauma caused to a woman, whom has experienced prior sexual abuse, and who is now subjected to a series of cervical exams—in labor no less!

We certainly have forgotten what this time means to a woman. Though a very special time, pregnancy and birth may be one of the most challenging, overwhelming things she will ever do. Strangely, in this culture it has been our practice to assign machines to watch her, and we depend on their output for information about her, rather than dealing with her as a *person; a woman birthing her child.* We leave her alone and *she* becomes a birthing machine; just another of the machines it takes to produce a baby. In other places, women are honored and the birth of a mother is celebrated as is the birth of the child.

The Importance of Letting Go

It is believed that there are two different parts of the brain in charge of two different kinds of thinking—that the left takes care of logic, reasoning, and analytical thinking, and that the right is responsible for such things as creative ability, artistic thinking, lovemaking, and labor.

As a woman progresses in labor, she travels from the more left-brained, analytical way of thinking to a more creative, inward, perceptive, fervent and emotional level of focus. She finds she must give heed to her body, to allow it do what it was designed to do. Her contractions and her immediate surroundings become her all. She progresses to being entirely immersed within the power that is bringing her child to her. So consumed with what her body is doing, she may cry, moan or sigh, and throw inhibitions aside.

Lovemaking and childbirth both employ the right hemisphere of the brain. And when in the midst of either, a woman becomes more emotional, vulnerable, and less socially-inhibited. Birth, just like making love, goes better if a woman can let go and surrender to it.

But some have been taught by well-meaning parents, in an attempt to protect their children, that making love is dirty and ugly. It is difficult for many people to see the beautiful, spiritual aspects in either making love or birthing a baby. Other women, those who have suffered abuse, may have difficulty surrendering and letting go. (See The Impact of Past Sexual Abuse in **this chapter.**) Some may specifically want an epidural or a c-section so that they can remove themselves as far as possible from any parallels to sex. Some women emphatically state that they don't want to feel anything, choosing also to miss out on the intense wonders of labor as well.

Birthing women who are willing and able to let go, and who are not disturbed or distracted, are much more able to do what women have instinctively and intuitively done for ages.

How do you feel about your body? What do you feel when you hear each of these words—menstruation, pregnancy, labor, giving birth, lactation? Are you uncomfortable? Confident? Empowered? What were you taught about the substances that come out of the body? Feces, urine, ear wax, mucous—do you see them as dirty? Were you taught that sex is dirty? Or that it is wonderful? Were you taught that your body is wonderful, miraculous?

Birthing women who are willing and able to let go, and who are not disturbed or distracted, are much more able to do what women have instinctively and intuitively done for ages.

What would happen if you lost control and just did what came naturally at the moment? Would members of your birth team be uncomfortable and encourage medication? Would they allow you the freedom to moan, rock your body, have a good cry, and otherwise "lose control" without feeling the need to intervene and "save" you? To give birth triumphantly does not have to mean giving birth with perfect control. Releasing and letting go are sometimes just what a laboring woman needs, to be able to surrender to the power of her body and *just let it happen*.

A woman needs to know that the environment that she chooses to birth in will not only influence the level of freedom she is allowed, but will also influence the freedom she will allow herself. It is wise to prepare a place where she feels comfortable doing whatever she feels like. Being able to be in an environment that she has made her very own, wherever that is, would logically assist her in being able to let go and have an easier and more comfortable birthing experience.

Some women would feel inhibited by having the whole family there. She may want to request that they wait in the waiting room or that those witnessing the birth stay with her at the head of the bed (assuming she is giving birth in the hospital's traditional stirrup position) and witness (or even record the birth with a camcorder—if she desires) from behind her shoulder. These things may help her to feel less self-conscious and be more able to open and give birth to her baby. It can help to remember that this scene is certainly not new to her doctor or midwife, nurses, or labor assistant.

A laboring woman can easily absorb the fear, anger, and those feelings of her caregivers and others she has invited to attend her birth. It is important to choose these people wisely. Too many *unnecessary* people may actually take away from the birth energy in the room. Not enough privacy or intimacy can also slow things down. The father or doula may need to encourage those in the room to be more quiet and focused.

Good feelings should exist among all those in the birthing room. The presence of loving assistance and confidence from her team is a valuable support for the mother. This can help her yield to psychological changes

It is wise to prepare a place where you feel comfortable doing whatever you feel like doing.

and to experience a more comfortable, efficient labor. A woman needs to feel love, communication, and participation from her support people. It's good for those who are close to the woman to tell her how incredibly beautiful she looks. (A laboring woman does look radiant and beautiful, as sweaty from the work of labor and as unkempt as she may be!)

Ina May Gaskin suggests that it is helpful for a birthing woman to act kindly to the people around her, giving positive energy, and that this will help her a great deal. (Gaskin, Spiritual) Likewise, discourteous exchanges, and anxiety (yes, other people's too) in the environment can influence her deeply.

It is very important to note, as a part of this discussion, that emotional sensitivity and vulnerability are increased in labor. **Not only is the laboring woman usually much more open to suggestions for procedures she has been, and would still be, opposed to in her usual frame of mind, but so is the father. This is a time of vulnerability for him too.** For examples, such things as propositions to speed up labor, unwanted suggestions for pain medication, or superfluous routine newborn infant procedures may be more easily accepted in this environment of dependence, than they would be ordinarily.

The Importance of Dealing with Negative Emotions

When considering the above then, it is most helpful when all fears and emotions have been dealt with *prior to* the birth. It is critical to carefully choose birth attendants and the birth place. Everything should be in place so that worries are gone and so that the woman can concentrate on the forces within. **It is time for her to allow her mind to get out of the way and let her body birth her baby the way she was made to do!**

There are some good childbirth class programs now that focus on psychological issues. Many others, however, still deal mainly with the latest technology, how it will be used, and how to be a good patient. The lack of discussion in some classes about the psychological factors of labor and birth is appalling. This topic is of immense importance.

Women, by nature, are emotional beings, and emotions and beliefs have much to do with progress in labor. Some women have had difficult past birth experiences or hospital encounters. Issues and fears often come forth during projects and discussions in effective childbirth classes. Now, instead of during labor or in early postpartum, is a good time for a woman to give attention to doubts about her ability to be a good mother, for example, or to unresolved feelings about the relationship between her and her own mother. These kinds of things can significantly affect the kind of labor a woman will have and the kind of mother she will be.

> *Not only is the laboring woman usually much more open to suggestions for procedures she has been, and would still be, opposed to in her usual frame of mind, but so is the father.*

Pregnancy is a good time to get those things that would hinder us worked out!

Especially if she has had a prior negative birth or other similar experience, **as part of her preparation work, it is particularly essential for a woman to be sure to deal with feelings she might unconsciously carry with her regarding any items that will be in her birth surroundings.**

Some women don't want to wear the hospital's gown because they don't like being clothed in the uniform of the *patients* of the hospital. They feel wearing the jonnie sends a powerful psychological message that says, in a sense, that they are the property of the hospital, that they are sick, and that they should succumb to anything that is part of the routine. Will the IV, electronic fetal monitor, and other paraphernalia in the room create anxiety because they seem to symbolize that giving birth must be terribly risky? Can any of these instruments or things be avoided? If not, perhaps assigning different symbolic meanings (such as a "protector") to each of these before the birth, would be helpful.

Since women labor in a more right-brained state of mind, it makes sense to approach labor and birth in a more right-brained way before labor begins.

Writing, creating art, sitting quietly with fears and questions, contemplating, journaling, analyzing your dreams, or talking are all "right brain" ways of figuring out what might be the barriers that stand in the way of our having the most satisfying birth possible.

What do you fear? What unfinished business do you carry with you that might cause "failure to progress"? Have you experienced previous negative experiences in the hospital? Does your blood pressure go up every time you go to a prenatal appointment? What about past sexual abuse? When growing up what were you told about birth? Do you feel ready to become a parent? Is there anything about the experience of birth that might trigger fear or negative feelings due to those past experiences?

Getting rid of your fears now is crucial as you prepare for your birth. When you're in labor you need to just be able to let go and let your body focus on having your baby. Fears are one of the biggest things that can keep us from doing that, and **fear creates adrenaline.** Adrenaline may play a role in whether a laboring woman experiences pain at her birth. It can cause her to have a long, difficult labor.

There are two kinds of fear, one that is counterproductive to labor and another that can actually be productive. **Fear can sometimes help us to make better decisions.** If we acknowledge it *before* labor starts, and because of it we figure out what we need and get everything in place before labor begins, fear may actually be beneficial.

Which of your fears are productive? Which are counterproductive?

Dealing with Difficult Emotions during the Birth

A knowledgeable birth assistant can help you to work through problems that might surface in labor so that labor can continue unconstrained. Doing birth art and working on things beforehand is best. Then by having the support of trusted, experienced people such as a doula around you to help you through anything that might come up during birth, you can cover both bases. **Many cesareans for failure to progress, due to emotional issues, could be avoided!**

Sometimes more intensive sessions with a professional counselor are necessary.

Ways to Deal with Fears

Parents are often surprised to find that other parents have many of the same kinds of fears that they do. There are now a number of extremely valuable resources and ways to help you prepare emotionally and mentally for your birth. Here are a few:

- **Hypnobirthing**—Take a hypnosis-for-birthing class. You *can* learn how to give birth comfortably. Many women have given birth with no pain. An invaluable part of the Mongan Method HypnoBirthing® course is the Fear Release sessions. Overall, taking a hypnosis-for-birthing class can help you to figure out what you want so you can make decisions to help you have a better birth experience. (See **chapter 13**.)
- **Craniosacral Therapy**—This is a wonderful, nurturing way to realize, come to terms with, and release fears and emotions prior to birthing your baby. (See **chapter 12**.)
- **EFT**—(Emotional Freedom Technique, sometimes referred to as "Tapping") This is a fantastic, effective way to release emotions and fears, many of which cause physical problems. In pregnancy, and when preparing for birth, EFT can be invaluable. The web has a great deal of information on the subject.
- **Journal Writing, Prayer, and Meditation**—These are some of the best ways to "figure things out" and find the peace you are seeking.
- **Connect with Your Baby**—In a relaxed place (perhaps a place in nature, or on your couch, in bed, or in the bath), get in touch with your baby. Ask your baby where he/she needs to be born, what he/she needs for this birth to be born easily and safely.
- **Talk It Out**—With a trusted caregiver, your doula, or a friend. This is one very good reason to have a doula.
- **Daily Affirmations**—What you tell yourself is very important to the outcome of many things in your life. These are statements that

are repeated to one's self daily, during a time that you set aside for relaxation, which can help to bring about a desired outcome. You are encouraged to write your own list of affirmations, words that you know will be most helpful to you. It is okay if they are hard to believe at first. Your subconscious mind believes what you tell it. What really is possible for you? Listed on our website, and in many places including books and other places on the web, are wonderful suggestions for affirmations.

- *Birthing from Within*—Writing, making art, picking up a ball of wet clay and playing with it until it becomes something, or just doodling—all of these are ways to connect with your inner "right-brain" mind and to figure things out. This fun book is a guide to all of this and much more. There may also be Birthing From Within mentors who offer classes in your area. (Look for this book in the books section of **Appendix E**.)
- *Creating a Joyful Birth*—A wonderful book worth investing in, you will learn a great deal to help you to have a better experience as you use this book and the other resources on the author's site at http://www.pregnantsoul.com/guided-imagery.php. (You can also look for this book in the books section of **Appendix E**.)
- *Write It Down, Make It Happen* by Henriette Anne Klauser is one of those great books, though not specifically about childbirth, which encourage the reader to create in their minds what they want before it ever happens. This book uses writing as a powerful way to do this. The mind, as we've been discussing, is very powerful. These sources teach that that which we believe, we can actually bring into being. What do you believe about your birth and what it can be? Can you actually make things in your life more of what you want by first conceiving them in your mind? Study of these principles as you prepare for your birth could be extremely helpful. This book is thought-provoking, comforting, and enjoyable.

We are given nine months to prepare and deal with what needs to be taken care of. **If we can face and resolve things before labor starts we have a better chance of a better birth—and father/motherhood as well.** What do you need to help you to do that?

The Impact of Past Sexual Abuse

It is believed that somewhere between 25 to perhaps 50 percent of women have been sexually abused, though gathering numbers can be futile as many cases go unreported.

Does past sexual abuse have any affect on a woman during her pregnancy and birth? Yes, depending on the nature of the abuse and other factors, she *may* experience some of the following challenges:

Sometimes a woman who has suffered abuse experiences will undergo difficulty with vaginal exams, needles, procedures invasive to the body, and nakedness. She may struggle, experience anxiety, tension, and resistance. And she may have flashbacks and even flee her body by dissociation.

She may have issues with bodily secretions, doctors' tools, and certain positions. She may also feel revulsion when watching movies of birth or breastfeeding.

She may have a strong preference for caregivers of a particular gender, as well, and may have trouble trusting anyone giving her care. Some survivors of abuse may choose a caregiver who is very authoritative, with whom she behaves very meekly and agreeably, and is unquestioning about the kind of care she receives. Or she may try to control her care, may have a long birth plan, and need lengthy appointments with a lot of discussion with caregivers in an attempt to control this frightening experience. She is also scared of her own vulnerability. Different aspects of her relationship with her caregiver, including that of who is in control, for example, can trigger strong emotions. Understanding this need can help caregivers realize why this seemingly excessive attention to detail, and control over the situation, is so important to her.

A woman may flee from her body in an attempt to escape certain circumstances and may appear as if she is in a trance. Others may not be able to communicate with her. Returning to present surroundings may be a painful experience for the woman, or she may just slowly come out of it.

She may have a prolonged, non-progressing labor. It may be harder for her to open to birth, and there may be a stalling of labor during the active stage. She may have difficulty allowing labor to become stronger. Progress during pushing also may be slowed or stopped.

She may be especially fearful of pain or injury and it may even be disturbing for her to hear her own verbal expressions during labor.

It is possible that she may also have a disinterest in the baby after the birth and an aversion to breastfeeding.

Of course, not all women who have symptoms mentioned here have been sexually abused. It is possible, too, that some women will have no problems in either labor or birth that stem from their past abuse.

Healing is an important thing for survivors to do before they give birth.

Abuse is believed to affect many different aspects of a woman's life, causing problems in a vast variety of areas from asthma to infertility, and from panic attacks to phobias.

As we can see above, women that have previously had negative sexual experiences, including previous difficult birth experiences, will sometimes have much more difficult labors and births. Why would pregnancy and birth be a time when past sexual abuse would become an issue? The answer is obvious when we realize how interrelated birth and sex really are. Even if a woman does not recall all aspects of the abusive experience(s) in her conscious mind, it is believed that a woman's *body* does remember, that her cells store these memories, and that when they are still unresolved prior to giving birth there can be problems.

It is frustrating that the psychological and sexual aspects of birth are, for the most part, still ignored today as a part of obstetrical training. If failure-to-progress in labor is one of the results of past sexual abuse, how many women could bypass a cesarean section, with all of its risks to her and her baby, if caregivers understood this and knew how to help her? What an important thing to add to the black bag!

In contrast, if a doctor/midwife/nurse is coercive, disrespectful, deceitful, or forceful to a woman who has survived abuse in the past, he/she may be perceived on a subconscious level by the woman as another abuser. After the birth, the woman can feel violated, embarrassed, and angry, and can suffer depression that can last for years.

During the birth, if a caregiver or doula suspects that a woman may be having difficulty with an emotional aspect of her labor, he/she can do a lot of good just by being patient with the labor and with the woman and encouraging her, if she is willing, to talk about what is going on in her head and what might be holding her back on a psychological level.

Of course *before* the birth is the best time for survivors to begin the process of healing and preparing for their births!

So what are some things a woman can do if she suspects any of the listed challenges above might be a problem during her birth?

A woman can avoid, when possible, triggers that bring up negative feelings such as a lot of vaginal exams, different routine procedures, and certain positions.

She can make birth art, journal or talk it out with a trusted friend.

It might be beneficial to see a reputable psychotherapist that specializes in sexual abuse or possibly attend a support group.

Having a sensitive, gentle caregiver who has training in how to care for a woman that is a survivor of abuse can be very helpful. Open communication with the caregiver can be very beneficial for assisting him/her in knowing just how to help. Hopefully the caregiver of a client that seems overly demanding, anxious, and resistant, will be sensitive and patient with her, giving her that extra attention and care that she needs.

But no one on a mother's team, except those she knows can assist her with it, needs to know of these issues if she would rather they didn't.

It is imperative that caregivers always be trustworthy, respectful, thoughtful, and patient with each of the women in their care.

Having at her birth a professional labor assistant (doula) that has training in this area can be one of the most valuable things a woman can do to prepare. A doula can be a true ally at this time.

Use other suggestions from the list for facing fears, above.

16

Roadblocks to a Better Birth

This chapter contains some very important points that would be wise to closely consider with an open heart and mind by those who truly want a better birth experience than most families in our culture are getting today!

There are many reasons women may choose an option that is not in the best interest of herself or her baby. In this chapter we will deal with eight of the most obvious or common ones. As you will see, this list is certainly not all inclusive. You can surely come up with others.

For simplicity purposes, the following focuses on the mother. Each of the below may apply as equally to the responsibility of fathers as well.

A False Sense of Security

Fears

Low Self–Concept

Lack of Information

Hesitancy about New Information

Relationship Issues

Lack of Effort

Choices Seem Impossible

A False Sense of Security

It is natural to take new ideas and judge them within the scope of what we already know to be truth. But what happens when the things we thought we knew are really false, or are somehow distorted? One of the first aspects of being a seeker of truth is to accept that many things we have always accepted as truth could very possibly be false. Secondly, it is important to acknowledge that there are still so many, many truths we have yet to learn that would greatly benefit our lives.

Pure, raw truths about the process of giving birth have been shrouded under veils of fear, self-interested intent, and misguided notions in a variety of areas. Because life is complicated and many people believe they don't have time to learn about everything that they need to make decisions about, they become used to accepting any advice from almost anyone who professes to be an expert, or who loves them. It seems easier not to have to make the effort to learn about the world themselves, from the foundations up. Too often, those who should know are actually functioning under passed-down, erroneous philosophies themselves.

And inherited fallacies can be very difficult to dispel because they appear to be self-evident. For example, we always hear, "Childbirth is painful and very dangerous for mothers and babies." This is something we have learned through the dramatized "horror story" or even just by inference in multiple conversations with other people, at the movies, from popular birthing shows, and on and on. This "fact" must certainly be correct in the face of all this evidence!

So what can one do as she begins to learn truths? Perhaps if she just studies and then gives her caregivers or birth place enough information those people will change what they believe and the way they do things in time for her birth—unlikely. Misconceptions about birth have grown much larger than that over the past one-hundred years. A woman who thinks she can change others' ways of doing things for her childbirth experience is like one who marries a man thinking she will be able to change him and make him the kind of man she wants. She eventually finds that such attempts are almost futile. She would have been wiser to move on and seek out the right kind of man.

Or she might believe that although a caregiver or birth place may not be as fully accepting of her wishes as she would like, if she just has a doula to help her "fight" for what she wants, then everything will be okay. A doula's job is not to be a savior for families who have wishes that are unlikely to be achieved at a certain birth place or with a particular caregiver. To put the doula in the middle can create problems for everyone.

As for writing birth wishes that state that something is wanted that is not typically "served" at a particular birth place, stop holding your breath. This is not to discourage families from writing a letter to, or visiting with, a birth place or caregiver about what they wished were offered and being able to state the logistics behind it. Families in the future could greatly

> A woman may think that if she just provides enough information, or brings birth wishes and a doula to help her "fight" for what she wants, that caregivers will change the way they do things in time for her birth.

benefit. But much experience has shown to too many families that simply writing a list of desires does not magically generate an ideal birth experience. In fact, presenting such a plan to an unsympathetic caregiver can produce results that are just the opposite. (See Tips as You Create Your Birth Wish List…**chapter 6**.)

Fears

The list of fears, ranging from illogical to logical, that a woman may experience during pregnancy, and that may hold her back from making the best choices for herself and her baby, is limitless. Following are examples of fears that prove to be roadblocks for many women.

Two Fears Based on False Assumptions

Like most Americans, women have watched a lifetime of reality birth shows on TV. We love to see the birth of a new baby. Although we glory in real births shown on TV and are privileged to witness this moment in a family's life, we need to understand that in these very births we see our own culture. We notice that the caregivers, not the birthing mother, are in charge even under normal circumstances. We observe the lack of faith from those caregivers that birth was *made* to work if they would only have enough faith in a woman's body and in the process. We see her hooked to machines that have not been proven helpful in normal birthing—quite the contrary. We see the mother on the clock, headed for a cesarean if her induction fails. We see other interventions imposed that, to someone who does not understand, seem necessary. And all too often we see the results of those interventions—results that seem to those who don't know any better to have taken place because birth just doesn't always work after all.

The family in the show may seem happy with the results. But is having a healthy baby all that matters? No, it can be so much more!

If you wonder if your birthing experience must be like ones you've seen on TV, watch birthing images from the recommended list of media in the back of this book for a refreshing change! The extent we have gone to in order to make birth perfectly safe, is ridiculous. Even sadder, is that all of these safety nets have not made birth safer.

Another example of fear based on false assumptions is that birth will be filled with unbearable physical pain. That's the first thing usually mentioned when the topic of childbirth comes up in a conversation, isn't it? Is that truly how it *must* be? Does childbirth really have to be a dreaded, horrible experience?

Many, many women around the world and throughout time have given birth comfortably and easily. It is unfortunate that the myths that

Is this a fear that helps me to recognize danger and avoid it? Or is this a fear that has been holding me back from doing something that would actually serve my baby and me?

childbirth has to be difficult, scary, and painful have been perpetuated for so long in our society. They do indeed set a woman up for this fear.

Fears about Possible Dangers

Sometimes women fear something that *could* indeed actually happen during her childbirth—that something might go wrong, that she might fail somehow, or that perhaps she will regret a decision she makes.

Fears that help us to realize danger and do what we can to avoid it are worth paying attention to and heeding.

On the other hand, we need to consider whether this fear is holding us back from doing something that would best serve us and our family, *despite some undesirable consequences.*

For instance, a woman may fear that someone will be angry at her for making a different choice than that person would like her to make, but she also fears the consequences of not choosing what she knows is best for herself and her baby.

Then the question is whether she is strong and wise enough to choose that which is best for herself and her baby.

Low Self-Concept

It is not uncommon for a woman to not believe she can actually give birth. Perhaps she believes her body has let her down before in some way. She may believe that her body probably won't work right, and that other women's bodies may work as intended, but not hers. She may conclude that a great birth just isn't possible for her.

Other women may have experienced being wrong before, and have continually berated themselves for those mistakes. They may second-guess that which actually rings true. Such a woman may wonder if someone is even trying to set her up for failure. She may be afraid of following along and then ending up looking stupid.

Some women may feel they don't deserve a good childbirth experience. Why even try?

What makes a woman think she is so different, so special from all of the other women that have come before her? Birth was made to work. If she was designed to hold generations within her body and grow each of her babies within that body, can that same body not also give birth in the way it was designed?

The empowerment a woman receives from succeeding at giving birth to her baby in her own way can provide a confidence in herself she has never known—an inner knowledge of herself that will give her strength throughout the years to come.

Birth was made to work!

Lack of Information

Many women want to know more but are not guided towards those opportunities. Their caregiver's office may provide only limited information that implies, "Don't worry your pretty head. We'll take care of everything." Often, information supplied is only what the caregiver or in-house educator thinks their consumers want to hear, or even worse, only what the professionals really want them to know.

Clearly, individuals must take the initiative and educate themselves by choosing from the best resources available, from worthwhile classes, books, and Internet sites.

Childbirth class educators who are employed by a hospital can only teach that which is approved by their employers—the administrators of the hospital. What a woman really needs to hear is all too often omitted from the discussion because the educator, though perhaps excellent in many other ways, cannot always give all of the information. Classes may be taught by a staff member such as a nurse whose only experiences with birth are those that have been medically managed. Many of these hospital workers have a great deal of medical knowledge but not a lot of training in normal labor and birth. Some of these classes are even called "natural childbirth classes," but they dwell a great deal on simply what to expect as others make choices for the couple. Families are often deceivingly reassured that drugs and other procedures will never harm the baby or mother. Classes such as these usually deal mainly with how the family can be good patients and how to "survive" until drugs arrive.

An independent instructor (who teaches classes outside of the hospital) is working for the consumer. She is probably an educator/mentor because she wants to make a difference, not because it is an assignment from her workplace. Her studies are usually specifically in pregnancy, birth, and infant care and so she may often be more knowledgeable in these particular areas.

Independent childbirth educators may lose clients whose caregiver or hospital tells their customers they must stop attending such a class. But independent childbirth educators continue to offer their classes for the benefit of all families because they know what they are doing makes a difference for babies, women, and families.

These independent educators are also not obligated to teach material they do not agree with or omit information they know will be very helpful to those taking their classes. (See What Should Quality Childbirth Classes Offer? **Appendix B**.)

Do you want to know the truth about what is really right for you? Are you strong enough to do the research and to birth in the way that you know is best for you and your baby—even if it means searching it out on your own?

Are you willing to do the research and to birth in the ways that you know are best for you and your baby—even if it means searching out "the how" on your own?

Hesitancy about New Information

Hesitancy about listening to and accepting new information may come from the following **six common pitfalls: distrust of new ideas, the belief that it's easier to let someone else decide, the assumption that one can't expect anything better, fear of making a mistake, not wanting to be convinced of anything that one did not think of themselves, and not wanting to face the fact that their previous experiences could have been much better.**

First, it seems to be human nature to distrust new information. And too people often simply want to believe everything is already taken care of. They would rather not have to make the effort to seek anything else out.

What's more, if something or someone challenges a long-held belief, human beings often avoid the new concept, particularly if they have deep, personal feelings about the matter. In the case of childbirth, most people do have opinions because, well—all people are born, and then a great many of those people *become parents* or they are closely associated with others who are. And many people do not have any desire to challenge what has "always been done" culturally. A great many are not willing, or have no interest, in looking at things from a different point of view.

Those few who will, usually find that new ideas can be of immeasurable assistance in a great many ways. And sometimes new ideas can be life changing.

The next stumbling block is believing that it is just easier to let someone else decide. Some women just want to hear, "Don't worry about a thing, Honey, we'll take care of the details!"

These women probably have never questioned why they believe what they do. They typically are unwilling to ask themselves what their beliefs really are concerning each of the following and more: doctors, midwives, hospital birth, homebirth, nurses, waterbirth, doulas, medical technology, spousal relationships, pregnancy, and birth itself.

Not studying and not making any conscious choices is, of course, a choice in itself. It may seem the easier option, but in the end is it really?

A third view is that that one cannot really expect anything better. After all, birth cannot possibly be gentle for a mother and baby.

Are there other women who have had a more positive experience than is typical today? Can you find some positive stories in books, on the Internet, and other places? What did these women/couples do to have a more satisfactory birth experience?

Fourth, there is the fear of making a mistake. We wonder what might happen if we were to do something different from everyone else and it

---

It is sometimes hard to accept new information when it means we will have to change what we've always believed.

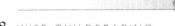

turned out to be the wrong step so sometimes people decide just to go along with everyone else.

Though women agree that childbirth could be better, they are afraid to try new things.

Putting one's head in the sand never kept a storm from coming.

It does take courage. But we will miss wonderful opportunities if we never try new things.

A fifth view of some women is that they do not want to be *convinced* by anyone to do anything. Unfortunately this can result in failure to listen to wisdom from someone who has been there, and in missed opportunities.

If you value self-reliance, you just want to find out for yourself. You want to figure out what you want to do, and find out what is best for you and your baby. The decision is yours, and nobody else's. Besides you don't want to be a copy-cat.

That is all well and good; keep in mind, though, that just because someone else has chosen something doesn't mean that they are the only one entitled to that choice. As you rely on yourself, it remains important to **listen to others, consider new ideas, challenge conventional thought, ask questions, and verify the answers.**

Sixth, some women don't want to admit that their previous births weren't the best. It is too difficult to face the truth. These women have tucked away their feelings about those previous disappointments and unmet needs. These emotions may have emerged as postpartum depression. These women may have felt detached or angry at their babies. They may even have believed incorrectly that it was the baby's fault somehow that the birth was a less than desirable experience.

If your previous birth experiences were not the best, it can be difficult to accept that. But for the sake of this baby, ask yourself what you are willing to give for a gentle and safe birth for this baby now and for yourself. If you fail to make positive changes as you prepare for this baby, it is very likely you will have another unfulfilling childbirth experience to add to the previous one.

You can use past experiences as a springboard to push you towards having a wonderful birth this time.

What concrete things can you do to deal with the challenges in the path to getting the kind of birth you want for this child and for yourself?

It does take courage, but we will miss wonderful opportunities if we never try new things.

Relationship Issues

While we love our husbands, friends, and extended family members, no one's family is perfect. We all face various difficult situations and have to deal with less-than-helpful people. Even the most well-meaning husband, friend, extended family member, or caregiver can become a roadblock to a better childbirth. Do you identify with any of the following? If so, try the suggestions in each section.

Husband

Does your husband disagree with you? Some husbands just don't see eye to eye with their wives when it comes to what she feels is best for childbirth.

It is instinctual for him to want to protect his family. He wants what is best for them. A father's objections are often based on being less familiar about birth options. It is natural to object to things that are unfamiliar. He has grown up with the same culturally-based fears as many women, and he knows less about a woman's anatomy and birth.

One of the best things you can do, if at all possible, is to study together from the beginning. This book is a good place to start. At the very least, tell him what you are learning and let him know how you feel about it.

Keep in mind that the less you butt heads, the more open and receptive he will be when he too comes to understand the same truth that you have. Sometimes all it takes are some loving conversations and a bit of time for fathers to also become advocates of proven, safe choices.

Friends and Extended Family

Are you afraid your friends and extended family members will think you are "weird" for wanting to make a different choice for your birth than they have made for theirs? Are you afraid they will reject you if you try a new way? What if they don't understand your choices?

Are you worried that it might seem like you are passing judgment about the way your own mother or other women in your life have chosen to give birth if you do something different? Are you afraid you might even hurt their feelings?

Remember the story about the woman whose mother always cut off the ends of the ham before she cooked it and so the adult daughter did the same? One day the daughter finally asked her mother about this. Her mother answered that the pan she used to cook ham was too small, so she cut off the ends so the ham would fit. Although the daughter's

Your first concern is your baby's safety and your own.

pan was adequate, she simply followed along assuming this was just the way it was done!

Rarely questioned beliefs are easily inherited from our parents and communities. Traditions are often rooted with unfounded beginnings (such as the all of the interventions that started with Twilight Sleep.) Most of those who influence our lives have good intentions. Yet frequently counsel about childbirth today comes from experience that has little to do with normal birth.

Many caregivers that lean heavily on "saving" technology, for example, have seen only a handful of normal births, if any, during their careers. They see a lot of problems occurring directly from unnecessary intervention into the birth process over their years in the business. These authorities then train the next generations of caregivers. Personal experience, seen through glasses of distortion, not facts and truth, are what has shaped much of today's birth culture in the US.

Some people may scoff at there being another, better way. But, "Those who say it can't be done are usually interrupted by others doing it!" —Joel Barker

Just because "everyone else is doing it" doesn't make it the best way. Why would anyone want to sign up for what the majority of people and babies are presently getting? U.S. birth statistics show that birth practices here leave much to be desired. By making different choices than are often presented, odds for getting a better experience for ourselves and our babies are naturally improved.

Why must a woman feel torn between wanting to fit in with friends and family and being excited that she really could have a wonderful birth? Does wanting more than what her friends are getting seem wrong in some way?

Why feel guilty about making different choices the women before us? Did they not do the best that they could with what they had available to them? Our choices, if different from theirs, are not a denouncement of theirs. We are simply choosing the best for us from among the choice and information now available to us.

Sometimes women fear that something may go wrong, and they will have to bear the responsibility for it alone. They know that they probably would get more sympathy from friends and family if an unforeseen circumstance were to occur if they were making socially-acceptable choices rather than trying something different.

John F. Kennedy said, "There are risks and costs to a program of action. But they are far less than the long-range risks and costs of comfortable inaction."

On the other hand could you handle it if an unforeseen circumstance, that you knew was preventable, were to occur and you could have prevented it by following the way you knew was better for your child? Imagine how angry you might feel at yourself and your relatives and friends if you allowed them to sway you and something did go wrong.

A myth is a fixed way of looking at the world which cannot be destroyed because, looked at through the myth, all evidence supports that myth.
—Edward de Bono

Some women find it difficult to stand up for preferred choices. Well-meaning individuals whom they respect, family, friends, and caregivers, may urge them to do something else. Discussions with loved ones and friends can leave some women angry, fearful, and worn out. Even strangers can be too free with their negative advice and horror stories. It's true that when a woman takes positive steps for her baby or herself that it can indeed change relationships. Those she loves might become angry with her and even take her choices personally. They may try to talk her out of her plans, causing her to doubt and feel guilty. They might tell her that she is selfish or that she is being irresponsible and obstinate. They might even insinuate or downright accuse her of wanting a "good experience" more than a healthy baby. This type of statement is manipulative, arising out of desperation on the part of concerned family members, friends, and even caregivers.

Is anything more difficult than contending with a myth that has grown so massively over many years and has left such damage in its path? It seems almost impossible to make a difference and to convince others, particularly those close to us, of what we have come to understand. When we, ourselves, have stripped a myth bare and the truths we have found seem so obvious that we may wonder how we couldn't have seen them before, we find it difficult when others do not yet see the ironies that are so plainly there.

While particular myths may have started with good intentions, and short-term problems are often solved, perpetuated myths often result in unintended long-term negative consequences. Many times myths begin in times of chaos and they appear to have saved the day. They grow strong in the soils of fear and of greed. Myths appeal to the baser side of human nature.

But in our world when one questions authority, particularly if it is a body of authority over a field of medicine, she is sometimes thought to be irreverent at best.

Winston Churchill said, "Men occasionally stumble over the truth, but most pick themselves up and hurry off as if nothing had happened." The fact is that there are some people whose minds are made-up.

It is possible that if in time others do come to the truth that it won't be before you have your baby. Do what you can to give concerned individuals the information they need to understand your choices. Their fears are often relieved when they realize why certain decisions are being made. Sometimes those most opposed to something become the strongest advocates of that very thing when they find out more about it.

But if they are unwilling to study it or truly listen to your side right now, you may need to let them know that you are unwilling to accept further input from them, although you understand that they care.

Sadly, you may even feel you need to make the decision to give up dreams and hopes for a better birth in order to keep the peace with those you love. You alone must decide what you think is the best course of action for yourself and your baby.

Caregivers

Many women are afraid even to approach their caregivers with something unusual for fear of appearing different or difficult.

But would you hire a painter that refused to paint your house the color you truly desired? Would you be afraid to express your wishes to any contractor or repair technician for fear of seeming difficult? You are paying your caregivers a lot of money for their skills and you deserve the best. You deserve what you pay for.

It is reasonable to expect that our care be well-researched, and it is our responsibility to look elsewhere for care if a particular caregiver is unwilling to provide us with that care. Caregivers should be expected to stay current on the scientific literature. Unfortunately, this is sometimes, and too often, not the case.

Good caregivers respect parents who are responsible enough to want to participate in their own and their baby's health. Caregivers should be expected to stay current on the scientific literature. This too often not the case, unfortunately. It is your challenge to find a caregiver who holds such philosophies.

Having good communication and exchanges with your caregiver about your options and care is of great importance. It is reasonable to expect that those professionals who are practicing evidence-based care will welcome this kind of relationship and be pleased that you are taking responsibility. **This type of caregiver is a keeper and is worth rewarding with your business and your recommendations to others!**

One who becomes angry about your wanting more information, defensive when you inquire about studies, or puts down your efforts to learn and understand is displaying a big red flag—a whole row of them, in fact. Do you ever hear words like, "Am I the only one here who cares about the safety of this baby?" If so, such phrases are meant to intimidate. If you are being manipulated during pregnancy, why would you expect any different at your birth? When a caregiver gives you service that you are not happy with, how much more proof do you need before realizing it is time to get out and not look back?

Parents who decide to look no further than their first contacted caregiver, although they know he or she is not ideal, are choosing the outcome being offered—good or bad. With the stakes are high, you don't want to be wrong about something so important, especially about who will assist you at your birth.

Some women stay with mediocre caregivers despite concerns because they don't think it would be "nice" to change. They want to be loyal. They may wonder, how bad could he or she really be anyway? It will all work out, they tell themselves. Besides, it's probably too late in the pregnancy to change. And who would take them now anyway, they wonder. Would word get around that they changed caregivers?

Sometimes those most opposed to something become the strongest advocates of that very thing when they find out more about it.

It takes a strong backbone to be a good parent.

If you are having these thoughts, do these things matter in the slightest when it comes to protecting your baby and making the best of your birth experience? Sometimes it takes a strong backbone to be a good parent.

Consider too whether you were brought up to fear authority. Despite the fact that we have been led over the years to believe that the medical profession is next to Deity, the profession is still made of men and women. Men and women are not gods, and human beings do make mistakes from time to time—maybe every day—just like the rest of us.

Search your heart. What does that inner voice tell you? You can know for yourself what the right choices are and what to do in certain situations. Don't leave it all up to someone else. (See Types of Caregivers in **chapter 11**.)

Lack of Effort

Another roadblock to a better birth is a lack of effort and initiative. Some women intend to make good choices. They think it would be nice to have a more comfortable, safer birth, and they would like to try. But they never find the time or get around to searching for a good class or checking out some worthwhile books. Maybe they have sort of prepared, but they feel it takes too much time to study.

"Trying" is different than "doing." When you try, you don't have to do your best. When you commit to "do," you do whatever is needed to reach your goal.

If you have learned what makes birth into a frightening medical event and you do nothing about it, just going along with the flow, don't be surprised when you get the ride you signed up for.

Do you find yourself making excuses for not doing what you know is best? Is it a matter of can't or is it a matter of won't?

Some parents have difficulty finding the time to attend a worthwhile set of childbirth classes. This period is of immense importance in your child's life. Make time for what is important.

Is your baby worth going the extra mile for? Is the making and carrying out of decisions pertaining to how she is born, cared for, and raised worth the sacrifice? Could staying in your own comfortable world right now actually be dangerous? Does anyone care more about your baby's birth than you do?

You are the one who has to do something about it. **You only get one chance to birth this child. A good birth doesn't just happen by hoping.**

Search your heart. What does that inner voice tell you?

Are you letting obstructions immobilize you from doing what you know is best for your child and you?

Choices Seem Impossible

Another roadblock is that some women don't believe their birthing experience can be any different than what they and their friends and family members have experienced.

Such women would rather have a comfortable, safe, and joy-filled birth but her friends only tell horror stories and talk about their sick or unhappy babies. It can start to seem that this is normal, just how it is.

What results are you looking for? Are they really unattainable?

Do you know a woman that raves about her birth, who had a happy, alert baby, who talks about what a wonderful experience and postpartum she had? Why not find out what made her experience different than everyone else's and do what she did?

Sometimes there really is a lack of opportunities. For example, perhaps there is no caregiver in your area whose services meet your needs and desires. Or maybe a free-standing birth center is your ideal place to birth, but there isn't one in your area. If so, must you give up your wishes?

Don't give up. How close is the nearest birth center that you would consider? Is it at all possible to travel there? Is there one in a parents' or favorite cousin's hometown? Are you willing to look outside of your area to make your dreams a reality? If this is impossible, you still have options although it may take a little creativity to discover them and bring them about.

Too many times plans are derailed and left at the side of the track simply because we let them be. Making choices and sticking it out, even under the toughest of circumstances, is certainly not for the weak-hearted.

Sometimes a low-interventive birth outside of the hospital is planned, but a serious health problem is diagnosed towards the end of the pregnancy. Such a diagnosis may necessitate giving birth in the hospital.

Certainly there are times in life when our wishes and plans must be changed midstream because of situations beyond our control. In that case we shift gears and continue to do our best with the new set of circumstances, even though we have not chosen them. If we can accept what is, if we can pick up the pieces and work with what we have left, then we can still be successful by doing the best we possibly can with what we have been given and what is still available to us.

What obstacles are standing in *your* way? Are you letting obstructions immobilize you from doing what you know is best for your child and you?

While it is good for a woman to exercise caution and make sure her choices are the right ones for her and her baby, she must not wait too long and risk losing it all by simple default.

> *You only get one chance to birth this child.*

When you commit to "do,"
you do whatever is needed
to reach your goal.

Obtaining Your Ideal Birth

Following is a summary of **some of the most important things that make the difference in whether a family's birth will be gentler, easier, and safer:**

- A caregiver (midwife/doctor) is secured who is more than happy to assist with a normal, low intervention birth. This is one of the top most important factors to consider. Wishes are discussed early on and often with the caregiver. If there are signs as pregnancy progresses that a particular caregiver is not truly offering this kind of care, one is secured who is accommodating of needs and desires. The woman and her family are in charge of, and a partner in, their care.

- The family's core belief about birth is that it is a normal and healthy function of a woman's body, and that the process can be trusted because it was made to work! They choose to not let fear and other roadblocks get in the way of a positive birth experience.

- More attention is focused on protecting and doing what is best for the baby and mother, than on pleasing others. Choices are obtained assertively (as opposed to aggressively or passively) when necessary.

- Truth is sought and studied, sound decisions are made, the courage to take the course that will lead to desired outcomes is found, and the responsibility to act in the best interest of the baby, mother, and family is embraced. Whatever is helpful for obtaining those wishes (books, classes, a doula and other support, etc.) is located and utilized with wisdom.

- Time and priority are given during pregnancy to preparing mentally, emotionally, physically, with comfort measures, and in all other ways for this birth.

- Good nutrition and healthful practices that benefit the baby and herself are followed by the mother so that both can function to their best abilities during the important times of gestation, birth, and postpartum.

- Positioning, of the mother and baby in physical relationship to each other, is carefully given the attention needed. The mother's body is aligned for the birth, and she is careful to keep the baby in an optimal position.

- A birth team of trustworthy individuals, who believe in the woman and in the process of birth, is chosen and fully utilized.

17

Ready? Set?

WE PLAN EVERY DETAIL of our weddings months, if not a lifetime, in advance. Career planning, building a home, decorating a room.... Many newborns' bedrooms are better prepared for than their births! The birth of your child is one of the most important things you will ever do in your lifetime and *for* your child in his/her lifetime.

Some of the things you choose will be different from what is on your neighbor's list.

Your choices belong to you and your baby. Your choices are for you to make. Take the time to carefully choose the best.

In the same spirit as a wedding organizer, we offer our **Before Birth Checklist**. It is an *incomplete* list of some things you may or may not wish to include on your own "things-to-prepare" schedule.

Your choices belong to you and your baby. Your choices are for you to make. Take the time to carefully choose the best.

Keep the following in mind:

- Some of the following are *simply fun*, a way to celebrate this time—like making a belly cast.

- Some are *fun and extremely helpful*—such as making birth art and taking a hypnobirthing class.

- Some are *essential*—like good nutrition and working through fears.

- Don't try to do all of the things on the following pages. On the other hand, avoid missing the ones most needed by you and your baby.

Let's begin...

Before Birth Checklist

EDUCATE YOURSELF

___ Read *Wise Childbearing* thoroughly, highlighting information that you want to remember.

___ Read books from the recommended list; use the Internet.

___ Take *quality* childbirth classes.

PREGNANCY: TAKE CARE OF YOURSELF AND YOUR BABY

___ Do what is necessary to avoid preeclampsia.

___ Get into the habit of drinking all of the water needed every day.

___ Eat well every day! Read about foods that are important to eat during pregnancy and keep those on your shopping list so that you will keep them in stock.

___ List, get, and begin to take the supplements and herbs needed daily after first checking with those who know about them and the pros and cons of their use during pregnancy.

___ Help to prepare your uterus with daily quarts of red raspberry leaf tea.

___ Start a daily routine of exercise (including perhaps walking, yoga, belly dancing, practice squatting, Kegels).

___ See a chiropractor for adjustments to help make pregnancy more comfortable and labor easier and more efficient.

___ Consider seeing a good Craniosacral therapist (massage therapists will sometimes be trained in Craniosacral therapy) for body energy work. Energy flows through the body during labor, and making sure that all of your body's energy is flowing normally can be beneficial both during birth and for a more healthy pregnancy and postpartum. Having your therapist work with your chakra energy can be especially helpful.

___ Seeing a Foot Zoner can be extremely helpful for treating physical as well as emotional difficulties related to pregnancy. Zoning can be very effective for assisting flow of healing energy within the body and within each organ and system, greatly benefitting health.

___ Keep fetal movement counts beginning several weeks before your "due time."

___ Try combating heartburn with raw carrots, peanut butter, or atomic fire ball candies. They've worked for other women!

PUT TOGETHER YOUR CHILDBIRTH TEAM AND PLACE

___ Study choices and interventions, together if possible, and write birth wishes including desires concerning newborn procedures.

___ Make a list of questions for interviewing caregivers and doulas.

___ Choose a caregiver and birthplace.

___ Choose a doula.

____ Discuss your choices with your caregiver and reevaluate.

____ Reassess—is this truly the birthplace and the caregiver for you?

PREPARE YOUR INNER MIND FOR CHILDBIRTH (See chapter 15)

____ Create some birth art.

____ Work through and eliminate fears.

____ Use EFT.

____ Schedule a Craniosacral session.

____ Take a hypnobirthing class.

____ Practice daily the techniques you've learned in your hypnobirthing course.

____ Find a quiet place (the mountains, beach, your bedroom) where you can go mentally during labor.

____ Take time to meditate, pray, and/or get in touch with your baby. "Ask" the baby how and where he/she would like to be born and under what circumstances, etc.

____ Keep a pregnancy journal.

____ Keep a journal by your bed to record those crazy pregnancy dreams.

____ "Talk it out" together as a couple, or with a trusted friend.

____ Write affirmations about what you want from your experience and carefully read them daily.

GET THINGS TOGETHER FOR THE BIRTH

____ Prepare homebirth kit (homebirthers).

____ Pack suitcase (hospital or birth center birthers).

____ Prepare a gentle welcome for your baby.

____ Buy or make snacks and drinks for during labor.

____ Plan your birthing clothes (something with easy birth and breastfeeding access that you will feel comfortable, beautiful, and confident in, and that is practical for laboring in, in different situations—such as walking around the halls in the hospital, etc. If you are laboring/birthing in the water, what will you wear (perhaps an easy-access skirt and tank top?) What will you wear after you get out of the water?

____ Decide whether to get a birthing stool.

____ Decide whether to get a birthing tub.

____ Decide who will use the camera and/or camcorder at your birth.

____ Assign jobs to any other members of your birth team.

____ Get a Strep B test. (See **chapter 7**.) If the test comes back positive, continue to build immune system and retest. Make decisions about how to handle Strep B.

____ Learn how to get and keep baby in a good position within the uterus.

____ Make a birth satchel to open during labor, with objects you have chosen as reminders of what you want to take with you on your journey into birth: perhaps a rock to represent strength and standing firm, a ribbon to represent flowing with whatever labor brings to you, a charm to remember the love of those around you, a flower to remind you of the *joy* that can be a part of every surge that brings your baby closer, etc.

___ Collect phone numbers of caregivers, doula, family, friends, birthplace, and pediatrician to have on hand.

___ Give thought and attention to your marriage relationship. (See **chapter 19**.)

PREPARE OTHER COMFORT MEASURES

___ Get a birth ball to use for labor. (Will your doula be bringing one?)

___ Choose and download or gather music for labor.

___ Prepare essential oils, such as clary sage, lavender, and peppermint with a carrier oil for massage during labor. Know the benefits and cautions of each oil you select.

___ Try different positions for labor and birth to see what you might like.

___ Practice your deep, abdominal breathing.

___ Prepare 1 oz. of red raspberry tea in a pint jar. When labor starts, add boiling hot water. Let cool until drinkable. This tea is said to make labor easy and efficient.

PREPARE BABY'S SIBLINGS FOR BIRTH

___ Prepare siblings for the new baby.

___ If they will be at the birth, prepare siblings for that experience. (See **chapter 14**.)

___ Choose siblings' doula(s).

___ Choose siblings' baby-sitter.

CELEBRATE/COMMEMORATE THIS SPECIAL TIME

___ Make a belly cast.

___ Take pregnancy pictures.

___ Have a celebration of Motherhood or Fatherhood. (See **chapter 12**.)

___ Attend your baby shower.

PREPARE FOR POSTPARTUM

___ Nurture your marriage relationship.

___ Learn infant massage.

___ Find a pediatrician for after your baby's birth.

___ Organize a diaper-changing area, and figure out sleeping arrangements.

___ Decide on household help after the birth, and find a postpartum doula.

___ Make and put meals in the freezer for after the birth.

___ Prepare for breastfeeding. (Contacting your local La Leche League leader now to get to know her beforehand and to learn about meetings in your area can be a smart idea.) Or prepare for bottle feeding if necessary.

___ Make "bath tea" bags to use daily in those first days after birth. (See **chapter 19.**)

COLLECT NEEDED ITEMS

___ Collect baby clothes, blankets, diapers, etc.

___ Get a car seat and learn how to use it properly.

___ Buy a baby carrier with which to "wear" your baby. (See **chapter 20.**)

___ Buy a new nursing bra(s) and breastfeeding pads (cloth or disposable).

___ Buy super-absorbent sanitary pads for after the birth.

___ Get Chux pads—helpful for protecting your bedding in the first few weeks from lochia. (See **chapter 19.**)

___ Gather night gowns or shirts easy to breastfeed in, and perhaps a robe for times when visitors stop by.

___ Have some food and supplies on hand so that you won't have to go out right away.

___ Get or make birth announcements and thank you cards.

___ Decide what to do for a baby book and first year calendar.

While reading this book and in your other research, you may wish to add other items to your list.

Signs Labor May Begin Soon

Some women have regular contractions, just as the textbooks say they will. Others do not. Both are variations of normal! Some babies are already engaged into the pelvis when labor begins. Other babies do not engage until well into labor. Both ways are normal. You will probably have some of the following signs. But remember, every woman and every labor (even for the same woman) is different!

- **Contractions**—Contractions may occur at any time during pregnancy. If you find that you are experiencing contractions that are just a strong pressure, you are most likely experiencing Braxton Hicks contractions, which may or may not have any effect on the dilation and effacement of your cervix and can occur throughout pregnancy. If the contractions are more intense, however, watch for signs that they are generally tightening the entire uterus. You may feel them as lower back pressure or pressure in the lower abdomen. You may have contractions, even strong ones, for days. Prelabor contractions just sort of do their own thing, when, where, and however they want. Generally, it is best to continue on with everyday life until you notice contractions becoming longer in duration (up to 60 sec.), progressively stronger in intensity, closer together, and regular in occurrence. If, when labor really starts, contractions are not very regular, it can be a sign that the baby is not in the most ideal position. For more comfortable, efficient labor, the Polar Bear and doing some belly lifting can be extremely helpful. (See **chapter 13**.)
- **Backache**—This can be from the contracting uterus pulling on your lower back. You may feel this intermittently in time with uterine contractions. This can happen at the onset of labor and during labor. (See **chapter 13**.)
- **Release of Membranes**—You might experience a pronounced dampness, a trickle of water, or a gush of fluid from the vagina. It may occur before contractions start, and—depending on your caregiver—you will be told either to wait until labor does start and keep a close eye out for any signs of possible infection (fever, etc.) or to come in to be induced. (For reasons why waiting may be the best choice, see **chapter 8**.) Let your caregiver know about the time it happened, about the color and odor, and the amount of discharge. Once your water has released, it is best to not a wear a tampon or have intercourse. It is also a good idea to have as few vaginal checks as possible, if any at all! Avoiding the tub until well into active labor is also probably best. Wearing a pad, or even a small diaper if necessary, can help to catch leaks.

There are many variations of what's normal for laboring women. Your body is wise and knows what it's doing!

- **Lightening or Engagement**—Baby settles or drops into the pelvis, sometimes around two to four weeks before labor. You may feel less pressure on your stomach and lungs and more pressure on your bladder. Sometimes the baby doesn't come down until well into labor. Either is normal.
- **Show of Cervical Gel**—A blood-tinged cervical gel, or cervical gel without blood, may be released as the cervix begins to dilate. This can happen during labor or perhaps a week or so before labor starts.
- **Flu-like Symptoms**—You may have soft bowels, diarrhea, nausea, or mild cramps for hours or days before labor begins, which is probably nature's way of cleaning out the system to make way for the baby.
- **Nesting**—An urge to clean or rearrange things, a sudden burst of energy—this can occur throughout pregnancy, but you may feel a particular urge to put everything in rightness a few days before labor begins. Be careful not to become overly tired just before your birth.
- **Intuition**—Either parent just knows that labor will start soon.

Ways Dads or Birth Partners May Be Supportive

Decide before the birth, what your role will be, and what the role of the doula and the other support people will be. You can decide how you would feel most comfortable assisting the mother. At the prenatal appointment with your doula, as a couple, discuss what Dad's role will be at your baby's birth, and what role you want her to play.

The lists that follow contain ways fathers and/or birth partners can be supportive to mothers. Lists are divided into categories according to stages of labor.

First Stage, Early Labor (about 0–3 centimeters)

Mild contractions may not be coming regularly; they may last thirty to forty-five seconds, and be five to twenty minutes apart. Every woman and labor is different!

The mother may show some or all of these physical and emotional signs:

- Appearance of cervical gel and/or vaginal discharge
- Water releases
- Frequent urination and looser bowels
- Pelvic pressure, cramps, gas, pressure or tightening in pelvic area, backache
- Flushed face
- Talks in a normal voice, usually even during contractions and may be sociable
- Excited, confident, or frightened that labor may be more than she can handle
- May feel labor is progressing faster than it is

Remind the mother of things she can do at this point:

- Continue regular activity. If it is night or early morning, though, get some sleep! It is important at this point for her to protect her energy! This may be the longest part of labor.
- Walking can help labor progress.
- Eat easily-digested food, to appetite.
- Drink plenty of fluids (non-acidic juices, raspberry leaf tea, water, etc.) and empty bladder often.
- Although it will probably not be necessary to use comfort rituals/routines at this point, you may want to start developing these with the mother so you are prepared when contractions get stronger.

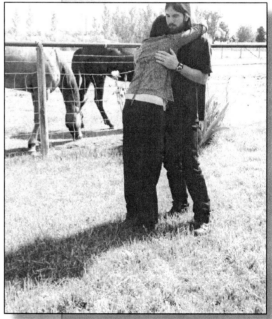

During early labor, this couple took a walk through the trees and out over a little bridge into a sunny pasture. When a contraction wave would begin its natural flow and then ebb, this father was ready to support his wife. Each time, she would stop walking and turn to put her arms around her husband's shoulders to "slow dance." Laboring mothers often find this position, of leaning into their husbands or another support person, extremely helpful. Moving her hips back and forth, the mother gives the baby room to move along.

- If contractions are not very regular, it can be a sign that the baby is not in the most ideal position. For a more comfortable, efficient labor, have her try the Polar Bear and do some belly lifting early in labor. This can be extremely helpful.
- She can call her caregiver and doula and update them.

You can help by doing these things:

- Get more sleep if it is in the middle of the night—unless she needs you.
- Stay calm and remember that it is best for labor to be well established and on its way before heading to the hospital. Your doula can help you to know when this is. Also listen to the mother. She has access to information that no one else does.
- Help her conserve her energy for the consuming journey ahead!
- Share the excitement. Talk about what is going through her mind during contractions (thoughts, images, feelings).
- Give your wife lots of physical affection, massage, and brushing her hair. *Now is the time to really connect with her!*
- Help her with belly lifting and to be as comfortable as she can be in the Polar Bear. (See Back Labor in **chapter 13**.) While she is in the Polar Bear position, you can make necessary calls and arrangements. But you can put on relaxing music for her, or if you have extra time, she might appreciate a massage.
- Walk together if labor isn't strong yet.
- Help her reduce tension and breathe deeply.
- Help to finish packing the bag, making the car comfortable for trip to hospital, calling work, making arrangements for your other children, etc.
- Get a good meal while *you* have the chance.

First Stage, Active Labor (about 3–8 centimeters)

Contractions may come on a more regular basis, three to five minutes apart, and be sixty to seventy-five seconds long.

The mother may show some or all of these physical and emotional signs:

- Doesn't feel like talking and moving through contractions any more
- Sweaty, feet may be cold
- Frequent need to urinate
- Backache
- Pressure in legs and hips
- Nausea

- Facial expression more serious, focused
- Flushed face, warm, sweaty, thirsty
- Body tension
- Quiet even *between* contractions
- Talks of discomfort, grasping hands of others, and pushing away of intrusive procedures, not wanting to be alone
- Detached from others, less social
- Becoming less inhibited
- Unsure if she will be able to do this
- May stop progressing at some point to integrate sensations, work through psychological issues, and prepare to go on

You can work with your doula to help by doing these things:

- Remind the mother to greet each contraction with a cleansing breath, and help her to get into her deep abdominal breathing.
- Give her lots of love, focusing on her throughout the contraction.
- Remind her to stay on top of the waves (the contractions), to ride them.
- Continue walking if she feels like it.
- Help her to change positions frequently (standing and leaning forward, sitting on or leaning over ball, sitting on toilet, walking, kneeling, sitting, straddling a chair, leaning over bed/partner, squatting).
- Remind her hourly to urinate and make sure she drinks some water or juice often.
- Help her to surrender to her body's power and follow her own instincts.
- Check for tension and help her release it.
- Give her a massage.
- Do not leave her!
- Alternate comfort measures (music, LOVE, encouragement, getting into water (not until five centimeters!), helpful words, cold washcloth on forehead, eye contact, massage).
- If she is having back labor, see **chapter 13**.
- Especially if she is a first time mother, don't be discouraged if she is not dilating quickly. Often first time mothers' cervixes efface (thin out) before dilating (opening). If she is only three centimeters dilated but 90 percent effaced,

This father and doula work together to support this mother who is well into active labor. Leaning into her husband's chest, feeling his strong arms around her, is very comforting to this woman. Their doula uses counter-pressure on the mother's hips. This feels great!

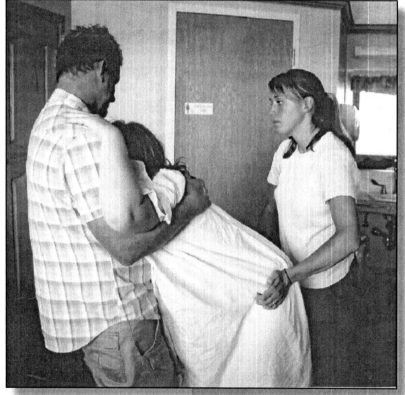

for example, take heart. Effacing is just as important to the process as dilating! Often when a mother becomes fully effaced, she will then dilate very quickly.

- If she panics and says she doesn't think she can do this, stay calm, stay close, be confident in her, hold her head or shoulders gently and firmly, hold her tightly, have her look into your eyes, guide her with deep abdominal breathing, encourage her to wait a few minutes, and don't give up unless she is very insistent. How strong was she about wanting to avoid/have medication? Sometimes when a woman says she can't do it anymore she wants encouragement and reassurance, and is actually asking for help. It takes strength not to follow your desire to "rescue" her. Have lots of tricks in your bag with which to help her through this time. Save a few of the best for later. (See **chapter 13**.)
- If contractions stop (as they can, even in transition) talk about fears, let her rest/sleep, shower, bathe, walk (outside if possible), help her to use a position that utilizes gravity—but not for so long that it reduces her energy, use relaxation, praise and encourage, utilize visualization, ask for privacy (so you can be alone with her to just love her for awhile). Be grateful for the break.

First Stage, Transition (*about 8–10 centimeters*)

Contractions may be one and a half to two minutes apart and sixty to ninety seconds long.

The mother may show some or all of these physical and emotional signs:

- Hot or cold flashes
- The "shakes"
- Nausea, vomiting
- Burping
- Flushed, social mask falls away
- Eyes may have far away look as she goes within to where she can best meet her labor, loses sense of time
- Sleepy, fatigue
- Complaining, irritability, restlessness, upset, discouragement
- Voice may be loud and demanding ("help me!")
- Uninhibited
- Pressure in thighs, bottom, and back
- Focused inward
- May panic or be fearful, feels like nothing is working
- Feels frustrated, helpless, physically trapped, unable to see the end, "I can't take much more. Do something!"
- Feels the power and tumultuousness of birth

- Fluctuates between desiring nearness of others and being intolerant of contact

You can work with your doula to help by doing these things:

- Remember that transition can be work, but it is doable! These contractions are getting the last of the work done. This is usually the shortest phase.
- Remind the mother to do just one contraction at a time and to rest in between.
- Use a variety of techniques.
- Ask only questions that require a "yes" or "no."
- Tell her how proud you are of her and love her (massage, hold her) and continue support even when caregivers are present.
- Screen out disturbances, such as that from other people.
- Encourage the mother to surrender to the forces of her laboring body.

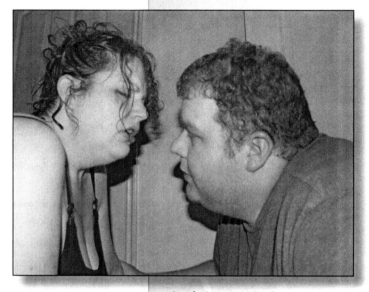

This father is right there for his wife, offering hugs, kisses, and sips of water. The mother expressed later how much it meant to have her support team, which also included their doulas and midwives, encircling her during her labor and birth.

- Remember how strongly she felt about avoiding pain medication. (See Pain Medication Preference in **chapter 7**.) Often a woman who says she can't go on actually wants encouragement, reassurance, and support—she isn't asking you to agree with her thought of giving up; she may just need you to hear how difficult this is. Stay calm, close, and be confident in her, holding her head or shoulders gently and firmly, holding her tightly, having her look into your eyes, guiding her with deep abdominal breathing, encouraging her to wait a few minutes. Do not give up unless she truly is insisting. How strong was she about wanting to avoid medication? Try everything you have prepared, reminding her that she is almost there.
- Remember that laboring in water is Mother Nature's epidural.
- Have some tricks you haven't used yet.

Second Stage, Birthing (10+ centimeters)

Contractions may be two to five minutes apart with contractions one to two minutes long. The actual birthing can last a few minutes or even a few hours.

The mother may show some or all of these physical and emotional signs:

- Feels low pressure
- Feels as if she needs to have a bowel movement (Don't let her go to the bathroom without being certain that what she's feeling isn't really the baby descending.)
- Has mucous or bloody discharge
- Burps or has catch in throat
- Feels fatigue or exhilaration
- Feels discomfort and/or relief
- Feels as if she is ready to burst
- Is emotional and loud
- Is glad she can finally *do* something
- Has an "orgasm" of birth
- Shows calmness and determination
- Experiences mental ambivalence
- Has vacillating emotions, loving or hating what she is feeling, at different times during the birth

You can work with your doula to help by doing these things:

- Help the mother change positions if needed.
- Bring water and ice.
- Place cool, wet cloths on her face, neck, brow, and chest.
- Apply warm/hot, moist packs and oils to aid perineal stretching.
- Remind her about opening her throat and relaxing her lower jaw to keep her vagina open; remind her to "open and release"
- Praise and encourage her.
- Remind her to trust her body and do what it tells her to do.
- Keep her informed about what is going on.
- Remind the caregiver of preferred birth position(s) already discussed with him/her, if necessary.
- Tell her when you see the baby's head. She *may* want a mirror to see it and may want to reach down and touch the baby.
- Encourage her to "breathe the baby down" through her chest and body, while allowing the baby to help himself be born. Unless there is a good reason to hasten this stage, things will often progress better if the baby is able to simply birth himself without the classic "purple pushing" that is so tiring and which is not very effective.

If she is birthing **with an epidural**, here are some things that might help:

- Delay pushing until baby's head is on the perineum (can be seen from the outside), unless there are reasons that the baby needs to be born quickly or if two hours have passed since complete dilation.
- If mother is lying down, have her lie at a 30-degree angle (sitting up farther pushes her tailbone into the baby's way). Have her hold her own legs if possible.
- With trusted assistance, have her try kneeling, leaning forward over the birth ball, squatting, or using a dangle squat (held from someone sitting higher behind her).
- Help the mother know where to push by putting warm compresses at perineum, encouraging pushing within the vagina, using a mirror, letting her feel baby's head, and encouraging her to push the baby to the person right in front of her.
- Let the epidural wear off.
- Avoid pushing on the bottoms of mother's feet as she will waste energy if she pushes with her feet. Avoid pulling way back on her legs as this may cause nerve damage.
- Don't forget to have mother empty her bladder before starting to push. Remind her to avoid prolonged breath holding.
- If progress seems to be impeded, the caregiver can check to see if the baby's head is in good alignment within the vagina. If not, manual positioning might be in order.
- If nothing else is working, suggest she try some "purple pushing."

Third Stage, Delivery of Placenta

Delivery of the placenta may last about five to thirty minutes. **The mother may show some or all of these physical and emotional signs:**

- More uterine surges
- Cramping
- Slight expulsive urge
- Hunger, thirst
- Discomfort if stitches are necessary
- Exhausted, excited, relieved, crying, talkative
- Increasingly aware of surroundings and events
- Scared of new responsibility
- Feeling of emptiness—may come as relief or shock
- Continues to need the support, focus, and attention of those around her

You can work with your doula to help by doing these things:

- Help mother to continue with breathing and relaxing if needed.
- Hold the baby where she can see if she cannot hold him herself.
- Give love, support, and reassurance.
- Use this time to fall in love with your baby.
- Go to the nursery, if birthing in the hospital, with the baby.
- If the mother must be separated from her baby at this time when she has just received him, she might appreciate having someone there that can help her to get washed up and brush her hair, or bring her something to eat, and listen to her as she debriefs about the birth. Perhaps it can be her doula—although doulas *may* leave a little before that. Someone besides the father, who is needed by the baby in the nursery, can help the mother to get positioned in bed and help her feel comfortable, clean, and settled. They can assist her with getting a shower, and offer support as she stands and walks to the bathroom. It is good to stand by once she is in, in case she begins to feel faint. They can also assist her with getting a clean gown to change into, making sure she has clean sheets, and an ice pack for her perineum. At home, this typically goes more smoothly because mother and baby are seldom separated. In the hospital, a nurse will probably take care of this task, but will probably not have the time to debrief about the birth and give much emotional support.

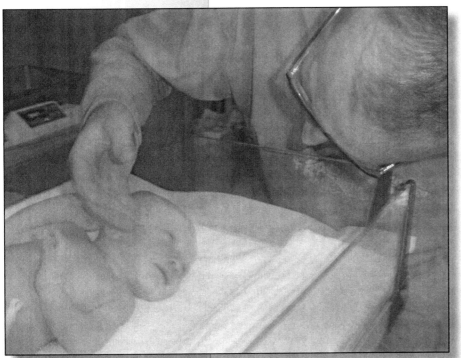

This baby turns toward a familiar voice. It is believed that if a father has bonding time with the baby for at least fifteen minutes within the first hours following the birth, that they will have a better chance of establishing a deep relationship that will last a lifetime.

What to Do for a Surprise Birth

Although a "surprise" birth happens only rarely, here's what to do:

1. **Don't transport if the baby's head is visible**—call 911 (or your homebirth midwife if you were planning a homebirth).
2. If you are enroute to the hospital when the baby crowns, **stop the car and make sure that mother and baby are warm. Follow the steps below.** Then resume your transport, carefully and safely, once the baby has been born.
3. **Remain calm. Don't leave the mother.** Just let the birth happen. *A woman's body was made to do this.* Comfort and reassure her.

   Sometimes what seems to be an urge to have a bowel movement is really the pressure of the baby about to be born, so it might be helpful to have help nearby when using the bathroom. You do *not* need to tear the bag of waters around the baby if it has not yet released.
4. **Let the head deliver slowly, by itself, without the mother pushing.** This gives time for the opening to stretch and prevent tearing. **To prevent infection, do not touch the mother's birth opening.**
5. If the umbilical cord is around the neck, slip it over the baby's shoulders.
6. Let the body deliver. The baby will be slippery (note the time of birth).
7. If cord is long enough, place baby on mother's bare chest, skin-to-skin with a blanket over the baby's body.
8. **Do *not* pull on the cord.**
9. Make sure fluids are draining from baby's nose and mouth.
10. **If baby is not breathing and is blue or limp, massage baby's back and feet.** Many babies look blue when they are first born. This is normal. He will probably pink-up right away. Feel for a pulse where his naval meets the umbilical cord. The pulse should be almost too fast to count and be staying steady.

    A baby does not need to cry. If his pulse is regular and is staying that way, he is breathing.

    If you did the above and the baby is still not breathing, see "If Resuscitation of Baby Is Needed" on the next page.
11. **Allow the placenta to deliver.** Transport the mother to the hospital if it hasn't delivered in half an hour.
12. **You don't need to try to cut the cord.** It can stay attached to the placenta for as long as you need.

    As long as the placenta is still attached inside the mother, he is receiving oxygen through it. You can wrap the placenta when it comes out, and put it next to the baby to take to the hospital.

    If there will be no help available, wait until the cord becomes slender and lighter in color and has stopped pulsing. With a string, tie a knot tightly around the cord an inch above where it enters the baby's navel. Tie another knot an inch above that and cut in between the two knots.
13. **Watch the mother's bleeding. It should be minimal.** The uterus, which you can feel when gently but firmly pushing your fingers into her abdomen around her navel area should be about the size of a grapefruit or orange once the placenta has delivered.

    If there is a lot of bleeding from the vagina, have the mother *firmly* massage the uterus from over the navel. Having the mother nurse the baby helps the uterus contract. And then transport to a hospital without delay.

If Resuscitation of Baby Is Needed

- **Avoid being rough, slapping, or shaking the baby if he still is not breathing.** *This will not help!*
- Call 911. If help is not immediately available, transport to a hospital, or to someone who can help. Do so swiftly but carefully while the mother or another person performs the following steps:
  - Keep baby warm.
  - If pulse has slowed greatly, begin resuscitation. Gently put a finger under the baby's neck so his head flexes back, opening the airway. Now cover the baby's mouth to block that airway, and *put your mouth over the baby's nose only*.
  - Gently blow air *only* from your filled cheeks, giving about six breaths.
  - The baby should be responding to attempts made above. If not, use the tip of your first two fingers on the baby's chest, and gently but firmly give three chest compressions and a breath.
  - Regularly evaluate respirations, heart rate, and color. Stop as soon as the baby begins to respond on his own.
  - **Keep the cord attached!** The baby is receiving oxygen through it as long as the placenta is still attached to the uterine wall.

18

More Choices at Birth and Beyond

THERE ARE SO MANY CHOICES for parents to make at their child's birth and beyond. First, let's step back for a few moments and **think more broadly about how babies may experience their births. How does our culture treat newborns** in its rituals, procedures, evaluations, immunizations, and feeding customs?

Now is a good time to study and think about routine nursery procedures typically performed and whether you want them for your baby.

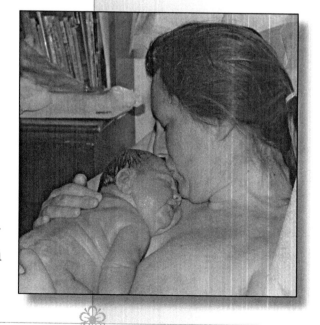

Exploring Our Culture's "Welcoming" Rituals

Although the custom of holding a baby by the ankles and spanking her is thankfully now history, we can still do much to protect babies from various painful, frightening, and unjustifiable procedures.

Dr. Frederick Leboyer's best-selling book, *Birth Without Violence*, was first published in France in the early 1970s. From there its wisdom moved rapidly throughout Europe and beyond, opening the eyes of the industrialized world. Leboyer had assisted at the birth of more than 10,000 babies and he had questions. Why, he asked, must babies be subjected to blinding lights and loud voices as they enter the world? Why do we separate them from their mother's arms? What are the reasons that we treat a baby not as an infant, but an object?

In his book, he challenged readers to consider the customs currently being employed. We can witness, in a detailed collection of black and white photographs, the terror experienced by newly-delivered babies being exposed to the routine birth practices of the day. These photographs are in sharp contrast with images of another group of babies. In this second collection of pictures, we can observe calm and serene expressions. These babies, unlike the others, have been received into their outer worlds with thoughtfulness, gentleness, and compassion. Some are shown being placed soon after birth into warm, soothing water—an environment much like the one from which they have just come.

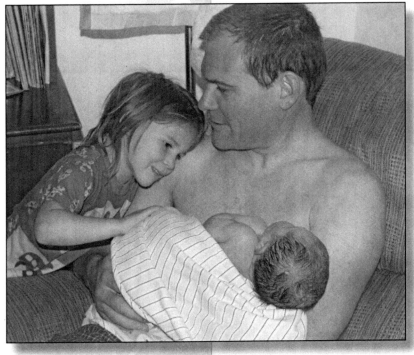

While her mother takes a refreshing shower, this baby snuggles up for some skin-to-skin bonding with daddy.

Considerations for Expectant Parents

Do we really need to give this newly-emerged little person shots and pricks, and sight-blurring ointment in his eyes during the first few hours after birth? And if circumcision is chosen, can it not wait at least a few days or weeks? Does a baby really need to be immediately stretched out of the position he has been in for so long, and weighed on a hard, unwarmed scale? How important is it that he is whisked away from his mother, off to the nursery for a bath, pictures, and other procedures?

Some hospitals still routinely suction babies with a tube down their throat directly after birth! This is horrific and incredibly unnecessary for most babies! Many caregivers allow the baby, as long as he is doing well, to expel birth fluids on his own, instead of using the uncomfortable suctioning of the old bulb syringe.

We must ask ourselves questions such as, whether newly-born babies really need to be given an efficient scrubbing right away, and to be placed wet and naked on the counter to await being dressed?

As long as the baby is normally healthy, would it be harmful to hand him directly into the warm and loving arms of his mother and to allow him to be *left alone* with his parents? Could not any necessary examinations be made at the bedside? The answer is yes! Many caregivers realize the *importance* of this. What of the others? Are they sometimes much too hurried? Is it so important to get the assessments and the paperwork done so that we can move on to the next "patient" or get back to the office? With the way the system is set up—yes, probably so.

Yet how much more gentle it would be to let him adjust in his parents' arms, to not have to leave them just so caregivers can finish up! **Most of the procedures, under normal circumstances, can certainly wait**—even until the next day—if they must be done at all. Under normal circumstances, the rest could be done without ever having to leave mother and father.

Even animal babies have kinder births than we as humans usually give our own babies! They are also usually left un-tampered with and are wisely kept with their mothers.

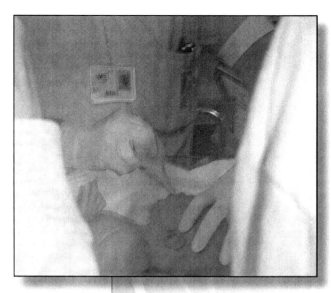

Many caregivers allow the baby, as long as he is doing well, to expel birth fluids on his own and do not use a bulb syringe to suction his air passages as is seen here.

Would it be harmful to hand him directly into the warm, loving arms of his mother and to allow him to be left alone with his parents? Many caregivers realize the importance of this.

In Mother's Arms or on Abdomen

How much better for both the baby and the mother's perineum when he is allowed to gradually emerge without frantic coaching, alarming (to him) cheers of "push!" and without being pulled out. Some hospitals and caregivers, particularly midwives, are happy to assist their clients with a tender, peaceful, warm, dimly lit, skin-to-skin reception.

Although you might meet with resistance in some hospitals, you can certainly

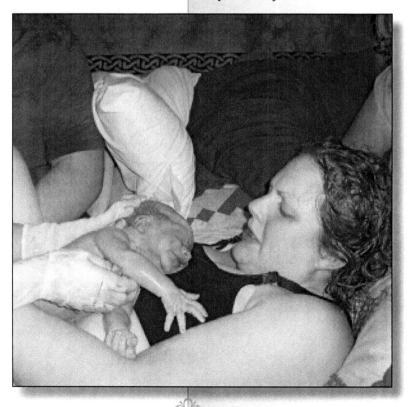

keep your baby just as warm, or warmer, cuddled against your skin with a blanket than under a heating lamp or in the nursery wrapped in a blanket. **In fact mother's bodies have been shown to actually be able to regulate the baby's temperature!** Fancy that. Perhaps there are a variety of measures already naturally in place to keep the baby safe— measures that we would do well not to tamper with.

How much better to simply let things be, and to hold his little body in the same position that he has been cradled in within your body for so long. Against your warm skin, covering him with a soft blanket, and allowing him to instinctively find the breast and to nurse, you can welcome him gently into this bewildering new world.

Rooming-In

Babies are aware, intelligent beings. To suddenly be separated from you can be distressing for him!

Experts now recommend that babies "room-in," meaning to keep them in the same room with the mother, rather than allowing them to

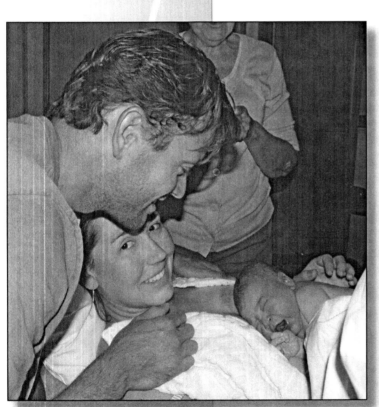

be taken to stay in the hospital's nursery. It also means keeping the baby near, and caring for his needs yourself.

You might hear moms say, "I was glad to have a baby-sitter so I could sleep!"

But your baby *needs* you and your attentive care. This period is the time for you to get to know each other and to show her that people can be trusted to attend to her needs right away. There is time to sleep when she sleeps.

She needs to be picked up and held and nursed and spoken softly to. It is often impossible for nurses to give a lot of care in a busy, packed, and bustling nursery. And more than that, she needs *you*.

When you room-in together, you are free to feed your baby whenever her body needs it, and to be sure that no "quiet down" bottles—which can sabotage breastfeeding—are given to your baby while in the nursery.

If you've ever had the opportunity to peek into the hospital nursery you may have seen newly born babies crying and not immediately attended to. If you haven't heard differently, you may assume that your baby must be okay when he may actually really need you!

Even when rooming-in, be aware that some hospitals require that the baby to be taken to the nursery during the shift-change of the staff. Some families choose to check out soon after the birth for a number of these kinds of reasons.

Effects of a Compassionate Birth

A gentle birth could have more far-reaching effects than we understand. It may well be the beginning of a nonviolent life. In fact, creating peace for our children, from the very moments of their births, could be the beginning of a more peaceful world. **The way we birth and raise our children has a tremendous effect on the kind of people they will become.**

Interestingly, after an extensive investigation on the causes of crime, **The Commission on Crime Control and Violence Prevention in Sacramento, CA stated that they endorsed natural birth, attention from parents, and family closeness, and they warned against over-utilization of intensive care nurseries and medications that are all too often used to induce labor.**

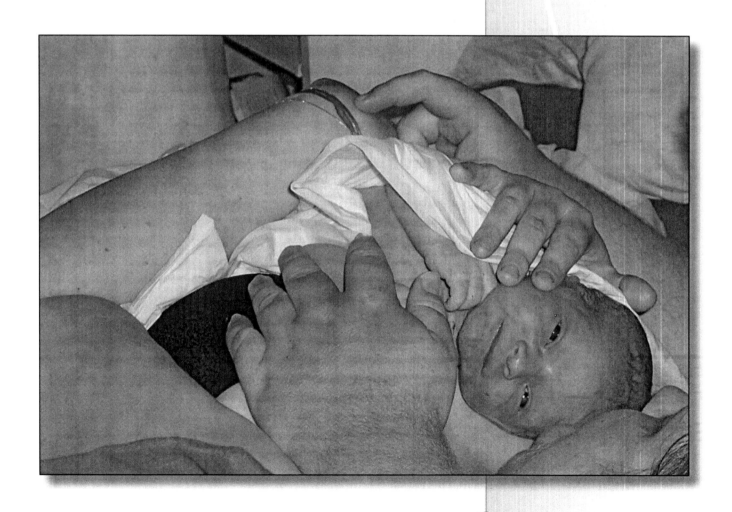

Babies are helpless little people who can only cry for what they need. As parents, *you* are the ones that care the most about your baby.

This is your baby to touch and to hold and to make decisions for. Don't let someone else tell you when you can and cannot hold your baby or that you can only breastfeed at certain times.

Follow your instincts. *It's okay to be a mother (or father) grizzly bear if necessary!* This can usually be done politely but firmly.

Nursery Procedures

Most nurseries have routine procedures for newborns. Some are given by law to all babies to protect the few that would actually need them. If you don't feel right about something, you may be able to sign forms that release those who would administer the procedures from responsibility. Following is an explanation of some of the main procedures carried out at birth.

Vitamin K

Most babies in our country are routinely given Vitamin K at birth. Vitamin K, which influences blood clotting, is naturally produced in the body. A baby, for reasons we still do not understand, doesn't begin making its own Vitamin K until after birth. In very rare cases an otherwise healthy infant develops a life-threatening hemorrhagic disease (HDN) which is characterized by unexplained bleeding or bruises. Bleeding may be external or internal. Vitamin K is given to prevent this minute risk. It is given intramuscularly or as a series of oral doses.

A label on the Vitamin K1 Injection strongly recommends, however, that the injection route be taken only if other routes (oral) are restricted. If given by mouth, it is important that each of the doses are given, and that if signs of HDN are seen, that the baby receives Vitamin K immediately, as babies with HDN are at high risk. Among other risks, keep in mind that with all vaccinations an anaphylactoid reaction may occur.

When Vitamin K began to be routinely given, babies received large doses of a synthetic type, which caused jaundice and other problems. This was soon cast aside and was replaced by a natural form, Phylloquinone which even in huge doses did not cause jaundice.

Early in the 1990s, researchers reported a heightened risk of childhood cancer in babies that had received the intramuscular administration of vitamin K. Later studies showed no correlation. Research continues and it is believed that oral administration of vitamin K is not

> As parents, you are the ones that care the most about your baby. This is your baby to touch and to hold and to make decisions for. Don't let someone else tell you when you can and cannot hold your baby or that you can only breastfeed at certain times.

linked to childhood cancer. Still, it has always been wise to use caution whenever science has attempted to improve upon nature.

Silver Nitrate or Eye Ointment

It is required by law in many places for babies' eyes to be treated at birth. This is done to prevent congenital blindness since the baby's eyes can be infected when passing through the birth passageway *if* the mother has Gonorrhea or Chlamydia, sexually transmitted diseases. Both can be asymptomatic in the mother.

Silver nitrate is caustic and it burns. It is painful and terribly irritating.

Erythromycin or Tetracycline are often used now and are just as effectual as silver nitrate without many of the side effects, but they still cause discomfort and make the baby's eyes blurry so that he can't see during his first hours of life. The makers of Erythromycin Ophthalmic Ointment USP, 0.5% say plainly that it is for "infants born to mothers with clinically apparent gonorrhea...." (Bausch & Lomb 1994)

In Great Britain, baby's eyes are watched during the first weeks of life. If no prevailing discharge is noticed, the baby's eyes are left alone.

If you've had Gonorrhea or Chlamydia and if you still have it, the ointment is important for your baby to get. If not, a release can generally be signed. Parents have run into problems with the hospital when declining this procedure as it is the law in some places. It is another routine procedure that is needed by a few and so it is given to the whole. What are the risks and benefits for you and your baby?

Follow your instincts. It's okay to be a mother (or father) grizzly bear if necessary! This can usually be done politely but firmly.

Newborn Metabolic Screening

Newborn metabolic screening is a blood test administered by pricking the baby's heel and is used to test for Phenylketonuria (PKU), Galactosemia and Congenital Hypothyroidism. Chances of getting any of these are very low, but occurrence can be devastating. One downside to agreeing to the procedure is that if your baby is hemophiliac or has a clotting disorder, bleeding from the hole punctured by the needle can be a serious problem. Also, whenever you break the skin there is a risk of infection. The test can also come back with the erroneous results and may have to be repeated. But, if you waited until you saw signs of the illness, it would probably be too late. If you decide to have the test, make sure your

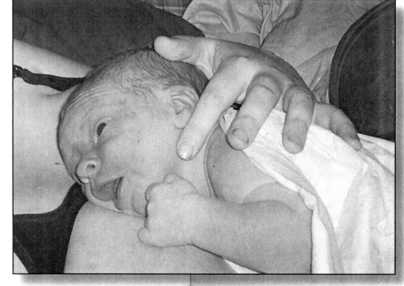

baby's foot is warm so that the blood flows more freely and so there is less of a chance of the staff having to prick more than once. Be there for your baby and hold him rather than having him go through it alone on the table.

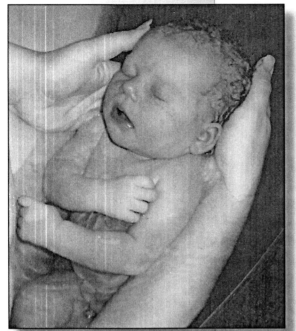

Blood Sugar Testing

Blood sugar testing is a procedure that may be done if a baby is a bit smaller (under five pounds) or larger (over nine pounds) than average, when the mother has diabetes, or when the baby has symptoms of low blood-sugar, such as trembling or shaking. If the baby shows signs of low blood-sugar, simply breastfeeding her can often remedy this situation. If not, glucose solution might *then* be given.

Treatments for Jaundice

A bit of jaundice is a common occurrence in babies, showing up about the third day. The baby will look slightly yellow. Very rarely does a baby have Kernicterus, which is a damaging staining of the brain cells by bilirubin. Kernicterus is more common in babies that have Rh negative problems and those who are premature, but has not been reported to happen at bilirubin levels below twenty.

It's best, if possible, to avoid Bilirubin lights as they are believed to cause skin rashes, anxiety, and vitamin deficiency. It is sometimes suggested that a mother give the baby water or even glucose water. This is not wise as it can interfere with breastfeeding.

Breastmilk and a little sunlight are two of the best things you can give your baby if he is experiencing jaundice. To give your baby sunlight, you can sit and hold him unclothed for a little while in front of a window. The window does not need to be open. Be cautious that he does not get too much sun and become burned or overheated, as this could happen easily on a hot day. Even a cloudy day provides sunlight that can help your baby to break down the bilirubin in his system. You still need to be cautious to not allow your baby's skin to get burned even on a day that is overcast.

There is also a good chance that when a cord has not been cut too early, that there will be no problems with jaundice.

Weighing and Bathing

When do you want the initial birth exams, weighing, and bathing to be done? Usually these are all things that can wait. Some families might even wish to delay the baby's bath for 24 hours, until he has had more time to adjust to his new world. When *you decide* that it is time for your baby to go to the nursery for weighing, bathing, and other procedures, parents can go too.

If you are birthing in a hospital that routinely separates mothers and babies, keep the baby as long as possible, an hour or more before they take him away. This is so important to bonding with and welcoming your baby into his new world. One hospital has allowed—even suggested—a mother be wrapped up and wheeled into the nursery in a wheel chair so that she could be with her baby. Even if for some reason only the father can go, it is a good idea for him to stay with the baby while procedures are carried out. He can continue to advocate for the parents' wishes concerning the care of their newborn. He may wish to record this period by camcorder or with photos for the mother to see later. But being there and reassuring your baby of your presence is important.

Some caregivers carry out procedures right at the mother's bedside. Some make sure that the baby stays with the mother and is not removed from her and the father's care at all during the first hours and days following the birth.

Considerations for Premature Babies

If your baby is born prematurely, the following may be of interest to you. Researchers at Brown's Institute School of Medicine asked mothers of premature babies to hold their infants for ten minutes a day. In one group, the baby wore only a diaper and cap and was held on the mother's bare chest with a blanket covering him. In the second group, the babies were dressed and had a blanket wrapped around them. Babies in the first group, who had skin-to-skin contact with their mothers, appeared calmer than the babies who did not. They also took in more oxygen with each breath. These babies who had skin-to-skin contact were more likely to breastfeed.

Pumping your milk for feedings, rather than allowing formula to be given, provides a premature infant with a wonderful advantage in many respects, as it gives them with the best possible nutrition available to them in their more fragile condition. The milk made by the mother of a premature baby, amazingly, is naturally formulated exactly for a premature baby! Pumping at this time also helps to establish your milk for nursing later when the baby is able to.

Apgar Scoring System

The Apgar Scoring system was created by Dr. Virginia Apgar to assist caregivers in assessing the state of a newly-born baby. A minute after birth, the baby is evaluated for **Appearance, Pulse, Grimace, Activity,**

Apgars go up when a baby is kept with his mother! Some caregivers make sure that the baby stays with the mother and is not removed from her and the father's care at all during the first hours and days following the birth.

and Respiration. Scores of 0, 1, or 2 are given for each, dependant on baby's color, heart rate, facial grimace (a cough or sneeze is great and a 2 would be given for **G**), flexion and motion, and respiration. The five scores are added together with ten as the top number.

If the baby's total score is a seven or above, he will probably end up doing very well at continuing to adjust. Those who are calculated to be between 4 and 6 total points may need some help—usually suctioning and some oxygen. Those who receive a number under 4, may need more assertive assistance and will probably need a little extra observation.

Apgar is assessed again at five minutes after birth. Typically, babies of mothers who have not had medication and a variety of routine procedures, and who have been under the care of a patient, watchful caregiver who trusts in the birth process, do well on the Apgar test.

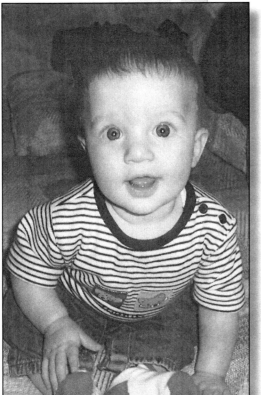

Circumcision

Circumcision is a procedure worth your careful study and choice. It is performed routinely in the United States on male babies after birth. Circumcision is the procedure of removing the foreskin which normally covers the head of the penis.

Circumcision originally began to be a routine course of action in our country in the early 1900s because it was believed that it would prevent masturbation. Throughout history a variety of other professed medical benefits, each just as absurd as the next, all had their day in the sun before being debunked as well.

Listed today as medical benefits, are claims that circumcision *very slightly* lowers the risk of urinary tract infections, that it lowers the chance of getting a certain kind of cancer which is *extremely* rare, that it *slightly* lowers the risk of getting sexually transmitted diseases, and that it makes genital hygiene easier. As for the latter, are men in the United States less able to keep their penises as clean as other men throughout the world and throughout history?

Among a variety of complications that are due to the operation itself, risks include loss of the penis, hemorrhage, and death. Babies have been known to develop gangrene and other infections from the surgery, and to have reoccurring infection at the surgical site, throughout their lives. When too much of the foreskin is sometimes accidentally removed, a skin graft may be necessary with the possibility of resulting complications. Penises can also grow crooked or become disfigured from the surgery.

Without an equal list of benefits, why risk such horrendous possibilities? The penis was made correctly the first time! Do we actually think we are going to improve upon it?

It may be surprising that as far back as 1971 the American College of Pediatrics stated, "There is no valid medical indication for circumcision in the newborn." In 1978, the American College of Obstetricians and Gynecologists also took a stand against habitual and customary circumcision as we had previously known it. But as we've seen in many different areas, old habits die hard, *especially when they bring in steady revenue.*

Thus, we perform this surgery now basically so that boys will all look the same—for cosmetic reasons. The United States is the only nation left, in fact, that routinely circumcises the majority of its newborn males for non-religious reasons. Circumcision is almost unheard of in Europe, South America, and non-Muslim Asia. In fact, only 10 to 15 percent of men throughout the world are circumcised. The vast majority of those are Muslim.

Sadly, in some places *girls* are circumcised (by removing her clitoris)! In those places, the notion of circumcising a boy is considered unthinkable.

Circumcision is an extremely painful procedure for the baby that takes about fifteen minutes. Sometimes pain medication is used with its risks and the painful injections to administer it, but this does not mean that it is a comfortable, enjoyable experience by any means.

The following days of recovery from the surgery, just when he is learning what the world is all about, are, as can be imagined, painful and distressing.

Some feel that infancy is the ideal time, because the surgery will not have to be done as an adult. This way it is done and over with, they argue, and babies forget. But do they really? Can any of us forget a traumatic experience fully? Do survivors of other types of sexual assault really entirely forget? Or do our bodies hold onto memories of such experiences within them? A great deal of research in other fields have shown that they do.

What is also often forgotten, as we see in many of the procedures our culture subjects our newborns to, is that babies are people *now*. They have no less feeling than we, ourselves, presently do. They are even perhaps *more* sensitive as babies, at this time of such vulnerability, when everything is so new and bewildering.

Registered nurse Terry Schultz wrote, "When I have to set up a baby for circumcision, I feel like crying and often do. I feel like I'm betraying that being behind those eyes, as I calmly and easily strap him on the 'circboard'.... After witnessing many circumcisions, I can say: 'Yes, it hurts. It's pure and simple torture.' As often as I can I leave the room....I've talked to parents many times about their babies' circumcision before it's been done. I see fathers just sort of shrug like...it's one of those things boys have to go through. And mothers who wince at the thought, and hope not to hear his screams, still sign the papers of permission. Parents ask, 'Does it hurt him?' and I tell them yes....But they always have

Do we really think that we can improve upon the way that the human penis was so brilliantly designed?

a good reason to go ahead…'He would be teased.' 'He wouldn't match his dad (or brothers).' 'We've always done it in our family.' 'It's so much worse if it would have to be done later.'" (Schultz 1979)

Some feel that if a man wants to be circumcised, that it should be his informed choice, as a consenting adult—when he is old enough to make that decision—and not as a baby (at a time of greatest helplessness when he is first learning to trust those who care for him).

The foreskin, just as all other parts of the body, is there for a reason. It is the most highly sensitive part of the penis, and was made to protect the glans just as the eyelid protects the eye. When it is excised, the glans becomes callused and its skin protectively becomes many times thicker, causing it to lose much of its sensitivity. A great difference in feeling has been reported by men that have been circumcised later in life. Women have also stated that they have experienced less sexual pleasure during intercourse with men whose penises have been circumcised.

How important is it for all men to "look alike"? More and more boys are now being left intact. In the future, most boys will probably *not* be circumcised. This may surprise American men who were born during a time when nearly 90 percent of boys were circumcised *without their parents' consent.*

Most of those of the Jewish faith circumcise for religious reasons, although some are beginning to opt not to have their babies circumcised or to instead hold a type of token ceremony that is still rich in symbolism.

Many Christians believe that ritual circumcision, as with other types of sacrificial offerings, was done away with by Christ who required the living of a "higher" law. (Acts 15:1–11; Galatians 5:1–6)

If you do opt to circumcise your infant, insist upon staying with him during the surgery, talk to him, and comfort him. Afterward, nurse, sooth, and cuddle him and be sensitive to his soreness in the days following.

Circumcision is sometimes performed the first day, although we recommend that if you choose this procedure, that you wait *at least* a week, rather than having it performed just when he is beginning to experience many of the wonderful sensations of life outside of the womb, and until the baby has made his own Vitamin K (see Nursery Procedures **in this chapter**).

When caring for a baby boy who has been left intact, you do not need to retract the foreskin. The foreskin is mostly self-cleansing (according to the American Academy of Pediatrics). At puberty, a boy can simply be taught the importance of cleaning beneath the foreskin as part of his daily shower.

See Resources in **Appendix E** for websites on this subject.

The foreskin is the most highly sensitive part of the penis. It was made to protect the glans, just as the eyelid protects the eye. When it is excised, the penis loses much of its sensitivity.

The Hepatitis B Vaccine and Other Immunizations

Hepatitis B and/or other vaccinations may be a part of the routine newborn procedures in your hospital.

Here are some facts and items about Hepatitis B:

- It is primarily an adult disease, transmitted through blood or the infected fluids of the body.
- Two to three percent of babies acquire it. It is most commonly passed from mother to baby.
- However, hospital-born babies are more likely to come into contact with it than are babies born at home.
- Symptoms may include nausea and vomiting, fatigue, low fever, pain/swelling in joints, headache, and cough. Jaundice, as well as enlargement and tenderness of the liver, may follow.
- Most of these symptoms do not require hospital care and 95 percent of those who contract it recover completely. Fatality rates are approximately *0.1 percent of those who actually get Hepatitis B*, according to Harrison's Principles of Internal Medicine (1994).
- Those who acquire it develop life-long immunity.
- Fewer than 5 percent of the low numbers of those that don't completely recover become chronic carriers with a quarter of that 5 percent developing a life-threatening liver disease later in life.
- However, the **risks of the Hepatitis B** *vaccine* include chronic fatigue syndrome, pain and/or damage to muscles, headaches, and death.
- Although lower than 10 percent of all doctors may report problems with vaccines, more than 16,000 injuries and deaths due to vaccines have been reported to the Vaccine Adverse Event Reporting System since July 1990.

This information was gathered from the National Vaccine Information Center. (Richardson 1999)

Become fully informed about vaccines. Don't let anyone intimidate you into doing anything.

The Association of Wise Childbearing is neither for nor against immunizations as a whole. We believe that **it is your responsibility to seek what is right, not only for your family collectively, but for each individual that is a member of it.**

It is the parents' responsibility and right to seek out what is right for each member of their family.

Study various
resources,
ask questions,
contemplate and
seek inspiration
about your
decisions.

There have been many campaigns in the past years to vaccinate all children with an ongoing regiment of immunizations throughout childhood. And what caring parent wouldn't want to protect their children? Of course immunization is the responsible thing to do—well isn't it? This all depends on a number of factors. There is in actuality a rather hot controversy on this subject.

Opponents maintain that it wasn't vaccinations that wiped out certain diseases; a look into the past shows that these diseases were already naturally dying out and that better public sanitation had a great deal to do with it. In other countries these diseases were also eliminated even though those populations weren't vaccinating for these particular illnesses.

A growing number of physicians and parent groups argue that we are trading one list of terrible things for yet another list of terrible things when immunizations are given. Although vaccinations can help prevent terrible diseases, there are many cases where vaccinations have actually harmed individuals or caused death. Very soon after receiving certain immunizations, a shocking number of children have become autistic, died of SIDS, developed cancer, and have actually come down with or spread the disease that they were just vaccinated for. The list goes on to include a vast array of other problems that have been developed upon receiving an inoculation.

Another factor that has given much cause for concern is the ingredient Thimerosal (mercury), a poison that has been contained in a number of vaccines in the past. It has supposedly been removed from many vaccines, but there may still be mercury in the vaccine that your child would receive, mercury in an extremely high dose. There have also been found to be other very serious contaminants in vaccines.

Scientists believe if 80 to 100 percent of the population were inoculated for measles, that epidemic would be eradicated. This theory is called "herd immunity." They believe that the risk to those individuals who would be susceptible to damage from those vaccines received is not reason enough not to immunize the whole.

After careful study of both sides, some families choose not to have their children immunized at all. Others choose only to give certain immunizations. This is called "selective immunization." These parents sign an exemption form at their public health department to meet requirements for public school admittance, etc.

Whether to immunize is a decision that isn't as clear cut as many others are. You want to be careful about what and whom you follow, even if it seems that everyone is doing it one certain way. Books and many other resources including the Internet offer literature about many aspects and various sides of the issue.

We strongly suggest further educating yourself about this and other issues. As always, think ahead. In the future will the push for particular practices always be as strong as now? In a few years or perhaps decades, when more information is collected, what will the general prescription be then? We don't know. But it is wise to use caution and seriously consider what is right for your own family and child when considering any situation.

As with other procedures and decisions, we recommend studying, asking questions, contemplating, and seeking inspiration about the risks and benefits of *each* individual immunization and any other procedure for *each* child.

Until you have enough information, perhaps it would be wise to consider waiting until you know for sure what you want to do.

For additional information about particular vaccines, ask for and read the package insert from the box of the specific vaccine.

Contact:

> Vaccine Reaction Information Center 1-800-909-SHOT
> www.909shot.com
> Health Department Immunization Programs 1-800-275-0659

Further reading:

> Vaccines, Autism and Childhood Disorders: *Crucial Data That Could Save Your Child's Life*, Neil Z. Miller

Breastfeeding

Breast milk is the perfect, unmatched food for babies. The American Academy of Pediatrics has stated, "Human milk is uniquely superior for infant feeding," and "Human milk is the preferred feeding for all infants, including premature and sick newborns, with rare exceptions....Breastfeeding should begin as soon as possible after birth, usually within the first hour." The Academy goes on to say, "Babies ideally should be exclusively breastfed for the first six months. Other foods are generally unnecessary for the breastfed infant." They maintain that breastfeeding is very important to continue "for at least twelve months and thereafter as long as mutually desired." When the mother or baby must be hospitalized, "every effort should be made to maintain breastfeeding, preferably directly, or by pumping the breasts and feeding expressed breast milk, if necessary." Pediatricians were encouraged to, "promote and support breastfeeding enthusiastically."

Both mother and baby benefit from the emotional aspects of the relationship created through breastfeeding. The closeness and bonding that a baby receives from his mother helps him to develop in diverse ways. And there are many other very important benefits.

Benefits to Babies

Babies receive many advantages from obtaining their nutrition from breast milk. Babies' brains grow at an amazing rate during the first two years. Very commonly, breastfed babies glow with rosy-cheeked health. They are easy to spot. Breast milk is more easily digested and better used by your baby than any substitute. Breastfed babies are believed to have fewer and less serious illnesses, including a reduction in SIDS, leukemia, childhood diabetes, and obesity later in life. Babies that are breastfed may also face a lower risk of ear, bladder, kidney, intestinal, and other infections, as well as protection from meningitis, reduced diarrheal diseases, and reduced RSV (a serious respiratory illness that, for small children, very often requires hospitalization). As breastfeeding continues throughout the first year and beyond, the infant is receiving antibodies against illness. Breastfeeding may provide protection from some effects of pollution in the environment as well. Research is also showing that breastfed babies have higher IQs as well as better development of brain and nervous systems. Mothers' milk provides the necessities to grow bigger brains with more neurological connections. It is even believed that a baby receives immunities that his mother has developed throughout her lifetime, as well as immunities to things that she is now being exposed to.

Breast milk is the perfect, unmatched food for babies.

Babies enjoy breastfeeding very much. The immense comfort that it can bring to the baby has been a big plus for many a parent.

"Breastfeeding is protective against SIDS, and this effect is stronger when breastfeeding is exclusive." (Hauck 2011)

Babies enjoy breastfeeding *very* much and the immense comfort that it can bring to the baby has been a *big* plus for many a parent.

Benefits to Mothers

Mothers who have breastfed have been shown to have decreased risks of breast and ovarian cancer, anemia, and osteoporosis. After giving birth, breastfeeding helps to contract your uterus and control bleeding. Pregnancy weight is more easily lost, especially when breastfeeding into the second year. Generally, breastfeeding is much more convenient than bottle feeding. There are no bottles to warm. Your baby's warm milk is readily available, anywhere you are, and it's always fresh. Night feedings are so much easier! Just pull your baby close, help him to latch on, and go back to sleep. Diapers smell much better. A substantial amount of money is saved (costs of bottle supplies and formula run $900 to $4,700 reported Lamaze clear back in 2001), and not only because breast milk is free. But so is that which might have been spent on costly doctor and hospital visits and medicines, since breastfed babies are generally healthier. Less childhood illness also means more sleep for Mom and Dad and less time off from work. And helpful for keeping stress low, hormones that help mom to relax are released during breastfeeding. Breastfeeding mothers have reported that travel is much easier if your baby is breastfeeding, and parents who enjoy camping have expressed how easy it was to take their babies.

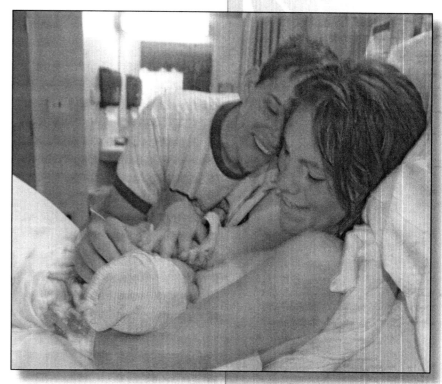

During the first few days, the breasts make colostrum. Colostrum is the perfect food, and provides great protection for the newborn.

Regular breastfeeding typically delays the return of menstruation for quite awhile. Despite what you may have heard to the contrary, breastfeeding really can be used as a form of child spacing *if certain practices are followed.* For more information, we recommend Kippley's book referred to in this chapter.

Other Benefits

Even **communities** reap the benefits of breastfeeding. Research shows less absenteeism from work. Breastfed babies have been shown to have higher IQs, as well as better brain and nervous system development. Because babies are breastfed, both babies and mothers are healthier throughout their lives—which means lower health care costs, reducing the burden on families and insurance companies and on community and government programs.

The **environment** also benefits when babies are breastfed. Nursing a baby doesn't require tin, paper, plastic, or the energy necessary for preparing, packaging, and transporting artificial baby milks. Since there is no waste, breastfeeding in no way adds to pollution and garbage disposal problems.

There's really no comparison between benefits of breastfeeding and formula feeding. Breast is best!

There are circumstances when breastfeeding isn't possible. Thank goodness there are other options. That is what formula was created for in the beginning.

Too many women, however, decide to quit breastfeeding due to misinformation and because they are unaware of where to get help. Proper instruction and help after birth are very important! Often mothers' concerns aren't resolved. Frequently mothers mistakenly think they don't have enough milk. Or they may have other problems they do not know how to deal with. **La Leche League** has been the solution for many mothers who have ultimately been successful at breastfeeding. Sometimes it just takes a little knowledgeable information and encouragement from a supportive someone, and some sticking with it to get breastfeeding off on the right foot. A visit about concerns, over the phone or in an appointment, with the local La Leche League leader has helped many a mother-baby pair.

Length of Breastfeeding

Some of the most significant benefits of breastfeeding during **the first few days** are the colostrum and the vital attachment that occurs between the mother and newborn. It may feel to the mother that in the first few days there is nothing to be had in the breast for the baby—but there is colostrum. Colostrum is the precious substance that the breasts miraculously formulate for the baby before the milk comes in—usually about the third day. It is pure gold, full of antibacterial properties, and exactly what the baby needs.

Breastfeeding in the **first few months** supplies the perfect food and perfect preventive medicine the baby needs, as well as comfort and security.

When your baby begins solids, about **six months to one year old,** she nurses more for security, comfort, and overall optimal health and very gradually less for nutritional reasons. Babies *love* to nurse. They know it is good for them and exactly what they need.

Breastfeeding **into the second year and beyond** continues to provide that comfort, security, and continued health benefits to mother and baby including what researchers believe are great benefits for the baby's brain.

Babies in many non-western societies breastfeed for three or four years. The World Health Organization recommends breastfeeding *at least* two years. La Leche League International promotes breastfeeding until the baby outgrows the need. There are even a number of women that tandem-nurse—nursing two babies, usually an older one and a younger one, at the same time.

Researchers have found that new mothers who were able to stay at home for at least three months were much more likely to be primarily breastfed longer than three months. (Gordon 2011)

Both mother and baby benefit from the emotional aspects of the relationship created through breastfeeding.

Facing Customary Challenges

Unfortunately formula companies use a variety of cunning advertising techniques, including giving out free samples through doctors' offices and providing pediatricians' offices with loads of free paraphernalia with their ads on the items. Just watch and see how many freebies you get—including free formula! Obviously, once families start to give formula to their babies, breast milk supply can decrease and pretty soon mothers *need* to supplement.

Perhaps it would be most helpful if doctors were to insist that formula be available only by prescription for babies that really need a substitute, as formula is considerably inferior to breast-milk. A system for better support for mothers and babies as they learn to breastfeed could be made more widely available.

As if facing formula sabotages weren't enough, some people still balk at women nourishing their children where others can see. It still seems to be socially unacceptable to do so in some places. The more women take a leadership role by refusing to be thwarted in nurturing their children in one of the healthiest ways possible, even in public, the more it will become an acceptable thing for others to do in public *as well as in the privacy of their own homes.*

With a bit of practice, you can discretely nurse practically anywhere. Modesty is an understandable issue for many women. Practicing, perhaps in front of a mirror at home, can be helpful. Some mothers use a blanket, but by simply and quickly adjusting with your baby in front of you, you may be able to breastfeed even more discreetly without a blanket. You may be able to feed your baby without anyone being able to tell whether you are feeding him or if he is just sleeping.

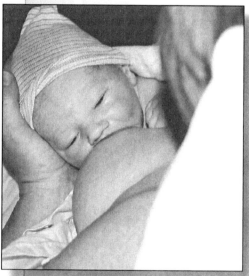

The closeness and bonding that a baby receives from his mother helps him to develop in diverse ways.

Breastfeeding Tips

- During the first few days, the breasts make colostrum. There won't be a lot, and this is just fine. This is how it is supposed to be. Colostrum is the perfect food, served exactly when your baby needs it. It was designed to give powerful protection to your baby against disease. It also meets the unique nutritional needs of your infant. The protein in it can help to prevent low blood sugar which is sometimes a problem at birth, and breastfeeding is a much healthier alternative to the glucose water that might be offered in the hospital nursery. *Colostrum is also two times faster than glucose water for raising glucose levels.* Colostrum also has laxative properties that help a baby to easily eliminate the meconium, the first bowel movements, from her intestines. This is very helpful, as the delayed elimination of the meconium is thought to contribute to newborn jaundice. Your baby will benefit from as much colostrum as possible. Feeding your baby colostrum by spoon is a very good alternative if nursing from the breast is impossible in the beginning.

- Taking care of yourself, getting enough rest, proper nutrition, and enough fluids are important for producing a good supply of milk and for providing the necessary care for your new baby. This isn't the time for a lot of housework, vigorous exercise, or entertaining. Too much stress can affect your supply. Napping when your baby does is a good habit to get into.

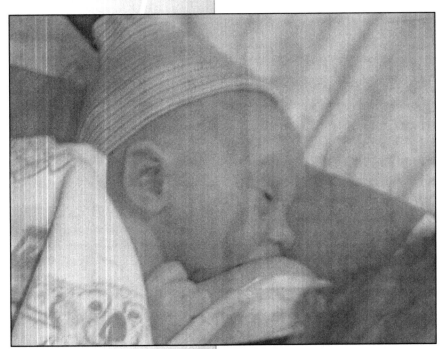

This little guy has his first lessons in breastfeeding soon after birth.

- Eating healthy foods can supply you with much needed energy. You need about 2,000 to 2,500 calories a day, depending on your activity level. More importantly, make sure that your foods are worthy of your baby's health and yours. Brightly-colored vegetables, nuts, seeds, and whole grains are some of the best to choose from—although do watch out for gas-producing foods such as broccoli, cabbage, and onions and things like chocolate as they are thought to possibly cause discomfort in the baby's tummy when passed through the milk. With luck, your baby will have no problems with any of these.

- Eliminating tobacco, alcohol, and caffeine from your diet, and running any prescription medicines you may take by your pediatrician is wise.

- Getting plenty of water is important when breastfeeding. Drinking a little every time you breastfeed is a good habit to establish.
- For babies with minor jaundice, breast milk can do wonders. (See Nursery Procedures in **this chapter**.)
- During the first few days, it may be necessary to wake a new baby every two to three hours to feed. If he is too sleepy, you may need to remove his clothing to help wake him and interest him in nursing. Even though he may not show signs of it, he *does* need to be fed and stay hydrated!
- Avoid the use of pacifiers and bottles for the first couple of weeks. This helps to avoid the common problem of nipple-confusion. Bottles and pacifiers can sabotage breastfeeding. Even in the hospital nursery it can be harmful for a baby to be given a bottle or pacifier. To avoid this, you may wish to put a note on your baby's bed politely indicating your wishes.
- It is helpful for mothers who have had a cesarean to ask to breastfeed as soon after the birth as possible. Mothers and babies are usually sequestered in separate recovery rooms unfortunately. The sooner you can get your baby back into your arms for bonding and nursing, the better. Don't be shy about asking to have your baby as soon as possible. When he is brought to you, ask for help in trying to nurse right there in the recovery room. Your husband or birth partner can also help you find a comfortable position for nursing.

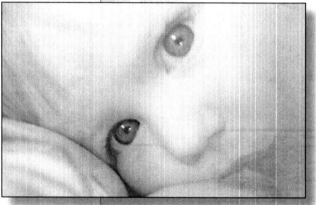

Breastfed babies glow with rosy-cheeked health. They are easy to spot.

- Begin nursing on the breast that the baby last nursed at. Nurse the baby at both breasts for at least fifteen minutes on each side. This will allow him to get the hind milk, which is the milk with a higher fat content that helps to hold him over to the next meal. When breastfeeding is well-established, you no longer need to keep track of time.
- Let-down happens as the mother begins to nurse her baby, or sometimes even when she hears a baby cry or is simply thinking of breastfeeding. (Breastfeeding is connected to a woman's psyche, just as labor is.) Leaking from your breasts between feedings is normal. So is leaking from one breast while breastfeeding with the other. Nursing pads to absorb the milk can be either bought, or made from cloth diapers. Pressing your arm against the breast when milk lets down can be helpful and can be done discretely in public when your milk suddenly decides to come in.
- One of the biggest contributors to how much milk you will produce is whether or not your baby empties the breast at each feeding. Correct positioning on the nipple is a part of this. Frequency is also important.

Seek assistance if necessary. There is help available.

- *Make sure the baby latches on correctly every single time.* This is the best thing you can do to prevent sore nipples. It is no longer advised to "roughen up" nipples in preparation to breastfeed, prior to giving birth. This can actually even remove protective substances.
- Breastfeeding doesn't always start out with ease. Sometimes a little help is needed. It is important to be patient and keep working at it. Seek help from your local La Leche League leader, your doula, or a lactation consultant if you have questions about sore nipples, flat or inverted nipples, plugged or infected milk ducts, how to establish your milk supply, correct positioning, latch on, what the signs are that your baby is receiving enough milk, engorgement, weaning, ways to continue breastfeeding if you must continue working or going to school, and other questions you might have. Your questions may actually be common concerns. Seek assistance— before you give birth if you are aware of any of these potential difficulties. There is help available. When faced with obstacles realize that desire, determination, patience, and endurance are some of your most valuable tools.
- Although you may have heard differently, breastfeeding really can be used as a form of birth control. *If you breastfeed as often as your baby wishes, aren't giving solids, have very limited or no use of bottles or pacifiers, are nursing often (including during-the-night feedings) and if your periods haven't returned,* breastfeeding is said to be 98 percent effective at six months after your birth. Of course it varies for everyone. After six months, ovulation is more likely to occur. But there still seems to be some protection. Breastfeeding is the most common form of birth control worldwide. *The Seven Standards of Ecological Breastfeeding: The Frequency Factor* by Sheila Kippley is an excellent, reader-friendly book on this subject. (See **chapter 19** for more information on birth control.)

The Womanly Art of Breastfeeding is an excellent book by La Leche League about breastfeeding. To find a LLL leader in your area contact La Leche League at www.lalecheleague.org

Note to those who must use or elect to use formula: It is imperative to follow the formula company's instructions for preparation. Also, be sure to sterilize bottles and other supplies.

19

Postpartum Care

TAKING CARE OF YOURSELF, your new baby, and your family is a big job. While your body can't recover overnight from nine months of pregnancy, there are ways to ease the process. Be sure to reach out to others for help when you need it. And don't forget the importance of nurturing your marriage. This chapter will give you some information and ideas about how to deal with all that this new experience will entail.

Recovery

Recuperating well during the early weeks of motherhood is important. Mothers who don't push their recovery generally fare better than those who try to do too much too soon.

Baby care, while wonderful, is a lot of work. Permit friends and family to help you with tiring and time-consuming tasks around the house. If people offer to help, say, "That sounds marvelous. What do you have in mind?"

People *enjoy* helping, and when you allow them to have the opportunity to help, you are *giving* something to them. Let them bring in a meal, care for older children, and help straighten up. If you have a baby shower or mother celebration, the hostesses might consider passing around a list for friends to sign up to be contacted later by the hostesses or another friend to bring dinner. Interestingly, people tend to like someone that they have done a favor for. Stock up with a box of thank you cards to send out later. Expressions of heart-felt gratitude never go out of style.

Take this opportunity, while others are helping out with household responsibilities and your older children as you recover, for you and your new baby to get to know each other. Your baby needs you, her parents. Don't let others with good intentions keep your baby away from you. Hang on to her and cuddle up together as much as you can.

Enjoy this time as much as possible! This wonderful time of "baby moon" goes by *so* quickly.

Something that can be very helpful is to hire a **postpartum doula** to help you during that initial period of mothering your new baby. Go online to learn more about the advantages of hiring a postpartum doula to give care to you and your family in your home. She does such things as light house work, making dinner, perhaps running some errands, helping to make sure breastfeeding becomes well established, and answering questions about infant care. Postpartum doulas can help to reduce risks of Postpartum

Recuperating well during the early weeks of motherhood is important.

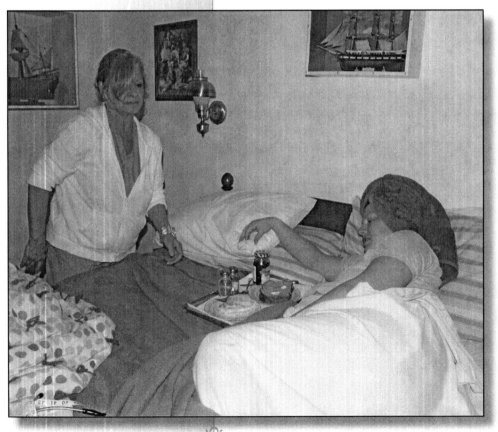

Depression. She nurtures a woman and her family, and is there for the new mother's emotional needs. For more information on postpartum doulas, look in the website section for the DONA website under "Doulas." There are also other fabulous organizations that provide postpartum doulas.

Psychological Recovery

It is important for a new mother to have people around her who are supportive, who will listen non-judgmentally as she talks about her birth, and who will lend an ear as many times as she wants to tell about it. This can help her to understand it herself and be able to move on to the other aspects of mothering. (See Postpartum Mood Disorders in **this chapter**.)

Uterus

Each day the uterus shrinks a bit. Sensations of uterine tightening may heighten with breastfeeding because the baby's sucking helps to stimulate the release of oxytocin, the hormone that helps the uterus to contract. These extra contractions are beneficial. Intense, unrelenting cramps can be a sign of infection, however. Keeping your bladder empty will help your uterus to contract.

Lochia

Vaginal flow after the birth is a bit like a heavy period. It isn't a regular menstrual period. It may last up to six weeks or be gone in a few days. If you soak two sanitary pads in a half hour or less, firmly massage your uterus. Your uterus should feel hard. Nurse your baby (this produces uterus-contracting oxytocin) and *immediately call your caregiver*. Offensive-smelling lochia, just a scarce amount, or heavy lochia that doesn't slow with rest isn't normal. Call your caregiver. Use pads, not tampons. Breastfeeding mothers may not menstruate until the child weans. Menstruation starts within six to eight weeks in mothers who bottle feed.

Breasts

Although it may seem like your breasts aren't producing much food for your baby at first, wonderful colostrum is provided for the baby during the initial few days. About the third day, the milk comes in. The fullness doesn't last too long, especially if you let the baby nurse often. A

Mothers who don't push their recovery, generally fare better than those who try to do too much too soon.

supportive, breathable bra is extremely helpful. Change nursing pads when damp. Use water, no soap on nipples as this can contribute to cracking and bleeding. Coconut oil, vitamin E oil, or lanolin can be helpful for dry, cracked nipples and doesn't need to be washed off before nursing. *Making sure your baby latches on correctly, with his mouth over as much areola as possible, can help you to avoid sore nipples.* If they do become sore, don't give up breastfeeding! The pain won't last forever, and they will toughen as the baby nurses. Severe and persistent pain, a warm area, redness, or a hardened area in the breast are signs of a plugged duct or breast infection. Very helpful is wet heat (a shower, or a rice sock hot pack—see **chapter 13** for simple directions for making one). So is massaging the lumps caused by plugged milk ducts (gentle but firm, from the outside of the breast toward the nipple). If your nipples are pulled flat from your breasts being engorged with milk, massage your breasts as described above, and then express enough milk out to relieve fullness. This can better help your baby to latch on. Try to nurse frequently to avoid engorgement.

Thrush is yeast that may also cause breast soreness when passed from the mother to the baby and from the baby to the mother during breastfeeding. Often antibiotics are a major contributor to this. Thrush can be extremely uncomfortable. A mother may also experience yeast internally in the breast, indicated by shooting, "toe curling" pain during the let-down phase of nursing. The sooner you can rid it from both yours and your baby's systems the better.

Your baby does not need to be weaned because of thrush! (See Diaper Rash in **chapter 20**.)

Drinking enough water is also important for a nursing mother to do.

Ice packs have a numbing effect, and help dry up milk for those mothers who won't be breastfeeding. Expressing some of the milk can relieve fullness.

Call the La Leche League leader in your area with other questions. There is help—don't be shy! The women that answer these calls help women often and without charge. The problems you are experiencing may be quite common. (See Breastfeeding in **chapter 18**.)

Bowels

Delicate episiotomy sites and hemorrhoids can make having a bowel movement painful. A diet of whole grains, fresh fruits and vegetables, and lots of liquids will encourage easier bowels. Labor can cause the bowels to slow. Consult your caregiver if you haven't had a bowel movement in a week. Hemorrhoids can be troublesome, but do shrink. Witch hazel compresses can be helpful until they do, as can ice packs. Using a finger to replace them can be effective.

Take this opportunity for you and your new baby to get to know each other. Your baby needs you, her parents.

Perineal Discomfort

The perineum (the muscular area between the vagina and rectum) may be a bit sore from the birth. Further discomfort may be the result of an episiotomy, tearing, and stitches. Ice packs the first twenty-four hours, and soaking in the tub as described below, can aid healing. Other remedies are walking to stimulate circulation, witch-hazel compresses, and numbing sprays. Urinating can be painful as urine runs over the perineum, so it may be helpful to squeeze a peri bottle with warm water over the area while urinating.

Avoiding an episiotomy, if possible, can greatly reduce recovery time and discomfort. (See **chapter 7**.)

Doing a Kegel exercise (see **chapter 7**) as you sit down, can make doing so more comfortable, as can sitting tilted slightly to one side with pressure on one buttock instead of the perineum. Getting the vaginal muscles back into shape using Kegels is even more effective when done early in the recovery period. Begin Kegels and abdominal tightening exercises as soon as the day after your birth and keep them as a part of your daily routine.

Daily healing herbal baths with your baby can be both nurturing and bonding and great for your perineum as well as your baby's umbilical cord area (it is actually helpful to let the cord area get wet under these circumstances). Before birth, in preparation for postpartum, some women prepare a healing mix and divide it into six separate bags (for six days). In a large bowl, they mix together approximately an ounce each of healing herbs such as the following which should be found easily at their local health food store: calendula (healing), uva ursi (woman's herb), thyme (antiseptic), plantain (bleeding), lavender (antiseptic, relaxing), and sea salt (water softener). In the days after the birth, they make a tea of the mix from one bag in water on the stove, let cool, strain, and add the "tea" to their bath water. Those giving birth at home can treat themselves and their new little one to one of these baths immediately following the birth as well.

Enjoy this time as much as possible. This wonderful time of "baby moon" goes by quickly.

Sexual Relationship

Let your body be your guide. As long as there is no pain or discomfort, you can resume intercourse when bright red bleeding has stopped. In the meantime, other physical affection can be continued. For more information about breastfeeding as a form of natural birth control, see **chapter 18**. *The Seven Standards of Ecological Breastfeeding: The Frequency Factor* by Sheila Kippley is an excellent, reader-friendly book on this subject. (See Resources in **Appendix E**.)

It is believed that other forms of birth control compatible with breastfeeding are barrier methods (such as condoms) and those with progesterone-only hormones. Those containing estrogen can lower milk supply among other negative side-effects. While the pill and mini-pill (neither of which should be taken during breastfeeding in particular) have been known to have high rates of side-effects, particularly alarming are the side-effects of implants, shots, IUDs and some other forms of birth control including high rates of infertility. Each should be very carefully researched concerning the high rates of health problems they are causing for women and babies without recall from manufacturers.

The mini-pill works by causing an already fertilized egg to not be able to implant and to be flushed out, presenting moral issues.

Understanding your body's signs of fertility (mainly vaginal secretions) can also aid you in both preventing and achieving pregnancy. This, when used correctly, can be one of the most effective forms of birth control. *Your Fertility Signals: Using Them to Achieve or Avoid Pregnancy Naturally* by Merryl Winstein is a good resource to consult. There are also teachers and classes that can help you to understand your own body and give you the information you need.

Weight

Remember, you most likely won't lose all the weight at the time of the birth. For both mother and baby, the periods of pregnancy and breastfeeding are important times when nutritious foods are essential. Certainly portion control is beneficial. And exercise for the mother is helpful for both body and psychological health. Getting out for walks with your baby or working out in your own living room with him nearby or even as a part of the routine can be fun for you both. Breastfeeding, especially when doing so into the second year, can also nicely aid the weight-loss process.

Reasons to call your midwife or doctor right away

- Heavy bleeding that increases instead of decreases, seems excessive, doesn't slow with rest, and is accompanied by large clots
- Flu-like symptoms
- Fever and chills
- Offensive-smelling discharge
- Severe abdominal pain or tenderness in abdomen
- Red, warm, painful swelling or a hard spot in your leg
- Pain with urination or a feeling of need to urinate even when there is no urine
- Acute pain in the vagina or perineum
- A red, warm, painful, firm area on a breast with or without streaking

If people offer to help, say, "That sounds marvelous. What do you have in mind?"

Post-Cesarean Discomfort

If you had a cesarean, recovery may or may not be a time of excruciating pain. The myth that a cesarean is the way to a pain-free childbirth is sadly ridiculous. Pain medication (pills) can be extremely helpful. The amount reaching the baby through breast milk is reportedly small.

Deep breathing and using imagery such as a healing light entering into the area of discomfort and healing it, as you breathe in, can be very helpful.

Coughing can hurt a great deal. You may want to press a pillow against the incision when you do.

Positions such as side-lying, the football hold, or using a pillow over the incision, may be the most comfortable for breastfeeding.

Walking can be painful, but a little at a time can be good, as can moving in bed often, rolling from side to side, and doing abdominal tightening. Lie on your left side, draw up your knees, and massage your abdomen from right to left. Hot fennel, peppermint, and ginger tea may be helpful.

Although it can be quite uncomfortable, abdominal gas is a good sign that digestive processes are getting back to normal. Rocking in a rocking chair can help reduce gas pain. Avoid soda, iced drinks, and gassy foods.

Blood collecting in the diaphragm can cause pain in one or both shoulders. The pain is carried through nerve passages to the shoulder. This may last a few days. If severe, medication may be helpful.

Relationships With Others

Has the time surrounding your birth changed the way you relate to others? It may be important to your own emotional health to work to heal those relations, building renewed bonds of love and even trust if necessary. To allow anger to get the best of you because of the behavior of another is only to punish yourself.

Going for postpartum Craniosacral sessions and chiropractic adjustments can each be particularly helpful for both you and your baby. (See **chapter 12**.)

Dad's Challenges

Typically, the father/child relationship doesn't really start until birth. Often a father may want very much to connect and to do his best, and then realizes when the time comes, that he does not really know how to care for all of the baby's needs. He sometimes feels pushed aside by well-meaning people who come to help after the birth. He also sometimes experiences jealousy, feeling unattractive, unloved, and abandoned. Sometimes fathers will withdraw from the mother and baby at this important time. There is a need for more truly excellent resources for fathers.

Don't let others with good intentions keep your baby away from you. Hang on to her and cuddle up together as much as you can.

Baby Blues

"Baby Blues" are pretty common. Symptoms may include insomnia; a depressed mood, or a depressed mood rapidly changing to elation; headaches; poor concentration; tearfulness; and confusion. These symptoms sometimes begin the third day after childbirth, last one day to two weeks, and disappear without treatment. A drop in hormones at about 72 hours postpartum could very well be the cause. Some mothers may feel disappointed over the fact that they have flabby bellies, feel tired, don't yet fit into pre-pregnancy clothes, or that their labors didn't go as planned. It's important to let moms talk it through. Simply getting out can do a world of good.

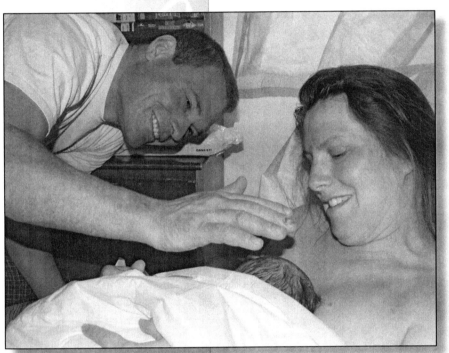

Postpartum Depression

Postpartum Depression is a mental disorder that is much more serious than the "Baby Blues." It may begin about two weeks to six months postpartum, and can last for weeks or months and require medication, psychotherapy, or both. Periods of excessive crying, despondency, feelings of inadequacy, poor self image, and inability to cope, insomnia, anorexia, and social withdrawal may all be signs. Women take pains to conceal their depression. Treatment is important because PPD can lead to destructive behavior and suicide.

Postpartum Psychosis

Postpartum Psychosis is an illness that is less common, but occurs in some mothers two to three weeks after the birth to as long as six to twelve months after. It is a very dangerous illness because the mother can be both suicidal and infanticidal. A woman loses her sense of reality. Medication and hospitalization may be necessary, and a mother should always be observed in her interactions with the baby when she's symptomatic.

Nurturing Your Marriage Relationship

Wise Childbearing would not be complete without discussing the importance of nurturing your marriage. Having and raising a family of children can be one of the most worthwhile and most fulfilling things you will ever do together as a couple.

Our children benefit greatly when our marriages are happy. They can suffer immensely when there are troubling conflicts between us. The atmosphere of our homes, into which we bring these little ones, is of profound importance. Every marriage has conflicts, but when considering the kinds of childhoods, lives, and future marriages we want for our children, giving thought to how we resolve problems and how we treat one another is essential.

It is important to learn how to handle disagreements and other problems that arise from these times. **Education and preparation are key. Strengthening your marriage now, and having specific relationship skills can be of immense help when conflicts arise.** There are many good books and other resources that can teach you what you will need to know—seek them out now.

Just as your baby needs food to grow, so does your marriage.

Adjusting to Changes

Parenthood, while wonderful and capable of drawing the two of you together, can also be one of the most challenging endeavors you will ever undertake. Many divorcing couples relate that the beginning of their discord commenced around the time they started having children. It can be helpful to know that other couples experience these kinds of things and have made it through.

Naturally, being parents carries with it increased responsibility. Though you still love each other, there will likely be a decrease in physical and emotional intimacy. Issues surrounding one's own childhood arise. Increased stress can lead to health issues. Sometimes unhealthy coping habits begin. Depression in both mother and father is not uncommon. Issues that are a concern now will almost certainly become more of an issue when the baby arrives.

Conflict in the relationship does impact both babies and older children. Blood pressure increases in children whose parents are arguing, and later emotional, behavioral, and cognitive problems surface. Subsequently, children will often withdraw from the father, which affects this essential relationship.

Having a postpartum action plan can be very helpful. Deciding beforehand how you will deal with challenges about division of labor, money, child-rearing philosophies, work, your sexual relationship, social life, and in-laws can alleviate misunderstandings and make adjustmends go more smoothly.

Take the time to assess the present health of your relationship.

What are some of the things you are going to do to preserve the relationship that started all this?

What can be done to prevent difficulties as much as possible, and to make the journey into, and through, parenthood a delightful and wonderful memorable experience?

Take Time for Each Other

Sometimes in your life, as your family grows, you will be tired and unbelievably busy, but just as your baby needs food to grow, so does a marriage. It's important to find time to enjoy each other and to love each other. Take the time to invest yourself in your marriage, and to keeping the "love cup" filled. Men, remember that those little romantic things go a long way with a wife! A husband appreciates a bit of loving care, given in his own love language, as well. A once-a-week date for the rest of your lives can be very helpful for staying unified as a couple. If you can't afford a babysitter, think about trading care. Paying a baby-sitter, though, costs less than an attorney! There are lots of inexpensive, fun things to do, just the two of you.

Try the Love Note Activity

For seven days, choose one topic a day. Husband and wife are each given 10 minutes to write on the same subject chosen from below. After you have both written, take another 10 minutes to read and discuss what you have written to one another. This is *not* a time for problem solving! It is a time to lovingly express your feelings to your spouse. See if you aren't closer as a couple by the end of just one week. It doesn't take a lot of effort, and done over time you should find that your relationship has been greatly strengthened and enhanced.

1. When I want to be with you and can't, I feel_____.
2. I feel _____ when you listen to me with your heart.
3. When I have done something to make you happy (or when you have done something to make me happy) I feel _____.
4. When we show love as a couple, I feel _____.
5. This is how I would describe you to someone else: _____.
6. I feel _____ when you reach out to me when I'm hurt.
7. When we plan things together, I feel _____.

Marriage & Family Enrichment, Inc. teaches a similar method.

Attend a Marriage Enrichment Weekend

A Marriage Enrichment Weekend may also be available in your community. During this weekend away together, couples are given valuable tools for creating a successful and satisfying marriage relationship. Instead of a buying a new crib set and nursery furniture, how about an investment in your relationship? What better welcoming gift could you offer your child as he/she enters your home than a loving, stable relationship between his/her parents? You do need to be careful about the kind of workshop you sign up for. Check it out fully before you do!

To find a seminar in your area you might try calling marriage counselors in your area. You also might try Marriage & Family Enrichment, Inc. in Utah at (801) 278-6831 or (801) 583-8371.

Commit to Sticking It Out

Not many years ago, it was the general belief that children whose parents did not get along, would be better off if their parents chose to no longer live with one another. It has since been shown that children suffer greatly when parents split up, that staying together and making the effort to create a better relationship is by far the better choice (except of course in such situations as where there truly is abuse).

Counselors have talked to many people in second marriages who say that if they'd only known what they know now they would have worked harder to keep the first marriage going.

Reaching Out

Birth can have an immeasurable effect upon the woman, baby, and family. This is a significant life event. You can expect that you will emerge finding yourself much changed.

And you've only just begun! With the birth of a child comes the birth of parenthood, and with the birth of parenthood comes a new kind of life for the whole family. Life as you've known it will change. You have realized already, more or less, some of the changes this new life will bring. At least for awhile you may be giving up getting enough sleep, some spontaneity, your marriage as you have known it, extra money, career and plans for education.

While it may be hard to imagine now, babyhood doesn't last long, and soon you have headed into stages you never dreamed of, and your child is doing things you told yourself your children would never do!

Who will help you to steer through this transition into parenthood? And as parenthood progresses, who will guide you when things get tough? There are many places to find that help and support; perhaps in family, friends, books, groups of other parents, at church, in parenting classes, or in an Internet group of like-minded parents.

Perhaps you will need to figure out how to get a group started yourself. The families you have met in childbirth classes may find that they want to keep in touch on an informal, if not regular, basis.

And don't overlook the wonderful, wise resource that might be available to you in your elders, those who have already been on this journey before you.

One place that women can find much strength as they ride the waves of parenthood is La Leche League. Those that attend local meetings (often held once a month) are either breastfeeding mothers or are proponents of breastfeeding. There is often a special bond between the mothers. This strength can then be carried home to the family.

Lean on each other, as a couple, for support.

Don't be afraid to reach outside your immediate circle and bring in other good things, from various sources, too.

20

Everyday Care of Your New Little One

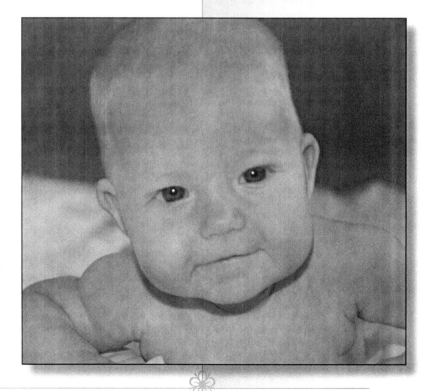

WHEN A BABY is attended to promptly and lovingly, it teaches this otherwise helpless being that someone cares and is there to meet his needs, whatever they may be, whenever there is a need.

Caring for Your New Baby

Caring for a new baby does take time. It is worth it all. When a baby is well cared for, he learns that the world is a good place to be and that he can count on his parents for dry diapers when he is wet and food when he is hungry—not just when they can make themselves available or on a schedule, but whenever he is in need.

Feeding

Babies need to eat about every two hours and will typically nurse fifteen to twenty minutes at a time. If your baby doesn't nurse this long, you probably will need to feed him more often.

Sometimes a baby is going through a growth spurt and it seems he needs to eat all the time. A good rule of thumb is simply to follow his lead and let him nurse as much as his body needs. Try to take it a little easier on these days if you can and let yourself enjoy his babyhood. These days of what seem full of nursing your precious little one will be over all too soon.

If you have had an epidural at birth, he will probably be much sleepier than if not.

You may need to awaken a new baby to eat, as sometimes babies are too sleepy to care a whole lot about necessary nutrition. Removing some of his clothing and massaging his skin gently can help him to waken enough to be interested in eating.

Giving your baby the colostrum that you produce until your milk comes in is one of the very best things you can provide for your newborn baby. The antibodies contained therein will help him to build a strong immune system. The milk thereafter is the perfect food for your baby. Nothing, no matter how "scientifically formulated" it is, can compare. If, after all you can do, there are insurmountable reasons you cannot breastfeed, infant formula is generally thought to be the next best thing. It is also recommended that cows' milk not be given until at least one year of age.

Warmth

During the first few days, babies are unable to regulate their body temperature. Make sure your baby is dressed appropriately—not too warm or too cool. If his hands and feet are cool, add a layer or wrap him in a blanket. Since most heat is lost from the head, you will probably want to put a hat on him when going out if it is chilly. Interestingly however, and contrary to common belief, babies probably do not need a hat right after birth if kept with their mothers. The practice of hats for babies, most

> *Research has shown that consistently answering a baby's requests for assistance actually helps him to become a more joyful child who is more compassionate of others and who is also more happily independent.*

likely, started when mothers and babies were routinely separated at birth, during the days of Twilight Sleep. Did you know that mother's chests are marvelously designed to actually regulate a baby's temperature?

Just like other mammals, mothers *need* to revel in the scent of their baby's heads! And babies and mothers *need* to be kept together.

Stools

Meconium is the first bowel movement a baby has. It is greenish-black and tar-like. You should see both urine and meconium within the first 24 hours. A rusty color to the urine is fine. Following your milk coming in, the consistency of baby's bowel movements will change to be a mustard yellow color. It will normally be rather runny with curds. Breastfed babies have less smelly diapers.

Diaper Rash

If the baby shows signs of yeast and thrush (small red bumps in diaper area and/or white coating in mouth) parents have found that both a good grade of coconut oil, and garlic oil from capsules can be very effective on both the diaper rash and for getting rid of thrush (give baby 1/8 tsp of coconut oil and squeeze a small amount of garlic oil from a capsule for the baby at each feeding). Certainly, as with all information in this book, consult your caregiver as to your and your baby's specific needs. Mother and baby can pass thrush back and forth until they are rid of it. Babies do not need to wean from breastfeeding. The case of thrush simply needs to be treated. (See Recovery in **chapter 19**.)

Diaper rash can also occur when the skin in the diaper area is subjected to moisture for too long. It is important to change diapers regularly, particularly in the case of loose bowels. It is important that the baby's skin is kept clean and dry. Particularly pay close attention to the area in between the folds that do not often get a lot of air. Regular baths and proper drying are important. Avoiding innocent-looking "baby care products" (baby shampoo, lotions, oil, and powder) that contain a myriad of strange chemicals is a good idea. Using a bit of organic soap to wash your baby and then massaging coconut or jojoba oil into your baby's skin after her bath, are much healthier for her. Though do avoid oils on the rash itself.

Cord Stump

The cord stump should be kept clean and dry. Daily herbal baths are helpful though, for healing the stump. (see Recovery in **chapter 19**.) Just have someone bring the baby to you once you are in the tub and

When you are nurturing a child, you are doing some of the most important work on the face of the earth!

have that person come get the baby when you are ready to get out. Dry the stump with a Q-tip, all down in and around it. This helps to keep it clean and free from goo. If it becomes smelly or red, call your pediatrician. The cord stump usually falls off within five to ten days although some take a little longer.

Jaundice

The third day, peaking on the fifth day, is usually when babies show signs of jaundice if they are going to get it. It will reveal itself with a yellowing of the face. Regular breastfeeding (not bottles of water as is sometimes suggested) and exposing a baby often, for a little while at a time, to sunlight from a *closed* window with the curtains open is commonly *all* that is necessary to take care of the problem.

If there is yellowness in the baby's torso, legs, arms, or eyes, if he is lethargic, doesn't waken easily, and/or becomes disinterested in eating, contact your physician.

Some babies require light therapy for more serious cases of jaundice. While this can sometimes be taken care of at home, hospitalization can be necessary for more aggressive therapy.

If jaundice appears on the first day, it is probably an indication of blood type incompatibility (ABO incompatibility). With this kind of jaundice, bilirubin levels can be high enough to be dangerous. Babies, in this case, may need special light therapy. Sometimes, under the supervision of a physician, this can be done at home.

Craniosacral therapy and Chiropractics

It can be very helpful for a newborn to have **Craniosacral therapy** and to be seen by a chirpractor after his or her birth. (See **chapter 12**.)

Danger Signs

Call your pediatrician *any time you have questions*, but immediately if your baby displays any of the following: is lethargic, is running a fever, has projectile vomiting, difficulty with breathing, or failure to urinate or have stools.

Protection

Don't be afraid to be a mother or father bear and protect your baby, the same as you are encouraged to do during pregnancy and at birth; in just the same spirit as a mother bear or other animal would do. Only you

Don't be afraid to be a mother or father bear!

can physically protect your little one from dangers. Some well-meaning people, perhaps even a physician, may encourage something that you know deep within is not right for *your* baby. You must be strong enough to stand up and not allow this to happen to your helpless, precious child.

Also be particularly cautious that you do not allow your baby to be subjected to dangerous kinds of germs or—particularly during the cold months—to viruses (many of which normally do not severely affect healthy older children and adults, but which can be life-threatening to babies). If your baby is in danger of any sort, it is up to you to take action to protect him in whatever ways are necessary.

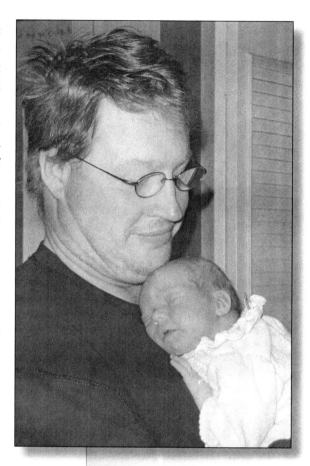

Parent/Infant Bonding

This is one of the most important things you can do for your baby and yourself. It may seem like there are so many important things you need to do now, but bonding with your child in the first year(s) of life is so important to his future well-being. You are needed. Do what it takes to be there for him. (See Attachment Parenting in **this chapter**.)

Self-Care

Don't forget about yourself. Taking care of yourself will allow you to be the best kind of parent you can be for your baby.

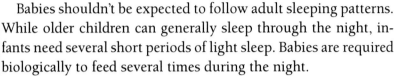

Nighttime Care

What new parent wouldn't agree that getting enough sleep would be wonderful? But sleeping through the night is actually unnatural for babies and could be dangerous. Any program that advocates any sort of "training" to make babies sleep through the night is best to steer clear of for a number of reasons.

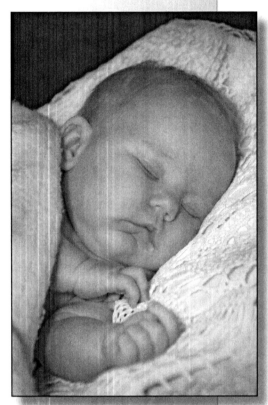

Babies shouldn't be expected to follow adult sleeping patterns. While older children can generally sleep through the night, infants need several short periods of light sleep. Babies are required biologically to feed several times during the night.

For a long time people advocated putting the baby in his own room away from the parents so that the parents could get their sleep. If the baby cried, parents were to let him cry himself back to sleep. They believed the baby would be spoiled if they responded to him every time he cried. Sadly, even now there are those who still believe this is best for a baby, and for his parents too, if they are ever going to get any rest.

With their first child, one family put their baby to sleep in his bassinet in another room. When he would cry they would get up, turn the light on, change his diaper, and then try to settle him back down by feeding and rocking him. By this time he was most often wide awake thinking it was time to play! It didn't take the new parents long to figure out that it was better to leave the ceiling lights off and to pick him up and bring him back to their bed for awhile where the mother would nurse him back to sleep. They also finally realized that babies are usually fine with just one diaper through the night, unless it is messy. By their third baby, they had learned about the benefits of the family bed approach, and so they decided to simply keep their new baby with them throughout the night. They were a little worried that they might not get enough sleep, but found the opposite to be true. They found that when the baby woke at night, it was easy to just nurse her back to sleep without even having to get out of bed. That postpartum period was a great deal easier than were those with the first two babies.

Those who grew up in their own bedrooms, braving the monsters under their beds and the shadows in the corner, might be a bit skeptical of the family bed approach at first. Probably one of the first things they think about is that intimacy would most certainly be hampered by children sleeping in the same bed. Or what about the baby being smothered? Also, how do people who sleep with their children even get any sleep at all with feet and elbows in their faces all night?

Advocates of the family bed reply that intimacy doesn't have to be squelched just because the bed may not be available.

They point out that families in countries around the world including Japan find it very natural to share sleep. Many parents feel that babies are too young to sleep alone, that they need continued body contact, and that they should be free to nurse without having to cry in the darkness until someone awakens and comes in to get them. They like to know they are nearby for their child in the case of nightmares, illness, a fire, or other unexpected occurrence. They have found from experience that co-sleeping enhances the bond between parents and child and between siblings. The closeness developed from sharing sleep, as well as awake time, helps a child to develop into a loving, balanced, self-confident, self-reliant person.

It is believed that incidents of sudden infant death syndrome may actually be *lowered* by co-sleeping. (Kibel and Davies 2000) Theoretically, this has to do with the baby's and parents' breathing patterns becoming related to each other, and the baby being roused periodically because of parents' sleep patterns, so that they don't lapse into a state where Sudden Infant Death Syndrome (SIDS) could be possible. No one knows yet exactly what causes SIDS. SIDS has occurred in both environments unfortunately. Incidences have been dramatically reduced by laying babies on their backs instead of stomachs or even sides. But leaving babies on their backs in another room when they are still working at coughing out newborn mucous from their lungs does not make sense. A parent needs to be available if the baby begins choking on the fluids. Many parents feel better about having their baby next to them in case something does occur. In either sleeping-scenario, putting your baby to sleep on a sturdy mattress that isn't too soft (nor should babies sleep on waterbeds), and keeping pillows, blankets, stuffed animals, and other things away from a sleeping baby is also important common sense. Not bundling up your baby and not smoking are believed to be other ways to avoid SIDS. Of course no one under the influence of alcohol or drugs should sleep with an infant.

To get your baby to sleep better, exposing him to a bit of morning sunshine is said to trigger brain chemicals that help him to get a good night's sleep. A warm bath, daily exercise, good ventilation, lullabies, and comfortable bedtime attire can all be helpful. Babies enjoy poetry, being read to, and the sound of your singing. They crave physical touch, so massage is wonderful.

Children certainly sleep better when their emotional needs are met.

Babies who are responded to, often learn that they do not even need to cry much and that all they need to do is "ask." They know they will be taken care of.

Attachment Parenting

The sacrifice required to create and foster a relationship that will allow you to be the kind of dedicated parent your child is depending on will be well-worth the effort.

Developing and Nurturing Strong Bonds

Babies need to have loving, caring relationships with their parents. The kind of relationship a child has with his parents has much to do with his physical health, cognitive functioning, the shaping of his capacity to love, and in managing his emotions and behavior later in life. If a

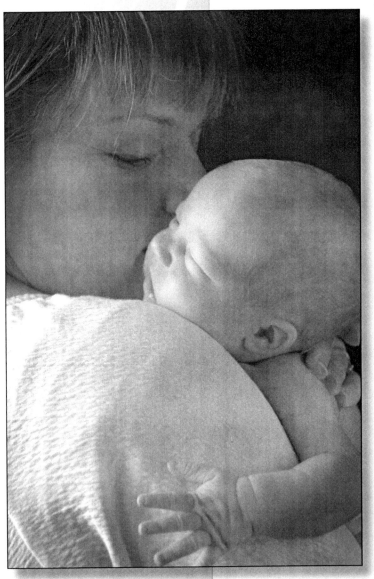

child has someone who is *there* for him, someone who responds to what he communicates, and if he feels secure in that relationship and in that care, a mutually satisfying bond results. He develops an assurance that he is worthy of loving care *when* he needs it, and that people are dependable. He learns that this is how things really can be. Perhaps he will begin, even now, to develop the skills it will take to be a leader of a better, kinder world.

If a child experiences unpredictable, inconsistent care from someone who is indifferent or even cold and unkind, though, it will be more difficult for him throughout life to attach securely and trustingly to others. Babies who are not securely bonded have been known to fail to thrive physically and may be at risk of death.

Insecure attachment as a child can even eventually lead to future emotional problems in life such as depression and anxiety, anger and aggression, addiction, and a variety of health issues.

Consistently Responding to Your Baby's Needs

Despite common belief, babies are really not trying to manipulate the adults who care for them.

How do you respond when someone asks if your baby is a "good baby"? Are they actually asking whether he is content and happy? Or is there really a common belief that some babies are good and some are bad?

Can a baby be bad? Of course not! Babies are not trying to coerce their parents by crying, by asking for help.

A few decades ago, it was thought that if you attended to a baby's needs every time he cried, you would spoil him. Some of that thinking remains today. Some adults are still adamant that parents should establish a routine, set a plan for control, and ignore their baby's cries until it is a more convenient time for the adults.

Parents *must* have time to care for their own basic needs of course. It only makes sense that parents who eat nutritiously; get the sleep they need (you have probably heard it said to, "sleep when the baby sleeps"); take some time to exercise and shower, get sun and fresh air and care for their spiritual needs will be happier and better parents. A lot of these things can be done with your baby nearby. While both stay-at-home parents and those who must work will probably find that a schedule for their day is extremely helpful, particularly with a new baby, let it be a flexible one. If at the end of the day it feels as if nothing has been accomplished with such a schedule, think again. Despite whatever drudgery caring for children may entail, you are doing some of the *most* important work on the face of the earth! So it is certainly critical that you keep yourself healthy.

But what parents have been told in the past is that if they cared for their baby immediately, it will lead to his being needy and manipulative. Ironically, the opposite is in fact true.

Research has shown that consistently answering a baby's requests for assistance actually helps him to become a more joyful child who is more compassionate of others and who is also more happily independent.

Not only this, throughout their lives people who have been properly attended to as infants and children will know better how to function interdependently with others in healthy relationships, and will be more apt to be resilient and successful in a variety of areas.

Crying is one of the few ways babies have to communicate their needs. Crying can mean they are hungry, wet, sick, lonely, in pain, fearful, sad, or have been startled. Perhaps all that they desperately need is some holding and reassurance. What if they've had persistent and distressing stomach pain for a week? Or a headache? What if their scalp itches terribly from having cradle cap or there is some other untold problem they cannot communicate?

Perhaps he will begin, even now, to develop the skills it will take to be a leader of a better, kinder world.

Not having the aid of verbal communication, in the form of words to express what is wrong, can be frustrating for both parents and baby. But if parents are patient and gentle, they can help to see their little one through what can be a difficult period in his life, that of being small, dependent, and helpless. If babies are responded to right away, they come to trust that their caregivers are there for them, and that there will be help available whenever there is a need.

When has a person been more in need of someone who really cares than as a baby? When, more than the helpless years of infancy and toddler-hood, does he need to be able to count on someone to be there whenever he has a need he cannot take care of by himself? What was it like for us when *we* were experiencing that vulnerable time in which we depended entirely upon others for food, water, dry clothes, warmth, or attention? What was it like to not have the words to let our caregivers know of our needs? His parents are everything to this little person.

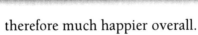

A baby has an instinctive, built-in need to be close to his parents. He *needs to be with them*, to depend on them. *No one* else can ever really take their place.

Interestingly, parents find that babies generally do not normally cry as fervently if their supplications are regularly and immediately answered. Such babies are usually more contented. They actually need to be consoled less often. Babies often learn that they do not even need to cry and that all they need to do is "ask" with particular cues that their caregiver is attuned to. They know they will be taken care of, and they are therefore much happier overall.

In contrast, babies who are generally not attended to right away often start off by crying much more intensely, because they know that they will not be taken seriously until they do. They are often then more difficult to calm.

Instinctively we want to care for a baby, especially our own baby, who is pleading for help. Trust your heart; **it is okay to let your child lead, to tell you what he needs, and to follow that lead.**

Amazing Benefits of Parents' Loving Care

Babies benefit emotionally, mentally, and physically when they receive the attached care they need. The first three years are critical. Babies' brains grow rapidly and make many neurological connections during this time. When babies are touched, soothed, and comforted, and when their needs are met, they grow to develop a stronger system of emotional health and function. Babies who are neglected are at greater risk later on in their lives for mental illness, disturbed cognitive function, brain damage, and behavioral problems. Beyond those first years, loving attention remains a crucial part of the healthy emotional, cognitive, and physical rearing of a child.

Moreover, we are learning that even *before* the baby is born, his relationships with the people around him, particularly his mother, make a significant impact on who he will become and on his future life. In fact, many women would tell you that they believe that their babies are tuned in to their thoughts. After all, there is truly a vast amount of territory in the study of human relationships, particularly that unique relationship between a woman and a baby developing within her body, that have yet to be tapped. Whether babies and mothers share a connection to this degree has not been scientifically proven at this point, but women have reported that their babies have turned from breech to a head-down position when they have simply visualized this happening. Or they have talked to or directed their thoughts to their baby concerning what was needed during birth and their babies have responded. There have also been numerous individual cases that would indicate that babies know if they are wanted. That knowledge alone can make a difference in physical development and even in the will to live and thrive.

A few decades ago, it was thought that if you attended to a baby's needs every time he cried, you would spoil him. Some of that thinking remains today.

Emotionally

Helping our children to feel safe and attached helps them to become well-adjusted, healthy children and adults. Again, it just is not possible to "spoil" a baby with "too much" love!

Parents who make themselves available, who respond when there is a need being communicated—whatever that need might be, and who offer that security and care, are helping to create securely attached children.

If a baby's verbalizations of his needs are continually ignored, he will learn to protect himself in this helpless state. He may come to understand that there is no hope and numb his feelings as well as learning other avoidance behaviors.

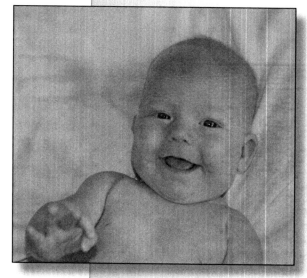

In fact, parents of adopted children who have attachment disorders have stated how much they wish their children had been able to bond with the mothers who gave them life, and how much of a difference they believe this would have made in their child's future ability to attach to others and function well in life. Those first relationships are of paramount importance.

One very important question is whether a baby should ever be left in a crib in a dark room to cry. Sadly, there are those who tell parents that letting their little ones "cry it out" in a play pen or in the next room is best. Best for whom? The baby? The parents?

Certainly, if the parent has been holding a crying baby and is becoming impatient to the point that they are thinking they might hurt the baby—then it would be best to lay the baby down in a safe place and leave for a bit until they have cooled down, are able to think clearly, and have returned again to a more compassionate state.

Otherwise, what if a parent were to throw off the conventional advice of leaving babies to cry themselves to sleep all alone by picking up their baby and rocking him for awhile, or bringing him to their warm bed for some nursing while they themselves get a little sleep too? Has it ever hurt a person to be held, to have someone there for them in a time of need?

Unfortunately, a great many parents do not truly understand their own early childhood experiences or their emotions concerning them. They may realize that some of what they experienced was not as positive and nurturing as it could have been and this can be saddening. They may feel guilty about some of the ways they have parented their children before they understood about the importance of such loving attention. Generations of parenting that was not very positive, kind, and nurturing may be in one's past. But new awareness can change the future.

Or there may be obstacles such as a parent's own physical health, unmet psychological needs, and postpartum hormonal difficulties that keep a parent from being as able to care for their child the way they would like.

Indeed, there may be some challenges to building this kind of relationship with our own children. But how vital it is to learn how to make it possible! Simply, we need to do the best we are able to—which may be more than you think possible.

Cognitively

In the last couple of decades, much has been learned about the human brain that we never before knew. We know a great deal more now, about how important early relationships and experience are in one's life. It has been found that when parents are positive and nurturing, that the

---

Some adults are still adamant that parents should establish a routine, set a plan for control, and ignore their baby's cries until it is a more convenient time for the adults.

systems of the child's brain that support attachment, regulate emotions, and help one to solve problems are all enhanced, as is growth of the brain.

Much of the way a baby's brain learns to manage stress is through positive, nurturing experiences. When a baby has a close relationship with his mother and when she responds when he needs her, he is easily calmed. But when a baby is purposely left to cry, his stress is amplified and he learns that his caregivers cannot be relied on for help and that he is alone. This is an unconscious belief he may take with him throughout his life, and it can leave him vulnerable to a lifetime of dysfunctional relationships.

It is also critical to understand that stress hormones are protective and meant to only be used for short amounts of time for surviving danger. It is damaging to the body to experience this state for an extended period, and health can actually be seriously compromised. It is a disheartening fact that, during a time when babies are learning about their world and growing cognitively in a safe environment, many must also learn to survive trauma.

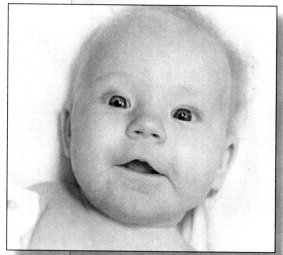

Modern society has suggested for much too long that caring for the family and home are insignificant, trivial tasks. On the contrary, all of those responsibilities of parenthood: the diaper changing, feeding, bathing, and rocking that sometimes make one look around and think they've gotten nothing accomplished, are actually central to the best brain building one can provide for their child. While scientists have been studying how to make smarter babies, mothers who have been carrying out the everyday jobs of mothering have been accomplishing just what has been needed all along. Eye-to-eye contact, skin-to-skin contact, holding, touch, interaction, warmth, love, play, comfort, and sensitive care—these are all foundational elements of brain development. They are the soil, moisture, sunshine, and minerals, so to speak, that are at the very center of what children need. **Flashcards and expensive toys are no match for your mothering and fathering—for lots and lots of loving interaction with your child, and for following what you know is best for your baby despite what you read or what others say.**

Physically

You will probably notice that if you set your baby down, he will soon cry to be picked up and held. He isn't trying to manipulate you or make you feel guilty. He is doing what babies do instinctively. He aches to be held and be close to you. It's simply how he was made. It makes further sense that he needs to be cradled next to his mother or father, when

While scientists have been studying how to make smarter babies, mothers who have been carrying out the everyday jobs of mothering have been accomplishing just what has been needed all along.

considering that he has been cradled for the first nine months of his life within his mother's womb. He does not suddenly give up his need for this closeness as he emerges into the outer world. It is still part of the nurturing necessary for his optimal emotional, cognitive, and physical development. Scientist still cannot fully explain why babies need to develop within the uterus for those initial months for basic development.

But they do, and for proper development a baby's need to be with his parents continues after he is born. Babies and children who have been unloved and uncared for, have actually been known to fail to thrive and even die.

Even adults who are in loving, caring marriages are healthier physically, mentally, and emotionally. It can take a great toll particularly on an elderly spouse when the other dies.

We need one another, and babies and children are by no means an exception.

Attachment Parenting is not really a new idea. It's quite ancient, in fact, and is about gentle parenting, bonding with and being there for your children on a "day in and day out" basis, and caring for them in a very personal way. There are not really set things parents must do to form close, caring relationships with their children. But there are many wonderful ways to be an attentive, loving parent.

The following are some tried and true practices that have been time-tested by parents throughout history—though culturally, Americans have abandoned many of them. For ages, these have been—and remain in many cultures around the world—the way parents have brought their children up and introduced the world to them.

Every family, parent, child, relationship, scenario, period in that family's life, etc, is unique. You are encouraged to try these things and take the best from other resources available to you too. Use your Inner Guide to implement what works; put aside what doesn't.

But remember that what may not be successful with one child, may be just the thing for another, or may be what is needed at a future time.

Start by learning your baby's preferences. What is important to him? Do you know what your baby needs even before others do, just by a look in his eye or his tone of voice? Do you understand his cues? These can only be learned well by consistent care and a loving, attentive, and attached relationship.

Tips to Assist Attachment

Here are a few simple things you can do to help with attachment: baby-wearing, breastfeeding, prompt nighttime comforting, and gentle effective discipling.

Babywearing, the practice of carrying your baby close in a sling or carrier throughout your day, is very comforting and bonding for both parents and baby. Though not widely used in our western culture, baby-wearing has been practiced around the world for ages.

Your baby naturally wants, even *needs,* to be a part of your environment. In fact, being with him and nurturing him is a crucial part of his every day education. Experts believe that a baby's brain soaks up information from everything around him. What happens then, if he is not picked up and his needs are not met? What impact does this have on his intellect and who he will become?

In the United States, we put our babies in seats to carry them, swings to rock them, and strollers to get them around. We purchase a plethora of other contraptions from cribs and play pens to plastic infant seat carriers and nursery accessories with which to welcome their arrival. Ironically, our babies couldn't care less about all these gadgets. They desire only to be held and cared for. They care little about what color the nursery is. What they do care about is a full tummy, the tenderness of their parents' arms around them, and gentle, soothing voices speaking to them.

How much better invested is money put into a comfortable wrap or sling for wearing of the baby, quality childbirth and breastfeeding classes, quality childbirth and baby care books, and having a doula at his birth. These things that usually do not cost a great deal, can make a real, defined, and wonderful difference in the kind of welcome that our children will experience as they enter and begin to learn about this world!

An added benefit of wearing your baby when in public is that people are less-inclined to touch, allowing her better protection from germs. And if your carrier allows, she can easily nurse inside it unnoticed, even when you are engaged in daily activities. Babywearing can be used by both Mom and Dad.

Breastfeeding, of course, naturally facilitates a close relationship. For a good, working breastfeeding relationship, mothers must be in tune to babies' cues that he is hungry or in need of closeness. A mother is more likely to develop ways for herself and her baby to stay in close contact with one another both day and night, because nursing babies need their mothers around the clock—interesting the way the plan works, isn't it? As a mother does this, the baby learns the security of always being sensitively nurtured and responded to, and at the same time helps the mother to establish an adequate milk supply. Eventually, the need for nutrition decreases, but the bond remains.

If babies are responded to right away, they come to trust that their caregivers are there for them, and that there will be help available whenever there is a need.

Prompt nighttime care is a vital need of an infant, as we've just discussed. Babies are not supposed to sleep for long periods of time. They need comforting care during the night. They do not understand if they are not responded to when there is a need.

The Harvard University Gazette published the results of a study conducted by Michael L. Commons and Patrice M. Miller, researchers at the Medical School's Department of Psychology. Commons and Miller found that the prevalent custom in the United States of putting babies to sleep in separate beds and rooms and not acting quickly to comfort them could actually lead to post-traumatic stress and panic disorders in adulthood. They stressed that parents need to know that leaving their babies to cry can have permanent consequences, such as being overly sensitive to future trauma. Those who teach parents that children might grow up to be too dependent if their needs are attended to immediately are on the wrong track, they say. Conversely, touch and reassurance will actually help children to be more secure and able to form better relationships.

Parents around the world share sleep with their babies and toddlers. Researchers have stressed how important it is to comfort a child in need of it. If children grow up feeling secure, they say, they will be more comfortable taking positive risks when they grow up. The pain a baby feels when left alone to cry is undoubtedly consequential. Beware of programs that tell parents to let their babies cry themselves to sleep. Commons reminds us that "punishment and abandonment has never been a good way to get warm, caring, independent people." (Powell)

Gentle Discipline is also an important part of Attachment Parenting. Kind, effective discipline, based on loving and respectful principles, is a key element in our relationship with our children.

In *The Baby Book*, William and Martha Sears discuss the above principles of Attachment Parenting in more detail, and other sound, loving, and gentle ways of parenting and nurturing babies and children as well as how to have a more comfortable, gentle birth, making love after the baby is born, potty training, soothing a baby, and how to swaddle (wrapping your baby securely to create a womb-like feeling which can be very comforting). This and other of the Sears' parenting books are a great addition to your library of childcare books.

Mothering.com is also an excellent resource of information on the subjects of considerate and nurturing parenting.

There are a growing number of resources about Attachment Parenting, including many on the Internet.

Raising Your Children Yourself

A Mission of Boundless Value

A large number of mothers are acknowledging that they really can't do it all, *at least not all at the same time.*

They are expressing that they do not want to miss the short and precious time of their children's growing up years.

Although dual-income households are in the majority today, a number of daring young mothers are looking back at the madness of the last decades. They are choosing to once again be the keepers of the hearth.

Their work is incalculable. Ultimately, those who rock the cradle nurture those who will "rule the world" by and by. They profoundly influence the values of the leaders of tomorrow.

What is "personal fulfillment" worth if a woman's children and spouse are neglected and if she fails as a mother and a wife? As David O. McKay declared, "No other success can compensate for failure in the home."

Our children know when other priorities come before them. Even babies know it. They are not fooled by the theory of "quality vs. quantity time." They want, and they need, both quality and quantity.

A question worth contemplating: If you personally were a child again, by whom would you rather be cared for—a nanny; a daycare worker; a boarding school teacher; or a loving, attentive, nurturing mother (and/or dad)?

Experts believe that superior mental development and future problem-solving skills can be traced to a child's loving interaction with his parents in the first years of life. These experiences impact a child so much more than brain-stimulating learning exercises some parents strive to provide their young children. If truth be told, simply being there on a daily basis is worth more than all the educational toys and the special schools and teachers we are working so hard to pay for.

In general *no one* can provide for a child's needs better than a loving, conscientious parent, no matter how much of an education that parent may have.

> *Those who rock the cradle, nurture those who will rule the world by and by.*

Is Staying Home a Real Possibility?

Certainly there are circumstances that demand that you work or your children don't eat. If your desires to personally raise your children are a possibility, what better way can parents show their love to their children than to see them through their growing-up years?

Mothers and fathers who decide to stay at home sometimes find that it isn't the easy thing to do and that there are sacrifices to be made for this privilege.

Perhaps it will mean that you will raise your children in a small house on chili from the crock pot and vegetables from your own garden. You might even need to move out of a more expensive housing area. Worthwhile things aren't always easy.

On the other hand, you may also be surprised at how difficult it is to leave your baby in someone else's care. These instinctive feelings are natural and shouldn't be disregarded.

When both husband and wife work there is usually more family income to show for a given year. However, much of this is eaten up by such things as child care, a second car, extra wardrobe items, more convenience foods, etc. It may be wise to step back and recalculate a bit!

Another thing to consider is the impact on the family that is had when both the mother and father work outside of the home. Families with dual incomes frequently experience less time for sleep, leisure, family togetherness, and household care. What is quality of life being exchanged for? Could less possessions really be *more* sometimes?

Some families have even arranged it so that both parents can be at home so that care of the children is shared. In times that were more agrarian, both parents were at home on the family farm and were able to work alongside their children, instilling in them good quality values. Having two work-at-home parents would be a beneficial situation for some families today.

Must you forget about having fun or taking on worthwhile projects if you have chosen to stay home to raise your children? Of course not; many at-home parents take a night class, meet with a group with similar interests once a month or more often, or find ways to give service to others in their churches, neighborhoods, communities, or otherwise. They might get together with other like-minded friends online. Continue to date one another as a married couple. But be careful, of course, not to let these *good* things take time away from the *best* things, those that you really want to make your main focus.

There are many excellent places, including books and the Internet, to find more information about how to make it possible and affordable to raise your own children and to do it well. (See Resources in **Appendix E**.)

Cloth vs. Disposable Diapers

Cloth diapers are becoming quite popular among many parents today. One need only search online to see how the dramatically the options available to cloth-diapering parents have grown.

Environment

Thousands of tons of plastic and millions of tons of wood pulp are used to make disposable diapers every year.

Cloth diapers use less than 50–70 gallons of water every three days to wash; about the same as a toilet-trained child or adult flushing 5–6 times a day.

The impact on landfills—8,000 disposable diapers per child, over an average diapering period, compared to a few dozen cotton diapers. An estimated eighteen billion disposables are thrown into landfills a year, taking as many as 500 years to decompose.

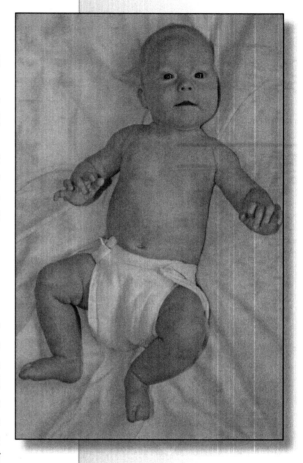

Convenience

Disposables win on convenience, although you'd be surprised at how easy cloth diapers really are. What is a couple more loads of laundry a week? Just as laundering takes a little time so does buying disposables, loading them in and out of the car, and hauling them out to the garbage. Some parents choose cloth for most of the time and disposables for outings or trips away. Others simply bring an airtight container along and take the diapers home with the rest of their laundry. This works well when camping, and leaves less trash in campsite barrels. Once you are used to the routine, cloth is not really a lot of extra worry at all.

Most cloth diapers do not need to be rinsed in the toilet. You can scrape soiled diapers off into the toilet, squirt with BacOut (a natural stain and odor remover), then put them right into the bucket. When the bucket is full, wash the load first in cold water to prevent staining, and then in hot. Avoid bleach and fabric softener! If you still get stains, try putting diapers out into the sun for safer bleaching action. You can experiment a little to see what works for you. If you plan right, cloth diapering is even possible if you use a laundromat.

Making sure your baby is changed often is crucial for preventing diaper rash. Either way, whether wearing cloth or disposable, a baby shouldn't have to sit in a dirty diaper.

However, for night sleep only, it is just fine to double or triple diaper; changing only if messy, thus avoiding the all-too-common nightly circus act that has put dark circles under the eyes of far too many new parents.

Diaper covers can often be used several times in a row before they really need washing.

Some parents report that their babies actually experienced fewer diaper rashes when cloth diapers were used. Other babies with sensitive skin may require cloth diapers that are better at wicking away moisture than are the less expensive tri-fold diapers found at large discount department stores. There are many companies easily found on the Internet that carry a myriad of choices in diapers.

Even if you decide to use disposables, you might want to keep some cloth diapers on hand in case you run out at an awkward time or you are waiting for pay day. However, switching back and forth from cloth to disposables may lead to diaper rash. Most day care centers require disposable diaper use while children are in their care.

Safety

Cloth breathes to let out ammonia.

There are toxic chemicals present in disposables. Also part of disposables is a substance called sodium polyacrylate, which was removed from tampons because of its link to toxic shock syndrome. No tests have been done on the effect of wearing disposable diapers twenty-four hours a day for two years.

Expense

Disposable diapers may cost around twenty-five cents each.

Cloth is approximately five cents a change. Using cloth can save you as much as $1,500.

Using a diaper service could cost approximately twenty cents a change. There is a wonderful array of cloth diaper designs on the market with assorted advantages worth researching.

Potty Training

Training may occur earlier with children that have been cloth diapered because they are more aware of being wet.

Getting Started with Cloth

Here's what you need to get started using cloth diapers:

- Three to five dozen cloth diapers—or—five dozen all-in-ones (covers and diapers as one)
- Five diaper covers per diaper size
- Diaper pail (A large, empty, airtight laundry detergent bucket with a tight lid works well.)
- Pins or clips (unless using pin-less diapers) See www.snappibaby.com.
- Two to three dozen washcloths. (You can keep a few wet cloths in a Ziploc bag at a time, tossing soiled ones in the diaper bucket.) Some parents make their own baby wipes or buy commercials ones. Using cloth works fine. If you wash the cloth washcloths with your diapers, make sure the cloths are colorfast.

Check out all the resources on the Internet!

Anti-Frustration Tips

There are times during parenting that can indeed be frustrating. Here are a few things you can do when things get hairy, so that you aren't tempted to take out your anger or frustration on your child.

- Stop, pace ten steps in the other direction (leave the room if necessary), and return when you are calm and rational.
- Plug your ears, close your eyes, and count to ten in another language.
- Call a friend.
- Flip through a photo album.
- Take them outside to play.
- Play uplifting music to change the mood around the house.
- Put the child in the bath, playpen, or yard with some toys and sit nearby with a good book you haven't had time for.
- Pull a stool up to the kitchen sink, fill with warm soapy water and some plastic pour toys (keep towels underfoot), and let them play while you work nearby. Never mind if a little water gets poured out on the floor. It can be wiped up. This activity gives you a break and water helps to calm the child.
- Write down your frustrated feelings.
- Take a bath or shower.
- Lighten up! Change your attitude and the situation.

Blow bubbles. Laugh!

- If your child really has tried but can't get to sleep, and your frustration is growing, would it really make things worse to just make up nachos and watch a movie for awhile with your child?
- Have a good cry, dry your tears, and try again.
- Remember, "This too shall pass." They won't be kids (or even in this stage) forever!
- Surprise them with a small gift.
- Don't forget your sense of humor! Surprise them by laughing and making a joke about it.
- Pray!
- Take little ones for a walk in the stroller.
- Blow bubbles with your kids—out of a bottle or with bubble gum.
- Read your children a story.
- Go brush your teeth.
- Spray on your favorite cologne or essential oil.
- Say "yes!" to your children as often as possible.
- If you've done something wrong, set the example by apologizing. Parenting isn't an easy job, but the longer you keep practicing more positive reactions, the easier it becomes!
- Take a parenting class. Along with good tips and advice, you'll learn you aren't alone.
- Order out or have sandwiches on those particularly stressful days.
- Fill a vase with fresh flowers. Cheery dandelions will do!
- Get enough sleep! Easier said than done some days, but the better perspective on life that a good night's sleep or nap can give is well worth the effort.
- Get a baby-sitter sometimes. Go out on a weekly date with your spouse. This benefits the whole family.
- Have a girls/guys night out now and then.
- Ignore others' negative comments and just do your best.
- Do something for someone else, and involve the kids.
- If you're afraid of really losing control, call someone who can help. Your child deserves the best you can give.
- Enrich your own life. Take time to learn new things and try something new. Take advantage of opportunities all around you.
- Build forts of blankets with your kids.
- If you can, change the pace a little by getting away, going camping, visiting grandparents, or staying at a motel for the weekend.
- Keep plugging away!
- What are other things that have worked for you that have made it a great day with your children?

Infant Massage

One of the first ways that we are able to communicate our love to our babies, in a language that they can understand, is through touch. So important is the stimulation of touch on a baby's skin, and the affection that accompanies it, that failure to thrive and even death may accompany the neglect of this universal need.

Infant massage is a wonderful way to love your child. As well, it may benefit your baby by improving his circulation, helping him to relax, to gain weight, to thrive, to release gas, and even strengthen his immune system. Just imagine what it can also do for premature infants and those with extra-special needs!

Finding a good infant massage book shouldn't be difficult. Better yet, set up a session with a professional massage therapist that can teach you to skillfully massage your baby using helpful motions and techniques. Perhaps you and a group of other parents and caregivers could get together with a massage therapist who is willing to show you a few things for free (or for a small fee that could be split between the group).

Simple touch allows for the expression of connection, warmth, sympathy, and love. It nurtures the bond of trust between parent and child. Lessons are learned that children carry with them, even throughout their lives.

Infant massage is a wonderful way to love your child.

Signing with Your Baby

You can communicate easier with your baby before he learns to talk if you and your little one have learned a few signs. Signing has actually been shown to help some children talk sooner. Here are a few tips to help you get started:

- Parents might begin by introducing just a few signs such as "more," "milk," "drink," "eat," "cat," "pain," or "diaper change" (signed "toilet"), in their daily interaction with their child.
- You may want to try signing with your child as early as the seventh month, though he may not produce a sign until he is eight or nine months or older.
- Sign while saying the word.
- Use repetition of signs often.
- Keep it fun!

Signing with your child is one among numerous gifts you can choose from to bless his life.

Check out these resources:

- *Baby Signs* by Linda Acredolo and Susan Goodwyn (based mostly on symbols)
- *Sign with Your Baby* by Joseph Garcia, a video and quick reference guide, (1-877-744-6263) www.sign2me.com
- *The Joy of Signing* by Lottie L. Riekehof (American Sign Language principles and signs)

Car Seats

Many people have been saved by wearing seat belts, and too many injured or killed from not. If you love your family, make sure they and you are buckled up *every* time.

Neither can the importance of the *correct installation and use* of your baby's car seat be stressed enough.

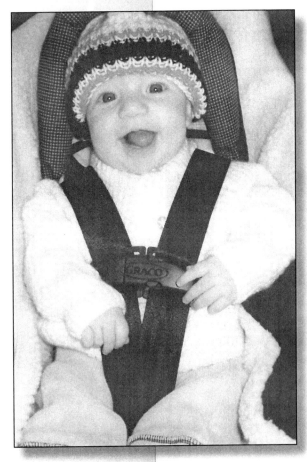

It's a really good idea to make it a family rule that the vehicle doesn't start until everyone is buckled up and children are in their car seats.

When your child graduates from the car seat, he is not yet old or big enough for a regular seat belt! Until he is, he needs to be in a booster seat.

Check on height and age regulations to be sure your child is properly restrained. These simple measures save children's lives!

A

The "What If?" Game: Test Your Birth Savvy

NO TWO FAMILIES are exactly alike, nor are two births exactly the same, even for the same woman. That is why there is not just one answer that fits every scenario. Weigh your decisions carefully. What is right for you? First, study it out. Search within yourself and seek inspiration through meditation. Have the courage to listen to and follow what you know is right.

What would you do in the following circumstances? For quick answers to these following common situations, refer to the listed sections. *Take the time to write down what you would do in the following circumstances, and why.*

Having your own list to refer back to, could be invaluable in helping you know what you would do and what choices you would make in these circumstances.

Dads and birth partners, if any of the following occurs during labor, the mother will likely not be up to fighting any battles right then. She may even be much more willing to accept things others suggest (even things she was formerly adamant she did not want). Will you be willing and able to stand up for her? The following test can be a good way to help both of you to examine as a couple how birth savvy you really are. Are you as prepared as you think?

Unfortunately, most of the following scenarios are not atypical.

Following each scenario, are places in the book that you can turn to for more information.

1. You are a week past your baby's estimated due date. At your prenatal visit today, your caregiver said she would like to induce labor soon. What do you do?

2. You have wanted to avoid pain medication in labor. The nurse shakes her head and says, "You're crazy." Whenever she comes into the room she says, "Are you ready for the epidural yet?" What do you do?

3. You have spoken with your doctor about laboring in water even if your water has released, and he is fine with it. The nurse, however, insists that it is the rule in the hospital that no one is allowed to labor in the water after their water has released.

4. In labor, you are dealing with intense back pressure. What can you do?

5. You return from walking in the halls and your nurse tells you it is time to get into bed so that she can monitor the baby. You remind her that you wanted to be monitored by the fetoscope. She says she has a hearing problem and cannot hear the heartbeat through the fetoscope, and the EFM would be much easier for her.

6. Your wife wanted to avoid an episiotomy, but the doctor is picking up the scissors, and is ready to cut.

7. Since getting to the hospital, your labor has slowed. Your care provider says she thinks it is possible that you may be dehydrated and that this is causing the slowing. She says she thinks an IV would be a good idea. She also thinks it would be good to rupture your membranes, although you wanted to avoid both of these. What do you do?

8. You wanted to try squatting as your position for the actual birth. You are fully dilated and the staff begins breaking down the bed and getting your feet into the stirrups. The doctor comes in, and you remind her of your original plans. She says it really would be inconvenient for her to have to get down on the floor to "deliver" the baby.

9. You wanted to be allowed to wait for the placenta to deliver spontaneously. Your caregiver has a meeting to get to, though, and begins to pull on the cord to get the placenta out. What do you do?

10. On the third day after birth, your baby is looking a bit yellow. Your caregiver suggests using a bilirubin light. Your baby's bilirubin counts are really not very high.

11. You had not planned on a homebirth and do not have a midwife. Your wife has gone into labor a week earlier than expected. She is has been hurrying around between contractions to get things together to leave for the hospital. Suddenly she calls out from the bathroom that she has to push and that the baby is actually, "coming out!"

12. Once he is born you wonder if you are producing enough milk for your baby.

13. At your 32 week prenatal appointment, you caregiver informs you that your baby is breech and that you'd better prepare for a cesarean.

14. Your nipples are starting to crack a little, just days after beginning to breastfeed. Who can you call to ask breastfeeding questions?

15. Dad, in labor, your wife loses her confidence that she can go without medication. Birthing without medication is something she has really wanted. What do you do?

16. A few weeks after the birth, you find that you feel sad a lot. You cry often and realize that you have a lot of negative feelings about yourself. What do you do?

17. You are fully dilated. It seems everyone in the room is yelling for you to "push!" Everything is progressing normally. There are no indications that the baby needs to be born quickly. Now what?

B

What Should Quality Childbirth Classes Offer?

WITH SO MANY different options for childbirth classes out there, which one should you choose?

This is a fun little quiz to use to see how the classes you have been considering actually rate. First, we dare you to test your own knowledge of what classes should provide! Good luck!

True or False Quiz

Questions

Childbirth classes should . . .

1. Tell you all you need to know to have the perfect experience.

2. Present information about how to have a healthier and more comfortable birth experience.

3. Teach you how to breathe.

4. Give you a vision of what the experience of birth can be.

5. Offer tips on how to birth within the birthing system you choose.

6. Allow you the opportunity to get to know others in the class.

7. Be fun.

8. Have you memorize terms.

9. Give you the knowledge of how to birth your baby.

10. Offer useful information about how to avoid medications if this is your choice.

11. Give you information and help you to prepare to make decisions beforehand, so that you will have the freedom to birth peacefully.

12. Be consumer-oriented.

Answers

1. **Tell you all you need to know to have the perfect experience.** False

   But your class should teach you how to have the best experience possible. Birth, just like most all other aspects of life, is unpredictable. It can't be planned. What you can do is become educated about the options and their pros and cons. You can learn how to make as gentle and safe a welcome for your baby as you possibly can.

2. **Present information about how to have a healthier and more comfortable birth experience.** True

   Certainly! In fact, you may find that after taking excellent classes that teach you about a variety of options for your birth, that you will decide to explore other kinds of classes, a hypnosis for birth class for example, or a breastfeeding class. There will probably be books and other resources on subjects you will want to study more about.

3. **Teach you how to breathe.** True and False

   What have you heard your friends say about the breathing techniques they learned in their classes? Were they able to totally get through with learned, patterned breathing? How many women have you heard say that they became frustrated with their husbands for counting wrong, and so on? These patterned breathing techniques take a woman out of her laboring mind, making her less able to work with what is going on within her body. Ironically, even though learning breathing techniques is one of the main things that couples expect from classes today, most classes that teach patterned-breathing don't have high rates of women that end up going without pain medication during their births. Of course, in other situations involving pain, these breathing techniques can be helpful because they are distractive. In labor, though, a woman needs to be able to naturally go within as instinct directs, to meet the sensations and work with them. This makes labor so much easier. Simple deep abdominal breathing can be extremely helpful to a woman who wishes to be able to relax and go to that "inner place." Deep abdominal and slow breathing are natural and help a woman to relax and allow her body to do what it was made to do. Classes that help you to prepare with deep abdominal breathing are teaching a worthwhile skill to prepare for labor. Regularly practicing this technique prior to labor can help you to find your way to that place within yourself in labor, where you can welcome the experience of labor.

4. **Give you a vision of what the experience of birth can be.** True

   As you attend your class, your vision of birth should come to include the spiritual and emotional aspects of birth and not just the physical. A woman's body takes care of the physical aspects of the process without any need for knowledge about it on her part. The spiritual and emotional elements of birth are misunderstood and largely dismissed in our culture's way of birthing. Women are taught to believe that as long as their baby is okay, that this is all that matters. Many women feel that their births were *at the least* what they would call unpleasant experiences. They are forgiving of pain and humiliation, believing that this is the price that must be paid for bearing children. Families need to know that under normal circumstances, they and their baby really can have a dignified, safe, and wonderful experience in which all of the elements of birth, including the spiritual and emotional ones are considered as important as the physical ones. Taking the same classes everyone else is taking will most likely get you the same kind of birth everyone else is getting.

5. **Offer tips on how to birth within the birthing system you choose.** True

Many classes do not deal with this subject at all. This is one of the most important reasons for taking classes. Families need to know about the current practices and procedures being performed, and their risks and benefits, so that they can make the decisions that are best for themselves. Some educators and caregivers don't want to scare you, so they do not give you all of the facts about every option. They may be educators for, or be affiliated with, a certain birth place that performs interventions routinely, so their classes may not necessarily be consumer-oriented. This is your body and your baby. You have the right to know the facts about what happens in various places of birth. You should be able to make decisions that are right for you and your baby, and say no to those that are not right.

6. **Allow you the opportunity to get to know others in the class.** True

Sharing the experience of preparing for your birth and new little one with others who are also preparing, can be a very beneficial and rewarding feature of a class for some. Many classes, especially ones that are large, do not give ample opportunity for this kind of interaction. Small classes that offer opportunities to learn together may even provide long-lasting relationships with others going through the same life experiences. To benefit, being willing to be friendly and reach out is important. Other women/couples would prefer to take a class, perhaps online, in the comfort of their very own home. It would be wise to research your options to find the type of class that is best for you.

7. **Be fun.** True

You bet!

8. **Have you memorize terms.** False

It isn't as if you have to pass a test to give birth and have the best experience possible. But it is good to have a basic knowledge *beforehand* of the different options and whether you would choose them or not. Studying this book and writing birth wishes as you go along, can help you to do this in an easy, efficient way.

9. **Give you the knowledge of how to birth your baby.** False

Your body knows instinctively how to have a baby. Women's bodies were made to give birth! You don't need anyone to teach you how to have your baby. As well, women do not routinely need anyone to take their babies out of them or "deliver" them. If you were in a cabin in the woods in a snowstorm that blocked you from getting out when you went into labor, chances are you would have your baby without any real problems. The knowledge is within your body!

10. **Offer useful information about how to avoid medications, if this is your choice.** True

Because teaching people how to birth without pain medication was an important part of childbirth classes when they first began, many people still believe that childbirth classes today are still about how to have your baby without medication. This is not the goal of numerous classes today, particularly those given by a hospital. Teachers of some classes assume that almost all women want epidurals, and so they spend less time on comfort techniques and more time on subjects such as when and how they will receive medication. One of the main roles of this particular type of class is to educate parents about what to expect at the hospital, how their birth will be managed, and what they can do to act in accordance with the requirements of the hospital. Seek out classes that have been helpful to people who have had the kind of birth you would hope to have.

11. **Give you information and help you to prepare to make decisions beforehand so that you will have the freedom to birth peacefully.** True

    Being given the opportunity to study about your different options can empower you to choose the kind of care you need. When preparations are in place, ideally you will be able to let go and safely birth in awareness and peace.

12. **Be consumer-oriented.** True

    This is one of the most important things good classes can offer you. Teachers that are working for, and are affiliated with, specific birth places or caregivers may not be allowed, or may be afraid, to give all of the facts—including all of the risks, alongside the benefits—of certain common procedures of that particular birth place.

    Good classes will give you the facts such as those you find here, or will point you in the direction of where to find them. As appalling as it might sound, you must know that some classes are designed not with families' best interests in mind, but to teach consumers for the benefit of the facility. Too many families are coming to their births unprepared, uneducated about their opportunities and choices, and less than informed about the decisions they will soon have to make.

Birth Wish Lists

THESE EXAMPLES of birth wishes might give you an idea of a format you could follow. Or you may wish to be less formal. Caregivers often will not necessarily remember all of the things each family discusses with them prior to labor. If your caregiver is really interested in helping you to achieve your wishes, it will probably be very valuable for you and the caregiver both, to have a list of reminders about what is important to you. Birth wishes that are no longer than a page are a good idea. If your plan is very long, it is probably because you are asking for a lot of things that are not normally offered in the place you are thinking of giving birth. In that case, you might ask whether you are really in your ideal place of birth.

These four example birth wishes are all labeled according to those for whom they are written.

Hospital Birth Wishes

Dear Nursing Staff,

We are looking forward to a quiet, serene birth with as few interventions as possible. As the moments surrounding the birth of our baby will remain with us always, we have given the details much study and thought. We hope that a nurse who is knowledgeable about natural birth will be assigned to our care. We are grateful for your caring assistance as we welcome our precious baby.

Thank you so much!

Special Circumstances

Mary is allergic to:

_____

Other:

_____

_____

Atmosphere

- Quiet, privacy, low lighting, freedom to move around room and L&D floor, and freedom to use sounding as wished

Comfort Measures

- Please don't mention pain medication—let us ask. Thanks!
- Shower and Jacuzzi after 5 centimeters (even if bag of waters has released)
- Thank you for not disturbing Mary during contractions. Instead, please talk with husband or doula who can then confer with mother.
- Caring assistance from our doula, Noel Karaboutte

Monitoring

- By use of Fetoscope or Doppler in positions chosen by Mary, instead of EFM or internal monitor (Our doctor has approved this and we have signed a release.)

IV

- We wish not to use an IV or heparin lock unless for use with medication.

Cervical Exams

- Minimal exams please

For Actual Birth

- Use of the birth stool and other positions as chosen by mother at the time, with floor covered by Chux pads, (bed, etc. moved back as far as possible)
- Low lighting, warmth, quiet

- Mary wishes to have the freedom to breathe the baby down to crowning as we learned to do in our childbirth classes; no coaching please.
- We wish to avoid an episiotomy, and prefer physical support of the perineum to allow it to stretch and to tear as little as possible.
- Delayed cord clamping until placenta has delivered, father to cut the cord

Welcoming Baby

- We wish that our baby be allowed to cough and expel his own mucous, with suctioning only if baby is having trouble getting started.
- Baby has immediate skin-to-skin contact on mother's chest, covered with a blanket, still attached to the cord, with freedom to breastfeed right away.
- We wish to delay our baby's bath, and would request that weighing and observation of the baby be done at the bedside rather than in the nursery. Along with the nursery staff, we will watch our baby closely and keep him warm skin-to-skin and with blankets.
- We are looking forward to bonding together during the first hour after birth as a family.
- We plan to room-in and then return home within twenty-four hours.

Placenta Delivery

- Spontaneous, with no traction on cord if delayed, freedom to stand and move around and to breastfeed
- Mary assisted onto bed after delivery of placenta, and once again given baby to hold
- Other

If Labor Has Slowed

- We wish bag of waters to be left intact until they release spontaneously, no AROM or Pitocin augmentation please. We plan to use walking, rest, privacy, etc.

Cesarean

- Please only partial shave
- Use of epidural
- Screen lowered so mother can see baby's birth
- Baby handed right up on mother's chest if baby is doing well, or as soon after birth as possible
- Free hands to hold the baby, oxygen mask removed so mother can talk to baby
- As many of the requests from Welcoming Baby as possible (Please refer to our wishes listed in that section, above.)

Death of Baby

- See and hold baby as long and as often as desired.
- We wish to have an autopsy performed.
- Recovery for mother in a separate place from regular postpartum area and early discharge
- We wish spiritual and grief counseling and contact from a support group.

I have read and approved the requests of Mr. and Mrs. Whitman on the above pages.

Caregiver's signature _____

Nursery Staff

We very much appreciate your assistance during the birth and immediate care period after our baby's birth. We have heard wonderful things about the nursery at Pine City Regional. The following are our desires for welcoming our child. Thank you for the gentle care of our baby!

Welcoming Baby

- Baby has immediate skin-to-skin contact on mother's chest, covered with a blanket, still attached to the cord, with freedom to breastfeed right away.
- We wish to delay our baby's bath, and would appreciate it if weighing and observation of the baby could be done at the bedside rather than in the nursery.
- We are looking forward to bonding together during the first hour after birth as a family.
- After that hour, the father will go with baby to the nursery.
- We plan to return home within twenty-four hours.

Procedures

- We want to avoid deep suctioning down the windpipe unless there is an emergency.
- We do not wish our baby to receive Vitamin K (unless there has been injury that would warrant its use), eye ointment, the PKU, or a Hepatitis B shot.
- We also will not be circumcising our baby.
- We wish our baby to receive breast milk only and no bottles or pacifiers.

Other

In the case of an unforeseen problem:
- It is important to us that the father is able to remain with baby during as many procedures as possible.
- If transport to another hospital is necessary, parents wish to accompany baby.

Death of Baby

- See and hold baby as long and as often as desired.
- Obtain a lock of hair, foot prints, if there are infant rings available, we would like one for the baby to wear to keep for a memento, wish to dress baby, and take pictures.
- We wish to have an autopsy.

Hospital Birth Wishes

(Yours and doula's copy)

Special Circumstances

Mary is allergic to:

_____

Other:

_____

_____

*Onset of Labor

- Spontaneous, no Pitocin or Cytotec unless medically warranted (and then only after tests for maturity of baby)

*Early Labor

- We will call you to let you know when we are in labor, and again when we need you to come over to our house to help.
- We want to use positioning techniques if labor starts out with irregular surges.
- Get more sleep if labor starts at night. If it is day-time make brownies for the hospital staff, go for a walk, get some rest, etc.
- We want to stay at home as long as possible (and want you to help us know when it is time.)

Atmosphere

- Quiet, calm atmosphere, *no unnecessary staff, low lighting, *music, *use of aromatherapy (lavender, peppermint, clay sage at appropriate times), *blinds closed, *low lights
- Freedom to move around room and floor, and freedom to use sounding as wished

*Clothing

- Own from home, extra changes in suitcase

*Comfort Measures

- Birth ball, massage, deep breathing, relaxation, imagery, hot and cold packs, upright positions, walking
- No mention of epidural
- Shower and Jacuzzi after 5 cm (even when bag of waters is broken)
- I am a -7 on the scale, please use encouragement and help us in every way to avoid medication. But if I am adamant, please help me to obtain medication.

Monitoring

- By use of Doppler in positions chosen by mother, no EFM or internal monitor (we're happy to sign a release)

IV

- No IV or heparin lock unless for use with medication
- For hydration, fluids will be taken orally, *please remind to use bathroom every half hour

*Nourishment

- Easily digestible food brought from home such as crackers, soup to warm in microwave, a banana, individual cups of apple sauce, juice, and red raspberry leaf tea.

Cervical Exams

- Minimal exams—*at admittance, at 5 cm for determining when to get in water (although we will hopefully be past this point before checking in), and before pushing

*Back Labor

- Hot and cold packs, positioning, stair climbing, counter pressure, belly dancing, shower, your suggestions

For Actual Birth

- Use of the birth stool/other position as chosen by mother at the time, floor covered with Chux pads, bed etc. moved back as far as possible
- Low lighting, warmth, quiet
- Mary wishes to have the freedom to breathe the baby down to crowning as we learned to do in our childbirth classes; no coaching please.
- No episiotomy please, prefer gentle perineal massage and physical support of the perineum to allow perineum to stretch and tear as little as possible.
- Delayed cord clamping until placenta has delivered, father cuts cord
- Mother announces sex of baby

Placenta Delivery

- Spontaneous, with no traction on cord—if delayed, freedom to stand and move around and to breastfeed to facilitate delivery
- Mother assisted onto bed after delivery of placenta, and once again given baby to hold

Welcoming Baby

- We would greatly appreciate it if our baby is allowed to cough and expel his own mucous, with suctioning only if baby is having trouble getting started.
- Baby has immediate skin-to-skin contact on mother's chest, covered with a blanket, still attached to the cord, with freedom to breastfeed right away.
- *Please help me to breastfeed right away.

* indicates wishes for yourselves and doula only; these would probably **not** be put on wishes given to staff

- We wish to delay our baby's bath, and would appreciate it if weighing and observation of the baby could be done at the bedside rather than in the nursery.
- We are looking forward to bonding together during the first hour after birth as a family.
- We plan to room-in and return home within twenty-four hours.

Other

_____

_____

_____

If Labor Has Slowed

- We wish bag of waters to be left intact until they rupture spontaneously, no AROM or Pitocin augmentation please.
- *Privacy to be alone, nap, walk, talk about feelings, open birth satchel, imagery, check out if necessary

Cesarean

- Please only partial shave
- Use of epidural
- Screen lowered so mother can see baby's birth
- Baby put right on mother's chest if baby is doing well, or as soon after as possible
- Free hands to hold the baby, oxygen mask removed so mother can talk to baby
- As many of the requests from Welcoming Baby as possible

Death of Baby

- See and hold baby as long and as often as desired
- We wish to have an autopsy performed.
- Recovery for mother in a separate place from regular postpartum area and early discharge
- We wish spiritual and grief counseling and contact from a support group
- Obtain a lock of hair, foot prints, if there are infant rings available, we would like one for the baby to wear and for us to keep for a memento, wish to dress baby, and take pictures

(Much of what is on the hospital wishes is not necessary to include in homebirth wishes because at home, avoiding these is the norm.)

Homebirth Birth Wishes

(for midwife and doula)

We are excited, Sherry and Kathy, to have chosen you as our midwives, and to have you, Noel, as our doula. We are so glad to have such a wonderful team. We are looking forward to a calm, serene birth experience. The following are our birth wishes. We would appreciate any wisdom you might have concerning them. We hope that you will feel comfortable in our home. Thank you so much for your loving care! Mary and Tom

Special Circumstances

Reminder: Mary is allergic to:

_____

Other:

_____

Early Labor

- We will call to let you know that we are in labor, and then when we need you to come.

Atmosphere

- Quiet, calm atmosphere, low voices, low lighting, music, use of aromatherapy (lavender, peppermint, clary sage at appropriate times), blinds closed, fire started in the fireplace, Chux pads nearby
- If anyone, even mother-in-law, comes to the door, please reassure them and tell them that we will call soon after the baby is born.

Comfort Measures

- We plan to use the birth tub as soon as Mary is at 5 cm. It will be set up by the fireplace in the den. We will leave birthing there an option.
- We look forward to using the birth ball, having our doula offer massage, assist with deep breathing, relaxation, imagery, hot and cold packs, upright positions, the use of different positions. We also may take a walk over to the park during labor.

Monitoring

- By use of Fetoscope, unless more frequent monitoring becomes necessary, then the Doppler is okay.

Nourishment

- We have easily-digestible foods on the cupboard shelf and in the refrigerator—crackers, soup to warm on the stove, bananas, apple sauce, and juice. Frequent cups of hot red raspberry tea would be great.

Cervical Exams

- Minimal exams—at 5 cm for determining when to get in water (although we will hopefully be past this point before you arrive), and only before "breathing the baby down" please

Back Labor

- Hot and cold packs, positioning, stair climbing, counter pressure, belly dancing, shower, your suggestions and help

Labor Has Slowed

- We wish bag of water to be left intact until it releases spontaneously.
- Privacy to be alone together, nap, walk, talk with Mary about feelings, open birth satchel, and use imagery.
- We may go for a walk outside.

For Actual Birth

- Either in the Aqua Doula tub or on hands and knees in own bed. We'll put the floor coverings and Chux pads from the kit you had us order both on the night stand by the bed and on the side table near the couch in the den.
- Low lighting, warmth, quiet
- Mary wishes to have the freedom to breathe the baby down to crowning as we learned to do in our childbirth classes; no coaching please.
- Physical support of the perineum and perineal massage
- Cord clamping after placenta has delivered, father cuts cord
- Mother announces sex of baby

Placenta Delivery

- Spontaneous, breastfeeding if placenta delivery is taking awhile, use of gravity if necessary

Welcoming Baby

- We would greatly appreciate it if our baby is allowed to cough and expel his own mucous, with suctioning only if baby is having trouble getting started.
- Siblings to be called from upstairs, where they will be with the baby-sitter, to see the baby (and perhaps the birth.)
- Baby has immediate skin-to-skin contact on mother's chest, covered with a blanket, still attached to the cord, with freedom to breastfeed right away.
- We wish to delay our baby's bath.
- We are looking forward to the bonding of our family after the birth. After Mary has had the chance to shower, we want to get into bed and rest. There will be fresh sheets in the closet in the hall.
- No eye ointment
- We have studied the following options in depth and have decided that we do not wish our child to receive Vitamin K, the Hepatitis B, or the PKU test.

If Transfer Becomes Necessary

- Refer to back-up hospital wishes—we understand, of course, that in an emergency not all of these wishes will probably still be possible.
- Doula will continue to accompany the mother.
- Father stays with baby at all times if possible.
- If baby needs to be transported to another hospital, parents go along.

D

Questionnaires

BEFORE HIRING A PROFESSIONAL to assist you in this most important event, you will want to find just the right individual(s). Does he/she have the same philosophies as you do? Is this the midwife/doctor that can help you to achieve your hopes and goals?

This is hard to know right off the bat. It might otherwise take a few months' worth of visits before you really begin to get a good sense of whether or not you are a good match. The sooner you can find just the right fit, the sooner you will be able to relax and move onto other things.

The following questionnaires contain samples of questions that would be worth asking. This process seems to work best when the caregiver simply fills out the page and then returns it. This allows you to then read over the answers on your own and bring up any further questions at future visits.

This way seems to work the best, as you want to be careful about seeming as if you wish to "take her on" with this questionnaire. You might let her know that you are interviewing a few different midwives/doctors to find just the right one, and perhaps that you are interviewing her because you have heard good things about her from friends.

The amount of time a doctor, in particular, can spend during a visit is limited. If you ask these questions one by one aloud it will likely take too much time and it might simply turn into a session in which it seems to you and your caregiver both, that she is being asked to defend her practices. Keep it as short and sweet as possible, but do make sure you get your answers!

Let her know how grateful you are for the time she has taken to fill out the questionnaire. Seriously re-think hiring anyone who doesn't have the time for your questions.

This is your birth and your baby, and you want the best. Follow your gut feelings about those you interview for your birth team.

Questions for Your Homebirth Caregiver

Name of midwife/doctor_____

Please take the time to fill out the following information and return this form to me at our first/next visit so that we can discuss it together. Thank you!

What are your rates of:

Episiotomy? _____ Tearing? _____

How do you avoid both?

_____

_____

_____

Infant mortality? _____ Mother mortality? _____

Transport to the hospital _____ Transport for c/sec.? _____

What is your philosophy of birth?

_____

_____

_____

Please explain your training.

_____

_____

_____

How many births have you attended? _____

Have you given birth yourself? _____ What were your births like?

_____

_____

_____

Tell me about you and your practice, and why you became a midwife.

_____

_____

Will we meet your assistant and back-up midwife? _____

What is the role of the mother, at the birth, as you see it?

_____

_____

_____

What do you see as being the father's role?

_____

_____

_____

How do you feel about VBAC?

_____

_____

_____

What would be the procedure if my labor took thirty-six hours?

_____

_____

_____

What would you do to encourage a slowed labor?

_____

_____

_____

How would you handle an emergency?

_____

_____

_____

Do you carry oxygen and drugs for hemorrhage? _____If not, what other things do you carry in their place?

_____

_____

_____

Do you have good relationships with hospital personnel so that if transfer became necessary it would be without unnecessary problems?

_____

_____

_____

How would you feel about our having a doula at our birth?

_____

_____

_____

Do you foresee a problem with attending my birth?

_____

_____

_____

How do you feel about my partner cutting the cord/receiving the baby at the time of birth if he wants to?

_____

_____

_____

Questions for Your Hospital Caregiver

Name of midwife/doctor_____

Please take the time to fill out the following information and return this form to me at our first/next visit so that we can discuss it together. Thank you!

What are your rates of:

Induction? _____

Episiotomy? _____Tearing? _____How do you avoid both?

_____

How many of your mothers have given birth without an episiotomy or any tearing?_____

What are your rates of:

Cesarean? _____Forceps? _____Vacuum Extraction? _____

Infant mortality? _____Mother mortality? _____

Women who give birth without medication? _____

Women who give birth with minimal medication? _____

What is your philosophy of birth?

_____

_____

_____

Please explain your training.

_____

_____

_____

How long have you been practicing? _____

Do you have children? _____How were they born?

_____

_____

How many births have you attended? _____

Tell me about you and your practice, and why you became a doctor.

_____

_____

_____

Do you practice solo or are you part of a group of other midwives/doctors? _____

Do you share the same philosophies with the others in the group? _____

Will we meet your assistants and/or back-up doctor? _____

How often will I see you during pregnancy? _____

If you are part of a group practice, can I choose which physician will attend me at my birth? _____

Will the others respect the agreements you and I have made? _____

Which hospitals do you have privileges at?

_____

_____

_____

Can I choose which hospital to give birth at? _____

Will you stay with me during labor? _____

What is the role of the mother, at the birth, as you see it?

_____

_____

_____

What do you see as being the father's role?

_____

_____

_____

Can he stay with me the entire time? _____

Can my older children be present during the birth? _____

Do you strip the membranes? _____Release the membranes? _____

What is the policy once my water has released?

_____

_____

_____

How soon do you like a woman to deliver? _____

Are there special guidelines from that point on?

_____

_____

_____

How long do you wait to cut the cord and allow for delivery of placenta? _____

How do you feel about my husband cutting the cord/receiving the baby at the time of birth if he wants to?

_____

_____

_____

E

Resources

Books

This is a list of excellent books that do not just tell you what to expect. They tell you why you can expect *more* from your experience and the how-to.

You are encouraged to read at least two of the following books during pregnancy.

Many of these books can be found at local libraries. Sometimes libraries have an Inter-Library Loan system with other libraries. Inquire about this as it may save you a great deal of money. Many of these may also be found at a local bookstore, or can be obtained by ordering through a bookstore or over the Internet. Your childbirth educator and/or doula may have many of these titles.

Alternative Birth, Carl Jones. Well-written and enlightening, discusses options available to birthing families that they may never have considered before.

A Wise Birth, Penny Armstrong and Sheryl Feldman. Compellingly, the author tells her own story. When she was first trained as a Certified Nurse Midwife she answered a call to assist Amish women at home. Little by little, the perspective that had become a part of her during her schooling began to shift and change. As she witnessed birth after relatively easy and uncomplicated birth, she began to wonder about the differences between these births and the births she had observed in the hospital during her training.

Birthing from Within, Pam England and Rob Horowitz. A popular book that dispels a lot of old myths. It reminds us of the importance of not overlooking the significance of the psychological components of birth that are all too often neglected. Suggestions and examples are included for wonderfully helpful self-discovery projects to assist you in really preparing, from within as well as outside of yourself, for your birth.

Birth Without Violence, Frederick Leboyer. There is still much room for improvement in the handling of newborn babies in labor and delivery units and hospital nurseries. The compelling photography and the poetic thoughts of this book are worth taking a look at, even now these many years later.

Born in the USA: How a Broken Maternity System Must Be Fixed to Put Women and Children First, Marsden Wagner, MD, MS. Wagner, who served for fifteen years as Director of Women's and Children's Health for the World Health Organization and was responsible for Women's and Children's Health in forty-five industrialized countries, contends that women today have been convinced that their bodies do not work. He discusses how a great many U.S. birth practices do not follow research.

Creating a Joyful Birth, Sandra Bardsley. A workbook designed to help you to have a less fearful, better experience.

Creating Your Birth Plan: The Definitive Guide to a Safe and Empowering Birth, Marsden Wagner, MD, MS. Excellent and user-friendly, this book can help you to create a birth plan that will assist you in working with your caregivers for a birth that is more like the one you hope for.

Gentle Birth Choices, Barbara Harper. Waterbirth, discussed by some of the top experts in the country, as well as other options for birthing families, is commendably introduced.

How to Raise a Healthy Child in Spite of Your Doctor, Mendelsohn, Robert S. M.D. Easy to read, this is one of the best books available to parents on their children's health. It discusses many child health subjects from pregnancy onward, and delivers much invaluable and common sense wisdom. Worth having in one's home library.

HypnoBirthing® The Mongan Method, Marie Mongan. HypnoBirthing®, quickly growing in popularity, challenges the common belief that pain has to be a normal part of birth. The HypnoBirthing® program has had much success helping women to have wonderful births in which, free from the fear that causes tension and pain, they are conscious and active participants.

Ina May's Guide to Childbirth, Ina May Gaskin. Author of *Spiritual Midwifery* and renowned midwife still practicing at The Farm in Tennessee, where the rates of positive outcomes far surpass those of our country's mainstream cultural norm, Ina May offers wisdom she has learned over the years. This is a powerful book comprised of birth stories as well as information that is so valuable to today's birthing woman.

In Praise of Stay-at-Home Moms, Dr. Laura Schlessinger. Offers perspective on the significance of raising your own children and how the sacrifices you make now as a SAHM can benefit not only your children, but also your marriage and family. This book provides advice and support to women as they experience the wonders and challenges of being at home with their children.

Having a Baby Naturally, Peggy O'Mara. Former long-time editor of "Mothering Magazine," Peggy shares her knowledge of what it takes to birth naturally in our society today. This book is full of wonderful insights and information about choices available to birthing families. It discusses a wide range of topics and issues including pain medication alternatives, nutrition, and health issues related to mother and baby.

Silent Knife and *Open Season*, Nancy Wainer Cohen. *Silent Knife* was a landmark book in the movement for cesarean prevention. Both books are well-researched, enjoyable to read, and very informative about many different aspects of birth, especially that of avoiding a cesarean. *Open Season* is a particularly delightful read for birth professionals.

Special Women, Perez and Snedecker. Explores compelling reasons for having a doula.

Spiritual Midwifery, Ina May Gaskin. This is the story of a large group of families, in the 60s and 70s, that traveled by caravan to Tennessee to establish a commune. Without the means to pay for assistance along the way, they began to birth their babies outside of the hospital and outside of the expected norm for American women. Ina May and other women in the group began to learn how to assist mothers in childbirth. This book is an intriguing documentation of many births that attest to the fact that birth works. The Farm, where the group eventually settled down, welcomes women even today as a place to birth. Their statistics for birth outcomes are some of the best anywhere. The Farm hosts trainings (such as on how to assist a breech baby) for birth professionals around the country. Many have benefited from her knowledge and wisdom.

The Act of Marriage, Tim and Beverly LaHaye. Tastefully discusses ways to enhance your sexual relationship, as well as teaching other ways to build a truly loving marriage. It frankly discusses such topics as sexual climax pertaining to both husband and wife.

The Baby Book, William and Martha Sears. Written by a pediatrician, highly recommended for a home library, most everything you need to know about raising a baby seems to be within these pages.

The Birth Book, William and Martha Sears. Also a highly recommended book by the same authors as above. William Sears and his wife Martha present different birth options with the pros and cons of those choices.

The Complete Book of Pregnancy and Childbirth, Sheila Kitzinger. This is one for parents who want to take an active role in their pregnancy and birth.

The Seven Standards of Ecological Breastfeeding: The Frequency Factor, Sheila Kippley. Excellent and reader-friendly enlightenment on the science behind how breastfeeding can be used as an effective form of child spacing if practiced correctly. References and books for more understanding are included.

The Thinking Woman's Guide to a Better Birth, Henci Goer. Well-researched and listing many studies and their outcomes, an intriguing discussion of birth options and common interventions, their pros and cons.

The Womanly Art of Breastfeeding, La Leche League International. Discusses how to establish breastfeeding, make sure you have ample milk supply, and position your baby to avoid sore nipples; teaches how to recognize and overcome common breastfeeding problems, how to breastfeed even if you work, how to express and store breast milk, and when and how to introduce solid foods; explains how breastfeeding helps keep your baby healthy, and how breastfeeding enhances parenting.

When Survivors Give Birth: Understanding and Healing the Effects of Early Sexual Abuse on Childbearing Women, Penny Simkin. Among a large library of groundbreaking literature written by Simkin is this book for survivors of childhood sexual abuse. The book discusses the common short and long-term effects that survivors may be dealing with. Subjects such as counseling, psychotherapy, and challenges that may occur within the caregiver-client relationship are covered in this valuable resource.

Your Baby, Your Way, Sheila Kitzinger. The author is a social anthropologist who has studied different aspects of the lives of women in different cultures. She writes about birth throughout time and how there is no right way for everyone to birth, only a right way for you.

Media

The following are just a few of the best birth education media on the market. There are many films about birth, some being better than others.

Many of the following on this list are sold to childbirth educators, so the prices may seem a bit high. To borrow some of these first, you might try getting them on Inter-Library Loan (a service which enables your library to borrow books and media from other libraries around the country).

Babies Know More Than You Think: Exploring the Consciousness and Capacity of the Unborn and New-born Child. This is a fascinating film about how babies know, feel, and remember much more than we imagine. Were you aware that the thoughts and feelings of both parents affect the unborn baby? How does this critical period affect your baby's development and his life now and beyond? This is a great one for caregivers to see too. *http://www.birthingthefuture.com*

Birth Day. Recorded in Mexico, this is an intimate view of one family's birth in their home. *www.homebirthvideos.com*

Birth Into Being. This amazing film, beautifully recorded by a Russian midwife and her husband, shows women birthing in water including in the Black Sea. It contains remarkable pictures of children and babies swimming with dolphins. To see birth in these settings is inspirational. *http://www.socalbirth.org/resource/books.htm#Videos*, 1-800-641-BABY

Blessing the Way. Viewers are introduced to Mother/Father Celebrations, or "Blessingways." See how two different women are aided through their own unique emotional challenges as loving friends share their gifts of the heart. *http://www.socalbirth.org/resource/books.htm#videos*, 1-805- 646-3893

Bonded Beginnings. This film features mothers, fathers, and professionals talking about gentle practices for birth. Topic discussions include circumcision, breastfeeding, co-sleeping, baby wearing, and the choices of birth place and birth professionals. It talks, as well, about the psychological and spiritual aspects that impact mothers and babies during the postpartum period. *http://californiawaterbirth.com/media.html*, 1-877-BIRTHING

Born in the Water: A Sacred Journey. This should dispel any fears about water birth, exquisitely filmed, featuring both English and Spanish-speaking families. This is a particularly good educational source for obstetricians and nurses. *http://www.yourwaterbirth.com/vhs-born-in-water-vhs-p-91.html*

Doulas: Making a Difference. Parents share their experiences of having a doula serve them at their births. Explores the complementary roles of doulas and dads *http://dona.org*

Gentle Birth Choices. Shows six women giving birth in the ways they choose, waterbirth, at home, standing, and squatting. This is a great companion to Barbara Harper's book of the same name. *www.waterbirth.org*, 1-800-641-BABY

Giving Birth. This is an eye-opening view of birth throughout history. It encourages women to take back their power and birth joyfully in their own way. *http://www.suzannearms.com/OurStore/videos/givingbirth.php*, 1-877-BIRTHING

Orgasmic Birth. Witness what is possible when birthing in an atmosphere that is safe and undisturbed, and how it can be a wonderful experience which enhances safety for both mother and baby. *http://www.orgasmicbirth.com*

Pregnant In America. View this humorous but sobering analysis of birth in the United States and how it compares to giving birth in the Netherlands where rates of positive outcomes are the best in the world. *http://www.sagefemme.com/dvds.html*

Special Delivery. Three couples speak about what they learned from their birthing experiences. They talk about what worked and did not work for them during their births. Home, Birth Center, and Hospital births are discussed in this classic. Injoy Videos 1-800-326-2082

Special Women. Shows the benefits of having a Professional Labor Assistant at birth, including how they make the birth safer, more satisfying, and less expensive. This film portrays doulas in action. Injoy Videos, 1-800-326-2082

The Business of Being Born. Birth is miraculous. It's an amazing journey of a lifetime for a woman. But birth is also about big business. Ricki Lake and Abby Epstein take you into the heart of childbirth in our culture today. *http://www.thebusinessofbeingborn.com/*

The Timeless Way: A History of Birth from Ancient to Modern Times. Presenting the history of birth throughout time, as recorded in pieces of ancient art, this film illustrates how women of the past have given birth, the kinds of rituals surrounded birth during other times and in various cultures, and how they contrast with our own. Injoy Videos, 1-800-326-2082

Information on the Internet

There are many valuable and trustworthy resources on the Internet that can be accessed by simply "surfing the web." Here are an excellent few that we can recommend to get you started.

Baby Sign Language
www.babysigns.com

Belly Casting
www.proudbody.com

Birth Centers
www.birthcenters.org
http://content.nejm.org/cgi/content/abstract/321/26/1804

Birthing Chairs/Stools
www.thebirthplace.ca/childbirth.htm
www.midwiferytoday.com/loves/birthstools.htm
email for plans to make a stool- phublou@innet.be

Birth Stories
www.thelaboroflove.com/directory/Pregnancy_and_Childbirth/Birth_Stories/

Breastfeeding
www.lalecheleague.org
http://aappolicy.aappublications.org/cgi/content/full/pediatrics%3b100/6/1035
www.childfun.com/breastfeeding
www.askdrsears.com

Cesarean Prevention and Vaginal Birth After Cesarean
www.ican-online.org
www.eheart.com/cesarean/oliver.html
www.caesarean.org.uk
www.vbac.com

Circumcision

www.nocirc.org

www.noharmm.org

Cloth Diapers

(Enter the words *diapers cloth,* and check out the choices!)

Doulas

www.dona.org

www.childbirth.org

www.members.aol.com/mrobyn/faqdoula.htm

www.birthpartners.com

www.cappa.net

www.alace.org

www.bradleybirth.com

www.birthingfromwithin.com

Ecstatic Birth

www.birthingthefuture.com

www.SarahBuckley.com/articles/ecstatic-birth.htm

Homebirth

www.mothering.com/pregnancy-birth/you-want-give-birth-where

www.gentlebirth.org/ronnie/homesafe.html

www.homebirth.org.uk/youcant.htm

www.birthpartners.com

www.changesurfer.com/Hlth/homebirth.html

www.midwiferytoday.com/articles/homebirthchoice.htm

Hypnobirthing

www.hypnobabies.com

www.HypnoBirthing.com

Infant Loss

http://www.nationalshare.org/

http://www.ldspail.com/

Infant Massage

http://www.makewayforbaby.com/massages.htm

Midwives

www.midwiferytoday.com

www.birthpartners.com

Mother-friendly Care

www.motherfriendly.org/pdf/MFCI_english.pdf

Nutrition For Pregnancy

www.pregnancydiet.com/recipes/

www.blueribbonbaby.org

Parenting Our Own Children

www.homebodies.org

www.familyandhome.org

www.homewiththekids.com

www.mommysavers.com

www.drlaurablog.com/category/stay-at-home-moms/

Placenta

www.placentabenefits.info/

Positioning Baby Optimally For Birth

www.spinningbabies.com

http://www.spinningbabies.com/techniques/activities-for-fetal-positioning/rebozo-sifting

www.midwiferytoday.com/articles/transcript.asp

Postpartum Depression

www.postpartum.net

TENS

www.babycaretens.com

www.tens-store.com/ems/

Ultrasound

www.aimsusa.org/ultrasnd.htm

www.midwiferytoday.com/articles/ultrasound.asp?q=ultrasound

www.midwiferytoday.com/articles/ultrasoundwagner.asp

Various Topics

www.babycenter.com

www.mothering.com

www.thehappiestbaby.com

Waterbirth

www.waterbirth.org

write- waterbirth@aol.com

birth tub rental- www.aquadoula.com phone- (888-217-2229)

www.tubsntea.com

The author accepts no responsibility for the information found on these sites. Also, sites do move and so there is no guarantee how long they will remain available into the future. Nor can we list all of the many wonderful available resources.

We invite you to visit us and become part of our community at:
www.AssociationforWiseChildbearing.com

Bibliography

ACOG Evaluation of Cesarean Delivery. The American College of Obstetricians and Gynecologists 2000.

American Academy of Pediatrics. *Breastfeeding and the Use of Human Milk.* PEDIATRICS Vol. 100 No. 6 December 1997, pp. 1035–1039 American Academy of Pediatrics. Newborns: Care of the Uncircumcised Penis, *Guidelines For Parents (pamphlet).* January 1994.

American College of Obstetricians and Gynecologists. *"Health department shows danger of home births."* Jan. 4, 1978.

American Journal of Obstetrics and Gynecology. *Magnesium. Sulfate* June 2002.

Amis, Debby, and Jeanne Green. *Prepared Childbirth The Family Way.* Plano, TX: The Family Way Publications Inc., 1982–2000.

Anderson, Kendra. Infant Massage handout. 2001

Anderson, Sher. personal interview. 2010.

Armstrong, Penny, and Sheryl Feldman. *A Wise Birth.* New York: Morrow, 1990.

Ashford, Janet Isaacs. *Sitting, Standing, Squatting In Childbirth, Mothering Magazine.* Fall 1986.

Backman, Carolyn. *Pre-eclampsia In Pregnancy. Utah Doula Association Newsletter,* Winter 2000.

Baldwin, Rahima. *Special Delivery.* Millbrae, CA: Les Femmes, 1997.

Banack, Connie. *Belly Casting Preparation, Creation, and Decoration. The International Doula,* Spring/Summer 2000.

Barger, Jan, Marsha Walker. *Is Your Baby Getting Enough Breastmilk? Mothering.* Summer 1995.

Barnett NM, Humenick SS. *Infant outcome in relation to second stage labor pushing method. Birth* 1982, 9:221–228.

Bausch & Lomb Pharmaceuticals, Inc. *Erythromycin Ophthalmic Ointment USP, 0.5% (drug insert)* 1994.

Beech, Beverley Lawrence. *Ultrasound: Weighing the Propaganda Against the Facts. Midwifery Today Issue 51.* Autumn 1999.

Berens, J. Michael. *A top cause of death: hospital infections contracted in hospitals kill more people each year than car accidents, fires and drowning combined. Chicago Tribune.* 2002.

Berg, Marie. *"A Midwifery Model of Care for Childbearing Women at High Risk," Journal of Perinatal Education 14, no.1, 19–21.* Winter 2005.

Birth 21, Sept 1994; cited in Colorado Midwives Association Newsletter, Summer 1994, p. 7.

Bishop, Sally. Breastfeeding Class handouts.

Booth, Trish, ICEA Study Modules, 1994, from McKay, S. 1986. *The Assertive Approach To Childbirth, 20–24* Minneapolis: ICEA

Buckel, Arcilla, Burnard, and James. *J Peds.* 67 (1965):239.

Butler, Hilary. *Delayed Cord Clamping. Mothering.* Fall 1986.

Caldeyro-Barcia R. *The influence of maternal bearing-down efforts during second stage on fetal well-being. Birth and the Family Journal* 1979, 6:12–21.

Caldeyro-Barcia (1978); M.D. Mauk et al., *"Tonic Immobility Produces Hyperalgesia and Antagonizes Morphine Analgesia," Science 213,*1981.

Childbirth Instructor, The.

Childbirth Instructor, The. Summer 1994. p. 8.

Childfun.com/breastfeeding.

Cohen, Nancy Wainer, *Open Season: A Survival Guide for Natural Childbirth and VBAC in the 90's*

Cohen, Nancy Wainer, Lois J. Estner. *Silent Knife.* South Hadley, Mass: Bergin & Garvey 1983.

Correa, Wendy. *Eco-Mama Why Breastfeeding Is Best For Babies...And The Environment. Mothering.* July-August 1999.

Cullen, Michael. *Important Drug Warning Concerning Unapproved Use of Intravaginal or Oral Misoprostol In Pregnant Women For Induction of Labor or Abortion. letter to health care providers.* August 2000

Davis, Elizabeth. *Heart And Hands.* Berkley: Celestial Arts. 1987.

De Marsh, Q. B., et al. *"The Effect of Depriving the Infant of its Placental Blood." Journal. A.M.A.* (7 June 1941).

Di Franco, Joyce Thomas. *Comfort Measures For Labor. Lamaze Parents Magazine.* 2002.

Doolittle, J. E., and C.R. Moritz. *Obstet. & Gyn.* (1996).

Dozer, Joanne and Baruth, Shannon. *Epidural Epidemic, Drugs in Labor; Are They Really Necessary...Or Even Safe? Mothering.* July/August 1999.

D.P. Ascher et al., *"Failure of Intrapartum Antibiotics to Prevent Culture-Proved Neonatal Group B Streptococcal Sepsis." Journal of Perinatology 13, no. 3* (1994): 212–216.

England, Pam and Horowitz, Rob. *Birthing From Within.* Albuquerque: Partera, 1998.

Enoch, Jennifer. *Misoprostol (Cytotec): A New Method of Inducing Labor. Midwifery Today Issue 49.* Spring 1999.

Enoch, Jennifer. *"Vitamin K: Is It Necessary?" Midwifery Today.* Winter 1996.

Eisenberg, Murkoff, and Hathaway. *What To Expect When You're Expecting.* New York: Workman, 1991.

Facchinetti F, Piccinini F, Mordini B, Volpe A. *Chlorhexidine vaginal flushings versus systemic ampicillin in the prevention of vertical transmission of neonatal group B streptococcus, at term. J Matern Fetal Med;11 (2) :84–8. Feb 2002.*

Fleiss, Paul, M. Advocating…Pillow Talk: Helping your Child Get a Good Night's Sleep. **Mothering.** Issue 96. September-October 1999.

Fleiss, Paul, M. *The Case Against Circumcision. Mothering. Winter 1997.*

Gaskin, Ina May. *Ina May's Guide To Childbirth.* New York, NY: Bantam Dell, 2003.

Gaskin, Ina May. *Induced and Seduced: The Dangers of Cytotec. Mothering. Issue 107. July/August 2001.*

Gaskin, Ina May. *Spiritual Midwifery.* Summertown, TN, 1990.

Giles, Vivian. *Waterbirth Facts: A Review Taken From Gentle Birth Choices. The Utah Doula. August 1999.*

Glezerman, Marek MD. *Five years to the term breech trial: The rise and fall of a randomized controlled trial. American Journal of Obstetrics & Gynecology. 194(1):20–25, January 2006.*

Goer, Henci, *The Thinking Woman's Guide To A Better Birth.*

Gordon, Serena. Health Day. *Pediatrics.* June 2011.

Grauer, Ann. *More For Doulas About Group B Strep. International Doula. 1997.*

Griffen, Nancy. *Avoiding An Episiotomy. Mothering. Summer 1995.*

Griffen, Nancy. *The Epidural Express, Real Reasons Not to Jump On Board. Mothering.* Spring 1997.

Harper, Barbara, R. N. *Gentle Birth Choices.* Rochester, Vermont: Healing Arts Press, 1994.

Hartmann, Katherine. MD. PhD. And Meera Viswanathan, PhD, et al., *"Outcomes of Routine Episiotomy," JAMA 293, no. 17 2141–2148. May 4, 2005.*

Hauck, Fern R., et al., *Breastfeeding and Reduced Risk of Sudden Infant Death Syndrome: A Meta-analysis.* American Academy. June 2011.

Haussmann, Robert and Kurth, Lisa. *Perinatal Pitocin as an Early ADHD Biomarker: Neurodevelopmental Risk?* Journal of Attention Disorders. April 28, 2011.

Haverkamp, A.D., Orleans, M, Langendouerfer, S., et al. *"A controlled trial of the differential effects of intrapartum fetal monitoring," American Journal of Obstetrics and Gynecology, 134, 4, 399–412, 1979.*

Health. United States. Table 25. Infant mortality rates and international rankings: Selected countries, selected years 1960–99. 2003.

Held, Nancy. *Myths About Second Stage. Childbirth Instructor Magazine, Winter 1994.*

Holland R, Smith D. Management of the second stage of labor: A review (Part I). *So Dakota J Med* 1989; 42:11–14.

Holland R, Smith D. Management of the second stage of labor: A review (Part II). *So Dakota J Med* 1989; 42:5–8.

Holy Bible, Acts 15:1-11, Galatians 5:1–6.

Holy Family Services Birth Center. *Fetal Movement Record.* Texas

Howell, Christina. manual for childbirth education classes. 1997.

Humphrey, M. et al., *"The Influence of Maternal Posture at Birth on the Fetus," J. Obstet Gynaecol. Br. Commonwealth 80, 1973.*

ICAN, questions for selecting a caregiver. ICEA. 2005.

International Doula Association Newsletter.

Jackson, Deborah. *Three In A Bed.* Mothering. Jan/Feb '00.

Johnson, Kenneth C. and Betty-Anne Daviss. *Outcomes of planned home births with certified professional midwives: large prospective study in North America.* British Medical Journal. 18 June 2005. 330:1416.

Johnston, Heather. *Taking Care of Your Baby.*

Johnston, Heather. *Information For After The Birth.*

Johnston, Heather. *Vitamin K: Information, Authorization and Refusal.*

Jones, Carl. *Alternative Birth, The Complete Guide.* Los Angeles: Tarcher, 1991.

Jones, Carl. *Mind Over Labor.*

Jones, Carl. *The Childbirth Companion.*

Journal of Nurse-Midwifery. pp. 89S–94S. March/April 1992.

Journal of Nurse-Midwifery. pp. 91–97. March/April 1994.

Kakuda, Kari. *Eating and Anesthesia.* HypnoBirthing® newsletter.

Keller, Trudy. *Labor Partner's Cheat Sheet.*

Kendig, Susan and Sanford, Diane G.. *Postpartum Depression, The Hidden Problem of New Moms. The Childbirth Instructor Magazine.* 3rd Quarter 1997.

Kennell, John, et al. *Continuous Emotional Support During Labor In a U.S. Hospital: A Randomized Controlled Trial.* JAMA. 265(17):2197–2201. May 1, 1991.

Kennell, John, et al. *Mothering The Mother: How A Doula Can Help You Have A Shorter, Easier, and Healthier Birth.*

Keslo, I. M., Parson, R.J., Lawrence, G. F., et. al., "*An assessment of continuous fetal monitoring in labor: a randomized trial,*" *American Journal of Obstetrics and Gynecology, 131, 5, 526–532, 1978.*

Kibel, M.A. and Davies, M.F., "*Should The Infant Sleep In Mother's Bed?*" *Program And Abstracts, Sixth SIDS International Conference,* Auckland, New Zealand, February 8–11, 2000.

King, Janie McCoy. *Back Labor No More.* Plenary Systems Inc.

Kitzenger, Sheila. "Second Stage," lecture given at Boston College, Boston, in November 1981.

Kitzenger, Sheila. *The Complete Book of Pregnancy And Childbirth.* New York: Knopf, 1996.

Kitzenger, Sheila. *Your Baby Your Way.*

Klix-Van Brummelen, Heidi. *Healing Waters For Labor And Birth.* The Utah Doula. August 1999.

Korte, Diana, and Roberta Scaer, *A Good Birth, A Safe Birth.*

La Leche League International informational handouts

La Leche League International. *The Womanly Art Of Breastfeeding.* New York: New American Library, 1987.

Lancent (11 May 1968).

Lamaze Parents. Spring/Summer 2001.

Leboyer, Frederick. *Birth Without Violence.* New York: Knopf, 1976.

Lewis, Mehl. *Women And Health.* "*Evaluation of Outcomes of Non-Nurse Midwives: Matched Comparisons With Physicians.*" Vol 5, 1980.

Lichtman, Ronnie. *Speedy Recovery, Childbirth.* pg 82–85

Lothian, Judith. *Trust Your Body. Lamaze Parents' Magazine.* 1998.

MacCorkle, Jill. *Fighting VBAC-Lash: Critiquing Current Research. Mothering.* Issue 110 Jan/Feb 2002.

March of Dimes Perinatal Data Center, August 2002.

Marieskind, Helen. *An Evaluation of Cesarean Section in the United States.* Washington, D.C. Dept. of HEW, 1979.

McKay, David, O. *Family Home Evening Manual.* Salt Lake City, 1965.

McKay, S. ed., "*Maternal Position During Labor and Birth.*" ICEA Review. Summer 1978.

McClure, Vimala Schneider, *Infant Massage: A Handbook For Loving Parents.* Bantam. 2000

McClutcheon, Susan, *Natural Childbirth The Bradley Way 1996.*

McConnell, Jane. *Diapering article, Mothering.* May–June, 1998.

Medical Association Journal 149, 1993.

Miller, Chris. personal interview concerning transfers from home to hospital. 1997.

Miller, F., et al., *Significance of Meconium during Labor,*" Am. J. Ob. Gyn., 122 (1975): 573.

Milos, Marilyn Fayre. *Infant Circumcision: "What I Wish I Had Known"*

Mongan, Marie F. *HypnoBirthing®A Celebration of Life.* Concord, N.H. Rivertree, 1998.

Mothering Magazine.

Mothering Magazine, pgs 72–73. Winter '94.

Nagourney, Eric. *Childbirth: Rethinking the Big Push During Contractions.* *New York Times.* January 3, 2006.

Newman, Diane K. *Stress Urinary Incontinence In Women, AJN, American Journal of Nursing 8/2003 Volume 103 Number 8 p. 46–55.*

Newman, Jack. *How Breastmilk Protects Babies. Mothering.* Spring 1997.

*Nurturing Magazine, Summer, 1998.*Odent, Michel. *Birth Reborn.*

Odent, Michel. "Birth under Water", 147.

O'Mara, Peggy, "*We've Come A Long Way, Babies*" *Mothering.* January–February 1999.

Pardue, Naomi L. *On The LAM (Lactation Amenorrhea Method). Mothering.* Fall 1994.

Perez, Paulina G. *Birthing Positions. Lamaze Parents Magazine.* 2002.

Perez, Paulina G. *Procedures Explained. Lamaze Parents Magazine.* 2002.

Perez, Paulina G. *What You Need To Know About Labor And Birth Positions. Lamaze Parents' Magazine.* 1998.

Perez and Snedecker, *Special Women*, The Role of the Professional Labor Assistant. Pennypress, Inc.

Pettiti, Diana, "*Have Increased Cesarean Delivery Rates Resulted In Lower Neonatal Mortality Rates?*" paper presented at Birth And Family J. Conference, San Francisco, 16 and 17, October, 1987.

Population Reference Bureau, 1990. United Nations, World Population Prospects: The 1996 Revision, Annex I. New York: United Nations 1996.

Porter, Lauren Lindsey. *Attachment Theory In Everyday Life. Mothering.* May–June 2009.

Powell, Alvin. *Children Need Touching and Attention, Harvard Researchers Say. The Harvard University Gazette,* April 09, 1998.

Prichard, Jack A., & Paul C. MacDonald, *Williams Obstetrics,* 16th ed. (New York: Appleton-Century-Crofts, 1980).

Procter & Gamble. *Childbirth Classroom. On Target Media Inc.* Cincinnati, Ohio 11022–2, 1991.

Pugh, T. , Ridd, K. , Smith, K. (untitled labor support for stages). 1991.

Rados, Carol. *FDA Cautions Against Ultrasound 'Keepsake' Images. FDA Consumer Magazine.* January-February 2004.

Richardson, Holly. Information received from the National Vaccine Information Center, Sept. 1998 *The UDA Newsletter vol. VII #1, Feb, 1999.*

Ridd, Kristi. *Labor Support Course.* 1997.

Schmitt, Laura. *Crazy for Cloth. Mothering.* 116 January/February 2003.

Schultz, Terry (1979). *A nurse's view on circumcision. Letter to the Editor. Mothering.* 26 (XII), Summer. 1979.

Scientific American. "*Brain Damage By Asphyxia at Birth.*" 1969.

Sears, William and Martha, *The Baby Book.* Little Brown And Company. 1993.

Sears, William and Martha, *The Birth Book.* Little Brown And Company. 1994.

Sears, William and Martha, *The Discipline Book.* Little Brown And Company. 1995.

Sears, William and Martha, *The Pregnancy Book.* Little Brown And Company. 1997.

Simkin and Klaus, "*Possible Impact of Childhood Sexual Abuse.*" 1994.

Simkin, Penny. "*Backache In Labor.*" 1979.

Simkin, Penny. *Clinical Challenges In Childbirth Related To Childhood Sexual Abuse (With Possible Solutions).*

Simkin, Penny. "*Overcoming The Legacy of Childhood Sexual Abuse: The Role of Caregivers And Childbirth Educators*" *Birth 19:4.* December 1992.

Simkin, Penny. *Pain Medications Preference Scale.* 1988, adapted from her *The Birth Partner: Everything You Need To Know To Help A Woman Through Childbirth.* Harvard Common Press. 1989.

Simkin, Penny. *Physiological Positions For Labor and Birth. Dona Doula Training.*

Simkin, Penny. "*The Take Charge Routine.*"

Simkin, Penny. "*Will You Have A Doula?*" *Lamaze Parents Magazine.* 2002.

Simkin, Penny and Klaus, Phyllis. *The Power Differential Between Caregiver And Client.* 1994.

Simkin, Walley, and Keppler, *Pregnancy, Childbirth and The Newborn.* (Deephaven MN: Meadowbrook Press. 1993.

Solomon, Suchi. *Where Sex And Violence Mix. The Sun.* 1995.

USP label, Vitamin K1 Injection Phytonadione Infection. *Utah Doula Newsletter.*

Wagner, Marsden. *Born in the USA: How a Broken Maternity System Must Be Fixed to Put Women and Children First.* University of California Press

Wagner, Marsden. *Choosing Cesarean Section. The Lancet,* vol.356, pp 1677–80. November 11, 2000.

Wagner, Marsden. *Creating Your Birth Plan: The Definitive Guide to a Safe and Empowering Birth.* 2006.

Wagner, Marsden. *Midwives and Cytotec: A True Story. Midwifery Today* Issue 57. Spring 2001.

Wagner, Marsden. Personal notes. February 18, 2008.

Wagner, Marsden. *Ultrasound: More Harm Than Good. Mothering.* Winter 1995.

Walsh, S. Zoe. *"Maternal Effects of Early and Late Clamping of the Umbilical Cord."*

Watson, Stephanie. *Preterm Labor Drug May Harm Baby. www.babycenter.com.* July 15, 2002.

Way, Kelli. *Anesthesia For Cesarean.* 1997.

Way, Kelli. *Characteristics of Effective Birth Plans.* 1997.

Way, Kelli. *If I Have An Epidural, Why Do I Need A Doula?* Kelli Way, 1997.

Way, Kelli. *Pushing With An Epidural.* 1997.

Weinhouse, Beth. *Hard Labor. Parents.* August 1999.

Wickham, Sara. *What's Right For Me? Making decisions in pregnancy and birth.* Aims. August 2002.

Wildner, Kim. *Mother's Intention-How Belief Shapes Birth.* Harbor And Hill. 2003.

Wilson-Davis, S. L., S. L. Tonkin, and T. R. Gunn. *Air entry in infant resuscitation: oral or nasal routes?. J. Appl. Physiol.*82(1): 152–155, 1997.

Winfield, June Hartman and Bull, Pat. *Summary of Policy Statement on Breastfeeding from the American Academy of Pediatrics.* May 29, 1998.

Wyckoff , Whitney Blair. *Home Births, While Still Uncommon, Are On The Rise In U.S.* NPR's Health Blog. May 2011.

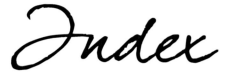

Index

Page numbers in bold indicate a worksheet, form or chart: Before Birth Checklist, **231–234**. Page numbers with a p following indicate a photo: birth ball, 103p. Book titles are italicized: *Baby Book, The*, 296.

A

ability to birth, women's natural, 9, 127, 145–146
abuse, sexual, impact of, 210–212
acidophilus, 114
acupuncture and acupressure, 111, 134
adrenaline, 207
affirmations, 208–209
American Academy of Pediatrics (AAP)
  on breastfeeding, 262
  on care of intact penis, 258
American College of Obstetricians and Gynecologists (ACOG)
  on birth place, 40
  on cesareans, 115, 118
  on circumcision, 257
  on Cytotec, 132
  on electronic fetal heart monitor (EFM), 93–94
  on episiotomies, 100
  on routine ultrasound, 96, 98
  on vaginal birth after cesarean (VBAC), 115
Amish women, 175

amniocentesis, 98, 147
analgesics (pain killers), 82–83
analogy
  cake, 126
  dinner ham, 220
  menu, 45
  mother hen, 76
  pediatrician babysitter, 116
  putting shoes on, 189
antibiotics, 112–113
Apgar score, 106, 118, 124, 173, 255–256
aromatherapy, 70, 134, 169
artificial rupture of membranes (AROM), 74, 127–128, 129, 132–133, 187
  and Strep B, 112
  why to avoid, 187
assertiveness, 69, 144, 149, 227
Association for Wise Childbearing (AWC), philosophies, 9–11
atmosphere surrounding birth, 10, 23, 32, 36, 168, 203
attachment parenting, 288–296

B

baby. see also position, baby's
  and bleeding issues, 252–254
  blood sugar screening, 254
  breathing at birth, 245
  crying, 289–290
  low birth weight, 127, 130
  metabolic screening, 253–254
  newborn care, 282–287
  respiratory problems, 108
  sex of, 98
  size of, 10, 17, 105, 128
  skull bones, 18
  stools, 283
  suctioning, 249
  temperature regulation, 250, 282–283
  turning from posterior position, 186–187
  and water birth, 182–183
  weighing and bathing, 254–255
baby blues. see also postpartum depression, 276
Baby Book, The, 296

About the Author

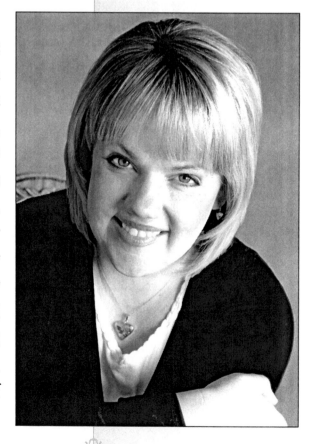

JENNETTA BILLHIMER is the Founding Director of the Association for Wise Childbearing, an Association for Wise Childbearing Childbirth mentor, a Mongan Method HypnoBirthing® Practitioner, and a doula of many years certified with Dona International. Jennetta Billhimer is a Personal Mentor and a speaker and writer on a variety of subjects involving childbirth, family development, and living a joyful and successful life challenges and all. She and her husband are graduates of Brigham Young University and are the parents of six children.

Find out what *Association for Wise Childbearing* has to offer you.

We invite you to join us on our website:

www.AssociationforWiseChildbearing.com

Make yourself a warm cup of herbal tea. Pull up a cozy chair, and make yourself at home at www.AssociationforWiseChildbearing.com, at our blog, and more. We have lots to offer you as you make this important journey. We hope you will visit often, and that you will acquaint your friends with our group too.

We'd also love to have you *join* the AWC. Bring your own unique traits and skills to our group and form meaningful relationships as you work together with other passionate people. Meet others who are determined to make a collective difference in how babies, women, and their families are cared for at this time of such far-reaching consequence.

The Association for Wise Childbearing offers childbirth education certification to qualified individuals as well. There are many ways you can make a difference in your own corner of the Earth.

If Wise Childbearing inspires you to do more, here are suggestions about how you can help:

1. Visit the www.AssociationforWiseChildbearing.com website for more information, to be inspired, share your own birth story, to join our group the Association for Wise Childbearing, and for ideas of ways that you can work with others to help make a collective difference. If you purchase books through this website, a percentage of your book purchases will go toward the Association for Wise Childbearing.

2. Suggest Wise Childbearing to a friend, colleague, book club, women's group, community group, university or high school class, or other groups interested in education and childbirth.

3. Check if Wise Childbearing is in your local library. If it is not, either donate a book or suggest to the library that they add Wise Childbearing to their collection. Ask your friends or family in other cities to do this also.

4. Encourage your local independent or chain bookstore to carry this book.

5. Write a Wise Childbearing book review for online bookstores such as Amazon.com, Barnes & Nobel, Borders, a blog, and places like Goodreads. Your candid comments will help the buzz of this book.

6. Ask the book editor of your local newspaper or radio to consider reviewing the book.

7. If you want to support our efforts, monetary contributions of all sizes to our organization, Association for Wise Childbearing, would be greatly appreciated.

8. Please direct media or Wise Childbearing inquiries to wise.childbearing@gmail.com.

CPSIA information can be obtained at www.ICGtesting.com
Printed in the USA
BVOW042011100612

292228BV00001BA/1/P